RENIN-ANGIOTENSIN SYSTEM - PAST, PRESENT AND FUTURE

Edited by **Anna Naidenova Tolekova**

Renin-Angiotensin System - Past, Present and Future
http://dx.doi.org/10.5772/63179
Edited by Anna Naidenova Tolekova

Contributors

Pantelis Zebekakis, Georgianos Panagiotis, Elias Balaskas, Rosa Marlene Viero, Luis Gustavo Modelli de Andrade, Ahmad Yarikhosroushahi, Elham Ahmadian, Aziz Eftekhari, Aleksandra Stankovic, Ana Kolakovic, Maja Zivkovic, Anthony César Souza Castilho, Patrícia Kubo Fontes, Fernanda Franchi, Priscila Santos, Eduardo Razza, Julie L. Lavoie, Émilie Pépin, Shahin Shabanipour Dehboneh, Nozha Raguema, Maedeh Talebi Esfandarani, Ozlem Sahin, Alireza Ziaei, Anne Pihlanto, Sari Mäkinen, Teresa Sousa, Manuela Morato, Marta Reina-Couto, Dora Pinho, António Albino-Teixeira, Jose Gabino Gerardo-Aviles, Patrick Kehoe, Shelley Allen, Eylem Taskin, Celal Guven, Carolina Baraldi A. Restini, Henrique Melo Natalin, Arthur Feierabend Engracia Garcia, Guilherme Melo Natalin, Elen Rizzi, Matilde Otero-Losada, José Milei, Mariana Nobile

Published by InTech
Janeza Trdine 9, 51000 Rijeka, Croatia

Publishing Process Manager Iva Simcic
Technical Editor SPi Global
Cover InTech Design team

First published July, 2017
Printed in Croatia
Legal deposit, Croatia: National and University Library in Zagreb

Additional hard copies can be obtained from orders@intechopen.com

Renin-Angiotensin System - Past, Present and Future, Edited by Anna Naidenova Tolekova
p. cm.
Print ISBN 978-953-51-3351-3
Online ISBN 978-953-51-3352-0

For EU product safety concerns:
IN TECH d.o.o., Prolaz Marije Krucifikse Kozulić 3, 51000 Rijeka, Croatia,
info@intechopen.com or visit our website at intechopen.com.

Meet the editor

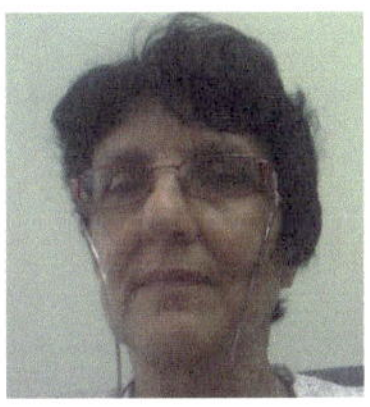

Anna Naydenova Tolekova was born on August 18, 1955. In 1979, she graduated from the Higher Medical School, Plovdiv, Bulgaria. From 1979 to 1983, she worked as the epidemiologist in Gabrovo. From 1983 until now, she has been working in Medical Faculty, Trakia University, Stara Zagora in the Department of Physiology. Since 2009, she has been an associate professor, and since 2016, she has been a professor. Since 2012, she has been the head of the Department of Physiology, Pathophysiology, and Pharmacology. From 2012 till the end of 2015, she was the vice rector of the Research and International Activities of the Trakia University, Stara Zagora, Bulgaria. In 1989, she earned her PhD degree in Physiology. The subject of the dissertation is "Investigation of plasma renin activity after some physiological and pharmacological effects." Her scientific field includes endocrine function of the kidney, neuroendocrine regulation of smooth muscle contractility, oxidative balance, and new mathematical methods in physiological research. She has authored 98 publications and 3 book chapters.

Contents

Preface

The renin-angiotensin system is a unique regulatory system by its nature and characteristic. Its main components have been discovered for the first time, in connection with blood pressure regulation. The historic pathway from Robert Tigerstedt and Gunnar Bergman to the discovery of the characteristics of individual elements and the study of their significance, including the first synthesis of the converting enzyme inhibitor, captopril, is described in the first chapter of the book by Otero-Losada et al. and José Milei. The accumulated data lead to qualitatively new knowledge of the whole system: local PAS (paracrine, autocrine, and intacrine system), new metabolites (angiotensin III and angiotensin IV, angiotensin 1–7 and angiotensin 1–9), new enzymes, and new receptors. In the second part of the book, the authors discuss the significance of the PAC for the functioning of the cardiovascular system. Restini et al. describe in detail the role of RAS main effector angiotensin II for the remodeling of the heart. A number of new studies, systematized by Kolakovic and Stankovic, clarify the importance of the two main types of angiotensin receptors in the pathophysiological mechanisms of atherosclerosis and interplay with other regulatory mechanisms. The importance of the first choice of antihypertensive therapy in the treatment of patients with chronic kidney disease is the focus of Georgianos et al. In the third part, the importance of PAC for the functioning of the reproductive system is described in the two separate chapters: the importance of classical and local PAS with the main effector angiotensin (1–7) for the development of pathological abnormalities in the progression of pregnancy (Pepin et al.) as well as the known facts about PAS and reproductive biology (by Castilho and colleagues). The fourth part contains chapters of varied content that systematize the latest facts in the respective topics. Morato et al. look at the new knowledge about the relationships between RAS and reactive oxygen species that are of great importance for a large number of disturbances. Newly discovered signal transduction pathways and their elements are also produced in the retina and are of great importance for the maintenance of the local homeostasis of the visual sensory system and for the control of the local inflammatory response (Ozlem). Ahmadian et al. systematize the interaction of stem cells and RAS as well as the importance of modulation of cellular interactions, including local RAS at different levels, which provides new perspectives for stem cell therapy. MicroRNAs (miRNAs) are posttranscriptional gene expression regulators, which can remodel brain RAS and act as mediators between local and systemic RAS. Gerardo-Aviles et al., systematizing all of these facts, address the challenges of using miRNAs for diagnosis and therapeutic interventions in the future. Viero and de Andrade analyzed the effects of RAS blockade on the development of renal fibrosis and rejection of allograft.

A new concept for a complete picture of the system is being created. From a system of blood pressure regulation, it becomes a complex system, extremely rich in feedback and regulating both brain functions and functions of all internal organs. It could be called "äutonomic" endocrine system. The central units of both autonomic systems converge on the level of the hypothalamus but interact not only on the central but also at the peripheral levels, making extremely precise regulation of body homeostasis.

Anna Naidenova Tolekova
Trakia University, Medical Faculty,
Stara Zagora,
Bulgaria

Section 1

History

Chapter 1

The Angiotensin Affair: How Great Minds Thinking Alike Came to a Historical Agreement

Matilde Otero-Losada, Mariana H. Nobile and
José Milei

Additional information is available at the end of the chapter

http://dx.doi.org/10.5772/67136

Abstract

In 1934, J. C. Fasciolo had to submit a thesis and Dr. Houssay suggested he investigate about nephrogenic hypertension. E. Braun-Menéndez showed interest in helping and Drs. L.F. Leloir and J.M. Muñoz from the Institute of Physiology joined them in their attempt to isolate and purify the pressor substance. In 1939, they extracted the substance "hypertension" from the venous blood from the ischemic kidneys. They proposed an enzyme-substrate reaction. They named hypertensinogen the substrate and hypertensinases the enzymes that break down the hypertension. Two months following the Argentine publication, the team in the United States, formed by I.H. Page and O.M. Helmer, published their findings, which were in agreement with those reported by the Argentine team. By 1940, they isolated angiotonin, the equivalent of hypertension, and called the renin substrate hypertensinogen. In 1957, in the conference held in Ann Arbor, Braun-Menéndez and Page agreed on a new nomenclature. As a result, the words angiotensinogen and angiotensin were born from the combination of the names originally set by both teams. The discovery of the renin-angiotensin system is an example that science should follow: Value the progress made by colleagues, collaborate side by side, and pursue the ultimate truth.

Keywords: angiotensin discovery, hypertension, renal disease, renin-angiotensin system, vasoconstriction, blood pressure, kidney ischemia, renal grafting

1. Introduction

A systematic review of both autobiographical and biographical documentation is provided, concerning with original experiments that change the course of hypertension treatment, along with a chronology of the major events which led to angiotensin discovery. This historical hit marked the evolution of antihypertensive treatment and later on gave rise to the development of a whole new family of drugs, the angiotensin receptor blockers (ARBs). At present, their main uses are in the treatment of hypertension, diabetic nephropathy, and congestive heart failure. By now, annual global sales of renin-angiotensin inhibitor drugs are estimated around US$ 27.3 billion, 24% in Europe. Actually, much of these come from single-sourced angiotensin receptor blockers (ARBs).

2. Discovery of angiotensin

Using relatively unsophisticated methods (in light of present technology), laboring hard and carrying out keen experiments, two teams of prestigious scientists identified the precise peptide called angiotensin, which induced experimental renal hypertension [1]. The discovery of the renin-angiotensin-aldosterone system (RAAS) was relevant in understanding a key mechanism involved in the maintenance and control of arterial blood pressure. As it would be revealed in time, this system indeed participates in other processes such as inflammation and oxidative stress as well. Years later, the characterization of the RAAS would render the synthesis of the presently used antihypertensive drugs. The development of angiotensin-converting enzyme (ACE) inhibitors proved that the RAAS is effective in controlling hypertension and heart failure, and in preventing vascular injury in chronic diseases.

2.1. Early investigation that led to the discovery of angiotensin

The nineteenth century was the seeding period where evidence and theories linking renal perfusion and blood pressure control in both physiological and pathological conditions were put forward [2]. It was not until 1936 when R Bright first reported evidence supporting the functional link between cardiac hypertrophy and renal disease [3]. He associated hypertrophy with an increase in small vessels resistance to blood flow as a result of an altered condition in blood. In 1868, G. George Johnson had indeed shared the outcome of his studies on nephritis and suggested that some kind of abnormal condition of the blood induced the hyaline-fibroid modifications he observed in renal vessels. Moreover, such particular condition of the blood was responsible for left ventricular hypertrophy as well [4]. Only 4 years later, FA Mahomed succeeded in measuring blood pressure using an interesting "ultramodern" device at the time, namely a sphygmograph [5]. He also reported the relationship between left ventricular hypertrophy and hypertension due to nephritis in patients not affected by renal disease [6, 7]. Later on, Riva-Rocci explained and depicted in detail the characteristics of another device, the sphygmomanometer which made possible to measure arterial pressure in humans. At the beginnings of the new century, the Russian physician Nikolai Korotkoff, at the time of his work at the Imperial Medical Academy in St. Petersburg, described the characteristic sounds which took his name in his honor [8, 9].

In 1898, the medical scientist and physiologist Professor Robert Tigerstedt (1853–1923) and Gunnar Bergman, one of his fellows at the Karolinska Institute (Stockholm), reported a dramatic rise in blood pressure following the injection of kidney extracts to rabbits, suggesting the presence of a vasoconstrictor substance which they called "renin" in renal cortex [10]. As to why Tigerstedt paid attention to the subject, inconclusive guesses had been put forward.

http://dx.doi.org/10.5772/67136

Perhaps the intertwining pathophysiology linking hypertension and renal disease established by Bright (1789–1859) or the discovery of an adrenal hormone by Séquard (1817–1894) awakened his interest. Yet, he abandoned the subject on his return to Finland later [11] and published no follow-up. Reproducibility of renin activity posed high technical difficulties. Tigerstedt may have felt discouraged and gave up trying any longer, as suggested by Professor Aurell [12].

The cardiovascular, renal, and central nervous systems are targets for hypertensive damage. In 1923, Franz Volhard (1872–1950) put forward the idea of a vasospastic substance causing malignant "pale" hypertension which characteristic symptoms as pale skin, decreased or blurred vision and headaches (ocular and central changes, respectively) [13]. Contradictory reports appeared regarding whether this vasoconstrictor substance was actually found in the blood of hypertensive patients or it was not [14]. Unsuccessfully, Volhard and his collaborators attempted to measure and characterize a circulating vasoconstrictive substance in hypertensive patients with acute glomerulonephritis [13], most probably due to technical issues and defective analysis techniques [15].

Many attempts were made to create an experimental model of hypertension, such as irradiating the renal parenchyma, reducing its mass by ablations, and occlusion of branches of the renal artery. These were not successful. In 1909, Theodore Caldwell Janeway (1872–1917) described an increase in blood pressure after occlusion of the renal artery branches and excision of the contralateral kidney [16]. However, it was not until 1934 that Harry Goldblatt (1891–1977) developed an experimental canine model of hypertension, known as "Goldblatt kidney." He reported that permanent hypertension induced by renal artery blockage that was neither prevented nor abolished by section of the vasomotor branch of the sympathetic nervous system in dogs [17].

2.2. Work performed by the Argentine team

In the 1930s, the lab of physiology at the Faculty of Medicine of the University of Buenos Aires, led by the Nobel Prize winner Bernardo Houssay (1887–1971), was about to live one of its most prolific periods. In 1934, J. C. Fasciolo (1911–1993), a student of the School of Medicine at the University of Buenos Aires, had to submit a thesis to complete his undergraduate degree. Dr. Houssay suggested he investigate about nephrogenic hypertension, a suggestion brought by the premature death of one of his most brilliant fellows called Juan Guglielmetti (1891–1922). He died at the age of 33 years from a malignant hypertension [18].

Carlos Alberto Taquini (1905–1998) was a member of the Department of Physiology who had the privilege of listening to F. Volhard in 1931. He proposed and discussed with Fasciolo and Houssay the humoral theory of vasospasm involved in hypertension. This theory considered the possibility that the substance released by the kidneys might act directly on the blood vessels. Taquini reported that following kidney ischemia, a vasoconstrictor substance appeared in the renal vein of dogs. Actually, perfusion with a blood of hypertensive animals induced strong vasoconstriction, while blood from normotensive dogs did not [19]. In the same line of work, he perfused the hind legs of toads with diluted plasma in the experimental condition known as Lawen-Trendelenburg preparation [20, 21]. During the same year, Taquini proved that the increase in blood pressure observed after restoring blood flow in ischemic kidneys was caused by the same vasopressor substance involved in the previous studies [22].

Fasciolo initially sought to destroy the renal cortex of rats to develop a model of experimental hypertension. However, he encountered methodological difficulties, and the results were not consistent. He came across the article published by Goldblatt, and after reading it, he began to apply the method described by him [23]. Being instructed in renal grafting by Houssay, now without failures and disappointments in the beginning, Fasciolo succeeded in inducing hypertension in dogs as shown by Goldblatt [24, 25]. Unequivocally, when the grafted kidneys were perfused, hypertension slowly and gradually developed [23]. This experiment confirmed that a pressor substance was actually secreted by the kidneys. Pharmacologically, induced hypertension was refractory to an administration of sympatholytic drugs, atropine or cocaine, while it was potentiated following bilateral nephrectomy [26].

Of course, they had to characterize, purify, and learn much more about the physiological role of this pressor substance to study its physiological activity [23]. Eduardo Braun-Menéndez (1903–1959) showed himself interested in helping, just after his return from England where he had obtained a grant and studied myocardial metabolism with Dr. Charles Arthur Lovatt Evans (1884–1968). Using a heart-lung preparation and perfusion of an isolated kidney, they observed that flow interruption for just a few minutes was enough to induce the presence of the vasopressor substance in the renal venous blood. This was checked by injecting the venous blood from that preparation into nephrectomized dogs. This finding would later become of huge importance. The preparation of hypertensive dogs was not simple, and large amounts of venous blood would be required to isolate the hypertensive agent [23, 27]. At that time, Drs. L.F. Leloir (1906–1987) and J.M. Muñoz were working at the Institute of Physiology and accompanied Fasciolo and Braun-Menéndez in their attempt to isolate and purify the pressor substance. Leloir and Muñoz worked mainly on the chemical aspects, and Braun-Menéndez and Fasciolo worked on the pharmacological aspects [23]. This group, perhaps one of the most brilliant that Argentine science has had, functioned in total harmony. In the words of Leloir: Good spirit reigned in the laboratory. Fasciolo pointed out the importance of the diversity in viewpoints of him and his colleagues stating that "Leloir and Muñoz are well versed in biochemistry, while Braun-Menéndez and I are better versed to physiology" [28]. Dr. Houssay was aware of the progress of their research and helped them with his advice and his constant support [23].

The group first tried working with the toad preparation successfully used earlier by Taquini in the characterization of various extracts. Later on, they decided to perform their research using the most reliable, though more expensive, dog model [23]. In 1939, they extracted the vasopressor substance with acetone from the venous blood from the kidneys that were subjected to periods of ischemia. This substance produced an increase in arterial pressure when it was injected in animals, although this effect only lasted a few minutes. A very different scenario occurred when ischemic kidneys were implanted to the cervical circulation, where the increase in arterial pressure was of a prolonged nature. The isolated substance was heat stable, dialyzable and had a brief hypertensive effect, characteristics that differentiated it from renin. The Argentine team named this substance hypertension. The next step was to elucidate the existing relationship between renin and hypertension. In the first instance, fragments of renal cortex were incubated with plasma in anoxic conditions. This, however, did not yield hypertension. It was explained by the possible presence of enzymes that metabolize it. In a second attempt, the extracts of renin were incubated at 37°C with plasma, obtaining through this method the vasopressor in vitro. Basing themselves on their findings, they proposed an enzyme-substrate reaction for the formation of hypertension. They named hypertensinogen the substrate, the enzyme renin, and hypertensinases the enzymes that break down the hypertension [29, 30]. The sustained hypertensive effect achieved through the implantation of ischemic kidneys would be caused by renin release of renin and continuous generation of hypertension in plasma, as they reported in the "Revista de la Sociedad Argentina de Biología" (Journal of the Society of Argentine Biology) in 1939 [23].

It is important to note that Taquini was not in Argentina exactly when hypertension was isolated. He had left to the United States to work at the Fatigue Laboratory at Harvard University alongside Dr. David B. Dill (1891–1986) and Dr. Paul Dudley White (1886–1973) within the frame of a fellowship in 1938 [31]. After 1 year working in Boston, Dr Taquini returned to Argentina and went on working as part of the team again, though he was not included in the work where the discovery was published [23].

2.3. The team in the United States arrives at the same conclusions

Only 2 months following the Argentine publication, Drs Irvine H. Page and O M. Helmer (Eli Lilly Research Laboratories, Indianapolis) published a full-scale study showing experimental evidence of the existence of a pressor substance, renin [32]. Their findings were in agreement with those reported by the Argentine team The Americans followed an entirely different approach: They dedicated themselves to concentrating renin from extracts of renal parenchyma and to study its vasoconstrictory function in dog tail and rabbit ear. These experiences showed that vasoconstriction was only observed when the animal tissue was perfused with plasma and did not happen when Ringer Lactate was utilized. In 1938, this led to the conclusion that there should be an activating substance for renin in plasma [33]. In 1939, this conclusion was presented by Page et al. at a reunion of the American Heart Association. Taquini, having been present in the auditorium and being aware of the progress of the Argentine team, refutes the arguments presented by Page saying it was not activated renin substance that caused vasoconstriction but an entirely different substance [20]. Page said that he was widely criticized for using the word activator of renin, but that he did so wanting to be wise, seeing as how the enzymatic reaction catalyzed by renin had not been demonstrated by that time [32]. By 1940, the team isolated angiotonin, the equivalent of hypertension that the Argentine team had obtained, through the interaction between the renin activator and renin [34]. Later, Page et al. reviewed the denomination called renin activator, hypertensinogen, or renin substrate [35].

2.4. Treaty between gentlemen

Braun-Menéndez et al. must have been very disappointed when a few months after their publication, Page and his team reached the same results utilizing another route. In 1957, 25 years after Goldblatt' successfully raised blood pressure by inducing renal ischemia in dogs, the Regional Conference on Basic Mechanisms of Arterial Hypertension of the University of Michigan was held in Ann Arbor in his honor. The Organizing Committee was chaired by Drs Sibley W. Hoobler and David F. Bohr [15]. It was then that, beyond and far from conflict, Braun-Menéndez and Page agreed on a new nomenclature. As the result, the words angiotensinogen and angiotensin were born from the combination of the names originally set by both teams [32, 36].

Edward D. Frohlich (Alton Ochsner Distinguished Scientist at the Alton Ochsner Medical Foundation and Editor in Chief of the *Hypertension* journal) commented that Page had pointed out to him, while he was drinking martinis with Braun-Menéndez at a lunch during the Michigan meeting. It was by then that the compromised to solve the differences getting to a common nomenclature for their findings. Then, a very short and concise report was published in Science and was the very proof of their settled agreement [1, 36]. Actually, as Page recognized, cooperation was so close that claiming priority from any part would have been nonsense and they should share either the blame of the congratulations [32]. In 1985, Page sent a letter to Fasciolo expressing his hope that their resolve on the nomenclature issue would serve as an example for future generations of scientists to come. He shared an interesting message for the future generations of scientists saying that they could not possibly leave unsolved a historical puzzle so anyone might speculate on an imaginary dispute which had never occurred. In his letter, he clearly stated that the hypertension story should well serve as a model to follow when dealing with difficult situations, for example, with gentleness and making alliances [23].

The following years were strange, in the sense that Goldblatt and Skeggs in the United States, and leading groups in Europe went on using the Argentine name [15]. In contrast, Taquini et al. emphasized on the need of accepting unified names [37]. In one of his publications, Leonard T. Skeggs Jr. (1918–2002, biochemist in Case Western Reserve University, Cleveland, Ohio) mentioned: "I must explain, parenthetically that angiotensin was known to us, being followers of Harry Goldblatt and Eduardo Braun-Menéndez, as hypertension. Merlin Bumpus knew angiotensin as angiotonin. This was natural because Merlin worked with Irvine Page, who had coined the name angiotonin. It was a number of years later that Page and Braun-Menéndez agreed on the name angiotensin, and all the rest of us used the new name" [38].

Both teams shared the merit of the discovery, proving that beyond being great investigators they were essentially remarkable persons.

2.5. What comes after this great discovery

Following angiotensin discovery, the Argentine team focused on studying the enzymatic origin and release of angiotensin from angiotensinogen, the peptidic nature of angiotensin, renin secretion from kidneys, hepatic synthesis of angiotensinogen, pharmacological profile of angiotensin, and so [39–41]. Researchers like Alberto Agrest, Pedro C. Blaquier, Alberto C. Taquini, Jr and Ignacio J. de la Riva, who had begun their scientific career working at the *Instituto de Investigaciones Cardiológicas* (School of Medicine, University of Buenos Aires) years ago, returned to work there [15]. Leloir et al. conclusively confirmed the hepatic origin of renin studying nephrectomized dogs with and without liver ablation [42]. This had been proposed earlier by Page et al. showing no convincing evidence though [43].

http://dx.doi.org/10.5772/67136

In the 1940s, a powerful mineralocorticoid called electrocortin was described by Grundy. In 1953, Russian-born English Sylvia Agnes Sophia Tait (1917–2003) et al. identified electrocortin by means of chromatography. This hormone was then renamed aldosterone. In 1955, Jerome W. Conn (1907–1994) described primary hyperaldosteronism, as a result of a single adrenal adenoma [44].

Skeggs et al. succeeded in the isolation of Angiotensin I (Ang I). Others like Lentz et al., Elliot, and Peart could elucidate the structure of Angiotensin II (Ang II). In 1950, Bumpu's and Schwyzer's groups reported the synthetic pathway of angiotensin. Skeggs and his group recognized the existence of two different forms of angiotensin and also identified the angiotensin-converting enzyme (ACE) which was later revealed as a kininase II enzyme by Erdös. Then, an intimate relationship between angiotensin generation and bradykinin destruction was demonstrated [45].

The contribution of another Argentine scientist the chemist Miguel Angel Ondetti (1930–2004) is also important. He synthesized captopril in 1975, the first of the ACE inhibitors, the same as the enalapril precursor and others of substantial therapeutic importance, showing the pathophysiological relevance of angiotensin [46].

The discovery of the renin-angiotensin system is much more than theoretical knowledge required for any physiology book. It undoubtedly represents one of the highlights of Argentine physiological discoveries, and what is even more important, an example that science should follow: Value the progress made by colleagues, collaborate side by side, and pursue the ultimate truth.

Acknowledgements

The authors thank Melisa Etchegoyen and Francisco Báez for helping with proof reading and language correction.

Author details

Matilde Otero-Losada*, Mariana H. Nobile and José Milei

*Address all correspondence to: molly1063@gmail.com

National Research Council, Institute of Cardiological Research, University of Buenos Aires, ININCA.UBA.CONICET, Argentina

References

[1] Frohlich, ED. Sixtieth anniversary of Angiotensin. Hypertension, 2001, **38**:1245.

[2] Wolf, G. Franz Volhard and his students' tortuous road to renovascular hypertension. Kidney Int, 2000, **57**:2156-2166.

[3] Bright, R. Tubular view of the morbid appearances in 100 cases connected with albuminous urine: with observations. Guy's Hosp Rep, 1836, **1**:380-400.

[4] Johnson, GI. On certain points in the anatomy and pathology of Bright's diseases of the kidney, II: on the influence of the minute blood-vessels upon the circulation. Med Chir Trans, 1868, **51**:57-80.

[5] Mahomed, FA. The physiology and clinical use of the sphygmograph. Med Times Gaz, 1872, **1**:62-64.

[6] Mahomed, FA. On the sphygmographic evidence of arterio-capillary fibrosis. Trans Path Soc, 1877, **28**:394-397.

[7] Mahomed, FA. Chronic bright's disease without albuminuria. Guy's Hosp Rep, 1881, **25**:295-416.

[8] Riva-Rocci, S. Un nuovo sphygmomanometro. Gazz Med Torino, 1896, **47**:981-1001.

[9] Korotkoff, NS. On methods of studying blood pressure. Izv Voennomed Akad, 1905, **11**:365-370.

[10] Tigerstedt, R. Bergman, PG. Niere und Kreislauf. Skand Arch Physiol, 1898, **8**:223-271.

[11] Hall, JE. Historical perspective of the renin angiotensin system. Methods Mol Med. 2001;51:3-21.

[12] Inagami, T. A memorial to Robert Tiegerstedt: the centennial of renin discovery. Hypertension, 1998, **32**:953-957.

[13] Volhard, F. Der arterielle Hochdruck. Verhandl deutsch Geselisch. Med, 1923, **35**:134-184.

[14] Bohn, H. Untersuchungen zum Mecbanismus des blassen Hochdrnks: I Mitt Gefassverengernde Stoffe im Blute beim blassen Hochdruck. Ztsckr klin Med, 1932, **119**:100-139.

[15] Basso, N. Terragno, NA. History about the discovery of the renin-angiotensin system. Hypertension, 2001, **38**:1246-1249.

[16] Janeway, TC. Note on the blood pressure changes following reduction of the renal arterial circulation. Proc Soc Exp Biol Med, 1909, **109**:5-6.

[17] Goldblatt, H. Lynch, J. Hanzal, RF. Summerville WW: studies on experimental hypertension: I. Production of persistent elevation of systolic blood pressure by means of renal ischemia. J Exp Mcd, 1934, **9**:347-379.

[18] Milei, J. Trujillo, JM. Historia del Instituto de investigaciones cardiológicas Alberto C. Taquini en su 60° aniversario. Medicina, 2004, **64**:163-169.

[19] Taquini, AC. Producción de sustancia vasoconstrictora renal en diversas circunstancias. Rev Soc Argent Biol, 1938, **14**:456-460.

[20] Milei, J. Alberto C. Taquini and the 'links' that led to the discovery of angiotensin: on the 100th anniversary of his birth. J Hypertens, 2005, **23**:1267-1269.

[21] Houssay, BA. Taquini AC. Acción vasoconstrictora de la sangre venosa del riñón isquemiado. Rev Soc Arg Biol, 1938, **14**:5-14.

[22] Taquini, AC. Braun-Menéndez, E. Liberación de substancia vasoconstrictora en el riñón completamente isquemiado. Rev Soc Arg Biol, 1938, **14**:422-429.

[23] Fasciolo, JC. The experimental observation that led to discovery of angiotensin. Hypertension, 1990, **16**:194-198.

[24] Fasciolo, JC. Acción del riñón sano sobre la hipertensión arterial por isquemia renal. Rev Soc Argent Biol, 1938, **14**:15-24.

[25] Fasciolo, JC. Papel de las glándulas adrenales en la génesis de la hipertensión arterial por isquemia renal. Rev Soc Argent Biol, 1938, **14**:25-30.

[26] Braun-Menéndez, E. Fasciolo, JC. Mecanismo de la acción hipertensora de la sangre venosa del riñón en isquemia incompleta aguda. Rev Soc Arg Biol, 1939, **15**:401-410.

[27] Braun-Menéndez, E. Fasciolo, JC. Acción vasoconstrictora e hipertensora de la sangre venosa del riñón en isquemia incompleta aguda. Rev Soc Arg Biol, 1939, **15**:161-172.

[28] Pasqualini, CD. Juan Carlos Fasciolo, discípulo de Houssay y descubridor de la angiotensina. Medicina, 2011, **71**:405-407.

[29] Braun-Menéndez, E. Fasciolo, JC. Leloir, LF. Muñoz, JM. La sustancia hipertensora de la sangre del riñón isquemiado. Rev Soc Arg Biol, 1939, **15**:420-425.

[30] Braun-Menéndez, E. Fasciolo, JC. Leloir, LF. Muñoz, JM. The substance causing renal hypertension. J Physiol, 1940, **98**:283-298.

[31] Basso, N. Schiffrin, L. Professor Alberto C. Taquini: 1905-1998. Hypertension, 1998, **32**:1-2.

[32] Page, IH. Hypertension research. A memoir 1920-1960. Hypertension, 1990, **16**:199-200.

[33] Kohlstaedt, KG. Helmer, OM. Page, IH. Activation of rennin by blood colloids. Proc Soc Exp Biol Med, 1938, **39**:214-215.

[34] Page, IH. Helmer, OM. A crystalline pressor substance (angiotonin) resulting from the reaction between renin and renin-activator. Exp Med, 1940, **71**:29-42.

[35] Page, IH. Helmer, OM. Plentl, AA. Kohlstaedt, KG. Corcoran, AC. Suggested change in designation of "reninactivator" (hypertensinogen) to "renin-substrate (α2 globulin)". Science, 1943, **98**:153.

[36] Braun-Menéndez, E. Page, IH. Suggested revision of nomenclature: angiotensin. Science, 1958, **127**:242.

[37] Taquini, AC. Jr. Taquini, AC. The renin-angiotensin system in hypertension. Am Heart, 1961, **62**:558-564.

[38] Skeggs, LT. Jr. Discovery of the two angiotensin peptides and the angiotensin converting enzyme. Hypertension, 1993, **21**:259-260.

[39] Leloir, LF. Muñoz, JM. Braun-Menéndez, E. Fasciolo, JC. La secreción de renina y la formación de hipertensina. Rev Soc Argent Biol, 1940, **16**:75-80.

[40] Muñoz, JM. Braun-Menéndez, E. Fasciolo, JC. Leloir, LF. The mechanism of renal hypertension. Am J Med, 1940, **200**:608-618.

[41] Taquini, AC. Braun-Menéndez, E. Fasciolo, JC. Leloir, LF. Muñoz, JM. Medición del hipertensinógeno. Rev Soc Argent Biol, 1943, **19**:500-506.

[42] Leloir, LF. Muñoz, JM. Taquini, AC. Braun-Menéndez, E. Fasciolo, JC. La formación del angiotensinógeno. Rev Argent Cardiol, 1942, **9**:269-278.

[43] Page, IH. Mc Swain, B. Knapp, GM. Andrus, WD. The origin of renin activator. Am J Physiol, 1941, **135**:214-222.

[44] Cherne, PN. Young, P. Historia del sistema renina angiotensina: grandes hombres, un gran descubrimiento. Revista médica de Chile, 2014, **142**:1210-1216.

[45] Robertson, JIS. Renin and angiotensin: a historical review. The Renin-Angiotensin System, 1993, **1**:1-18.

[46] Ondetti, MA. From peptides to peptidases: a chronicle of drug discovery. Annu Rev Pharmacol Toxicol, 1994, **34**:1-16.

Section 2

RAS and Cardiovascular System

Chapter 2

Involvement of the Renin-Angiotensin System in Atherosclerosis

Ana Kolakovic, Maja Zivkovic and
Aleksandra Stankovic

Additional information is available at the end of the chapter

http://dx.doi.org/10.5772/67137

Abstract

The renin-angiotensin system (RAS) is a well known for its role in the regulation of the blood pressure (BP). Angiotensin II (Ang II), the main mediator of the RAS, may act either, as a systemic molecule or a locally produced factor. Within the vessel wall it has significant proinflammatory role by inducing the oxidative stress, secretion of inflammatory cytokines and adhesion molecules. Ang II could trigger proliferation of vascular smooth muscle cells (VSMC) and its migration to the outer layer of the vessel wall. It could induce the release of matrix metalloproteinase (MMPs), from human VSMC and thus increase susceptibility to rupture of atherosclerotic lesions. Binding of Ang II to AT1R/AT2R could have opposing actions in vascular injury. The ACE2/Ang (1-7)/Mas axis of the RAS also opposes the unfavourable actions of ACE/Ang II/ATR1 axis. Inhibition of RAS could reduce inflammation-associated processes in vasculature, independently of lowering BP. RAS is significantly modulated by the genes coding for this system. Certain genetic variants (SNPs) in the RAS genes have been denoted as the functional ones and have been associated with hypertension, cardiovascular phenotypes and atherosclerosis. Also, the genetic components of the RAS interfere with the regulators of gene expression by microRNAs (miRs).

Keywords: renin-angiotensin system, atherosclerosis, genetic variant, micro RNA gene expression

1. Introduction

1.1. Short overview of the RAS

The renin-angiotensin system (RAS) is a cascade well known for its primary role in the regulation of blood pressure (BP) and sodium homeostasis. It has a significant role in regulating fluid and electrolyte balance by exerting its actions on the heart, blood vessels and kidneys.

The circulating RAS comprises liver-secreted angiotensinogen (AGT) that is enzymatically converted into angiotensin I (Ang I) in the bloodstream by kidney-derived renin. In the next step, Ang I is being converted by angiotensin-converting enzyme (ACE) to form Ang II. Ang II is the main effector in this system that acts either as a systemic molecule or as a locally produced factor.

The RAS is probably one of the most investigated biological systems over past 30 years. Given its pleiotropic biological effects, it is expected. Its complexity underlies the fact that research involving RAS molecules and actions in health and disease is still very active and intriguing. In the past decade, a substantial expansion of our knowledge of the RAS was emerged. It is verified by newly discovered components. One of them is a homologue of ACE, angiotensin-converting enzyme 2 (ACE2), which exerts a role as a negative regulator of the RAS [1] by cleaving Ang II to Ang-(1–7) [2, 3]. Namely, Santos et al. demonstrated that Ang-(1-7) is the ligand for the G-protein-coupled receptor Mas, and that the ACE2–Ang-(1–7)–Mas axis is the counter-regulating of the actions of classical RAS [4, 5]. Also, a variety of biologically active peptides, novel components of the RAS have been found recently: proangiotensin-12 (angiotensin-(1–12)) [6], angiotensin A (Ang A) [7, 8] and alamandine [9, 10].

1.2. Tissue and intracellular RAS

Our knowledge of the RAS has undergone substantial revision in the past few years. The existence of local (tissue) RAS systems that are independent of those stimulated by the classical RAS made it evident that the RAS is more complex than originally thought [11]. In that way, RAS is experienced substantial conceptual changes. Local (tissue) RAS represents tissue-based formation of angiotensin peptides that operate separately from the circulating RAS [12]. Tissue RAS systems are located in all major organs, including brain, heart, large blood vessels, adrenals and the kidneys [13]. Local RAS systems exert various actions depending on the type of cells involved and play crucial role in the maintenance of cellular homeostasis.

In order to identify a tissue-specific RAS at least one of the following criteria have to be fulfil [14]: (1) mRNAs for all components required for biosynthesis of a biologically active Ang II are present, (2) a biologically active angiotensin peptide is synthesized, (3) receptors for the biologically active angiotensin peptide are present, (4) the biologically active angiotensin peptide in the tissue is regulated, independently of the circulating RAS and (5) reduction or elimination of the action of the angiotensin peptide produces a physiological response.

There are other components of local RAS that are contributing to tissue-specific mechanisms of angiotensin peptide formation. They are participating in the progression of disease, or contrary, in mechanisms that protect from tissue injury [12]. These components include the (pro) renin receptor [15, 16], renin-independent mechanisms of Ang peptide generation from Ang-(1–12) [17, 18], intracellular RAS [19], previously mentioned ACE2/Ang-(1–7)/Mas receptor pathway [20] and they all may possess therapeutic potential.

Although different concepts of local RAS have been described, its key characteristic is a synthesis of AGT and enzymes, such as renin, that cleaves AGT to produce Ang I independently of the circulating RAS [12, 21, 22]. The presence of ACE, Ang II type 1 (AT1R) and type 2 (AT2R) receptors and Ang II in different cells supports the concept of local RAS [23]. The local RAS seems to be regulated independently from the circulating system in a specific manner depending on the cell type and extracellular stimulus [24]. Despite that it can interact with the circulating system and complement it.

Some of the attempts to define local RAS that are independent of the circulating RAS were made in animal models [12]. One of the approaches to studying the functional importance of locally synthesized RAS components is to demonstrate their targeted overexpression or deletion in specific tissues. The evidence shows that in most tissues, local RAS enhances the actions of circulating Ang II, which has important implications for the pathophysiology of cardiovascular diseases.

In addition to classical and local tissue RAS, there is an intracellular RAS. This system is characterized by the presence of a functionally active RAS within the cells that can intracellularly synthesize Ang II [19, 25]. This means that Ang II is involved not only in an endocrine but also is a paracrine and an intracrine signaling system within tissues [26]. For example, intracellular delivery of Ang II leads to increase in intracellular calcium, growth of vascular smooth muscle cells (VSMCs) and regulation of muscle tone [27, 28]. This suggests that the intracellular Ang II has different functions compared to extracellular Ang II.

2. RAS and atherosclerosis

2.1. Molecular processes in atherosclerosis through the prism of RAS actions

Ang II, the main effector peptide of RAS, participates in all phases of the atherogenesis. It is proposed that the activation of RAS, and particularly Ang II, is involved in the initiation and progression of atherosclerosis in the absence of hemodynamic influences [29, 30]. Moreover, activation of RAS in the vascular wall has important modulatory activities in the development of atherosclerotic plaques, by stimulating a series of coordinated cellular and molecular events observed in the lesions.

2.1.1. Role of RAS in atherosclerosis development

The initial steps of atherosclerosis include endothelial dysfunction, which allows the migration of inflammatory cells and lipid droplets into the damaged part of the vessel wall, where they accumulate and form a "fatty streak". Oxidative stress is one of the main factors that promote vascular endothelial dysfunction. This is initial phase of vascular damage, when elevated levels of reactive oxygen species (ROS) that might be caused by Ang II induce impaired endothelial relaxation and vascular function [31]. ROS are free radicals involving oxygen, such as superoxide anions, hydroxyl radicals and hydrogen peroxide. These are mainly generated by mitochondria as by-products of cellular metabolism in the vessel wall by all vascular cells, including endothelial cells, VSMCs and adventitial fibroblasts. However, the imbalance between ROS generation and antioxidant protection leads to a state of oxidative stress, which can have deleterious effects as it modulates numerous cell signaling pathways. This is manifested as increased expression of pro-inflammatory genes, cell migration and proliferation, extracellular matrix production and apoptosis in the vessel wall, all of which play an important role in vascular injury [32]. RAS activates NAD(P)H oxidase by enhancing Ang II/AT1R signaling which leads to increase in ROS production in both vascular endothelial cells and VSMCs [33, 34]. Ang II may traffic to mitochondria and AT1R could be expressed on outer mitochondrial membranes [35]. This way Ang II may stimulate an increase in mitochondrial oxidative stress, thus leads to VCMC senescence. Also, mitochondria may endogenously produce Ang II [36–38]. Several animal studies show that Ang II causes and contributes to aortic endothelial dysfunction [39–41]. It promotes abnormal vasomotion, a procoagulant state and transmigration of inflammatory cells into the vessel wall [42]. Within the vessel wall, Ang II increases vascular permeability via activation of vascular cell adhesion molecule-1 (VCAM-1) [43], intercellular adhesion molecule (ICAM)-1 [44], and endothelial growth factor (VEGF) [41, 42, 45, 46]. The key step in the formation of the initial lesion in atherosclerosis is the inflammation at the site of plaque formation caused by monocytes recruited from the blood stream by VCAM-1 [47]. Additionally, Ang II stimulates apoptosis of endothelial cell and VSMCs [48, 49].

The next stage in fatty streak formation is oxidation of low density lipoprotein (ox-LDL). Ox-LDL has important atherogenic properties as it penetrates the endothelial layer and gets taken up by macrophages and VSMCs, which results in the creation of lipid-containing foam cells. Ang II increases the interleukin-6 (IL-6)-mediated uptake of oxidized LDL by macrophages [50]. Moreover, Ang II upregulates lectin-like oxidized low-density lipoprotein receptor-1 (LOX-1) and 12-lipoxygenase (12-LO) and 15-lipoxygenas (15-LO) expression in human VSMC. Thus, these two actions are accelerating LDL oxidation within the cell and enabling the internalization of exogenous ox-LDL, which could increase the susceptibility of human VSMC to transformation into foam cells [51].

The exposure of vascular cells to excess lipid (modified LDLs) with concomitant endothelial dysfunction/activation and the internalization and lipid deposits in the intima of vessel wall leads to further progression of atherosclerotic plaques [52]. Since advanced lesions predominantly consist of inflammatory cells, it is considered that at this stage progression of atherosclerosis is inflammation-driven. Modified LDLs enhance a broad range inflammatory responses, including activation, recruitment and infiltration of different immune cells (monocytes, neutrophils, natural killer cells, mast cells and dendritic cells) although the contribution of circulating monocytes is the most important [52]. When monocytes infiltrate and reach the sub-endothelium they differentiate into macrophages, under the stimulation of macrophage colony-stimulating factor (M-CSF). Macrophages are very adaptable cells that can undertake different phenotypes and functional characteristics, depending on the local microenvironment, which is a process known as 'polarization' [53, 54]. Distinct macrophage subtypes (M1 and M2) have been detected depending on the stage of atherosclerosis. Once differentiated, macrophages express high levels of pattern recognition receptors on their surface. These receptors have the ability to take up modified LDLs. Macrophages, then become lipid-laden and convert into foam cells. There is a potential role that Ang II provoking recruitment and activation of both macrophages and T cells into the vessel wall, by stimulating the expression of pro-inflammatory chemokines and cytokines, since both macrophages [55] and T cells express the AT1R on their surface [56, 57]. Ang II also increases monocyte chemoattractant protein-1 (MCP-1) expression in culture VSMCs as well as monocytes [58].

http://dx.doi.org/10.5772/67137

Importantly, Ang II induces the activation of several pro-inflammatory transcription factors. One of them is nuclear factor kappa B (NF-κB). Ang II activates NF-κB via AT1R in vascular cells and mononuclear cells, both *in vivo* and *in vitro* [59, 60]. The increase Ang II activates NF-κB by phosphorylating IκBα and p65 [61], which induces enhanced matrix metalloproteinase 9 (MMP-9) expression [62]. The AT1R mediates most of the actions of Ang II, but experimental data suggest that AT2R is also involved in Ang II-mediated NF-κB activation in inflammatory cell recruitment [63]. Recently, both an increase in AT1R and ACE levels and activation of NF-κB in heart have been reported in rat a model of a metabolic syndrome known as an inflammatory condition associated with accelerated atherogenesis [62, 64].

On the other hand, Ang II-induced activation of NF-kB could downregulate peroxisome proliferator-activated receptors (PPARs), PPAR-alpha and -gamma. This may diminish the anti-inflammatory effect of PPARs, thus contributing to enhanced vascular inflammation, leading to the acceleration of atherosclerosis in mice deficient for apolipoprotein E(ApoE -/-) mice [65]. Also, Ang II is inducing inflammation and remodelling of the vessel wall via activation of transcriptional mediator, Ets-1, member of ETS family of transcription factors [66]. Recently, inflammatory actions of Ang II were diminished by sirtuin-1 (SIRT-1) activator SRT1720. Treatment with SRT1720 decreased expression of TNF-a, IL-6, MCP-1, VCAM-1, ICAM-1, activation of NF-kB, STAT3 and infiltration of inflammatory cells in atherosclerotic plaques, induced by Ang II [67]. In order to inhibit Ang II signaling, SIRT-1 activation is a promising atheroprotective mechanism.

2.1.2. Role of RAS in atherosclerosis progression and acute complications

Over time continued plaque growth causes thickening and stiffening of the vessel wall and destabilizes it. This process results in a plaque rupture, which manifests as an occurrence of acute complications and development of ischaemic syndromes. Furthermore, the release of growth factors and cytokines by foam cells stimulates VSMC migration from the media into the intima. Upon arrival, these cells divide and produce extracellular matrix (ECM) components that contribute to the formation of the fibrous cap covering the plaque lipid core [68]. Also, Ang II triggers VSMCs to proliferate and migrate to the outer layer of the atherosclerotic plaques, where they produce growth factors and extracellular matrix proteins [69, 70]. The deposition of ECM components secreted by VSMCs in the plaques increases their size and eventually become occlusive. The interaction between exposed atherosclerotic plaque components, platelet receptors and coagulation factors from blood leads to platelet activation, aggregation and the subsequent formation of a thrombus, which may compromise the arterial lumen [52]. The thrombogenicity of the plaque is favored by a disturbance in the balance of coagulation and fibrinolysis. The role of Ang II, as a mediator of thrombogenesis has been also supported by animal studies [71, 72]. Namely, models of elevated Ang II levels, elicited both genetically and via chronic Ang II infusion, have demonstrated increased tissue factor (TF) expression and increased plasma plasminogen activator inhibitor-1 (PAI-1) level [73–75]. *In vitro* studies confirmed that Ang II induces the expression of TF in rat aortic endothelial cells [76] and human monocytes [77]. Chronic Ang II infusion induces platelet-endothelial cell adhesion [78] and accelerates thrombus formation in both large arteries [71, 79] and arterioles [74]. TF in atherosclerotic plaques initiates blood coagulation, directly stimulates SMC proliferation and activates

MMPs capable of degrading collagen. MMPs digest ECM scaffold, including the overlying fibrous cap, increasing plaque susceptibility to rupture. Moreover, Ang II induces release of MMP-2 in murine VSMCs via p47phox cytosolic subunit of the NAD(P)H-oxidase. Therefore, the activation of RAS contributes atherosclerotic plaque remodelling and potential destabilization via a NAD(P)H-oxidase-dependent activation of MMP-2 [80]. Laxton et al. demonstrated *in vitro* that MMP-8 cleaves Ang I to generate Ang II, and that MMP8-knockout mice have a substantial reduction in formation of atherosclerotic lesions [81]. Moreover, an association between MMP8 gene variation and extent of coronary and carotid atherosclerosis [81, 82] was observed. Significant upregulation of MMP-8 gene expression in carotid plaque tissue was observed in patients carrying haplotype G(-381)T(-799) of two MMP-8 promoter polymorphisms rs11225395 (-799 C/T) and rs1320632 (-381 A/G) [82]. Recently, it was shown that Ang II treatment *in vitro* causes increased collagen I synthesis and galectin-3 (Gal-3) expression in mouse HL-1 cardiomyocytes via protein kinase Calpha (PKC-α) pathway [83]. Gal-3 is involved in all processes active in atherosclerosis: cell adhesion, cell activation and chemoattraction, cell growth and differentiation [84]. An increase expression of Gal-3 mRNA in human carotid atherosclerotic plaque tissue may be affected by rare genetic variants of the haplotype block, previously associated with Gal-3 circulating levels [85, 86]. Diverse cellular processes in atherosclerosis are affected by microRNAs (miRs) and their expression are often tissue and disease-specific [87, 88]. Recently, the prediction algorithms and computational methods were applied to identify novel miRs important in pathogenesis of early and advanced atherosclerosis [89]. Amongst a number of miRs upregulated in atherosclerotic plaque, miR-155 shows dual properties in atherosclerosis and has particular interactions with RAS. Its activity could suppress Ang II-induced extracellular signal-regulated kinase (ERK1/2) phosphorylation and activation and regulate AT1R expression in different vascular cells [90, 91]. Moreover, it is shown that miR-155 downregulates AT1R expression, but not other RAS components [90].

2.2. Main RAS molecules in atherosclerosis through the magnifying glass

It is evident that Ang II, as a main mediator of RAS, promotes the formation of atherosclerotic lesions. In animal models of disease, AT1R deficiency in ApoE -/- and LDL receptor (LDLR-/-) atherosclerotic mice attenuates progression of atherosclerotic lesions, suggesting that AT1R mediates most of the Ang II functions [92, 93]. Hyperlipidaemia upregulates AT1R whose activation augments vascular oxidative stress and accelerates atherosclerosis [93], particularly as oxidized lipid becomes a neo-antigen that attracts components of the adaptive immune system to the vascular wall [94]. Consistent with this, AT1R deficiency causes a marked decrease in atherosclerotic lesion size in both the aortic root and arch of female and male mice, without a discernible effect on the composition. Also, aortic ATR2 mRNA expression is not altered in AT1R deficient mice, and AT2R deficiency is not affecting the lesion area or cellular composition [93].

Pharmacological inhibition of endothelial dysfunction and diet-induced atherosclerosis in ApoE AT1R-deficient mice dramatically attenuates the severity of atherosclerotic lesions [92, 95]. It is believed that the protective effects of the AT1R blockade with its antagonists (ARBs) include reduction of oxidative stress, reduction of inflammation and improvement in endothelial function [92]. Pharmacological blockade of AT1R reduces lipid accumulation and

http://dx.doi.org/10.5772/67137

increases the level of collagen within the atheroma and thereby stabilizes the formation of atherosclerotic plaques in ApoE-deficient mice [96] and in those with disrupted AT1R gene in bone marrow cells (BM) [97]. BM chimeric mice with disrupted BM AT1R show a reduced number of atherosclerotic lesions in the aorta and more stable plaques with reduced accumulation of BM-derived cells compared to AT1R-positive BM chimeric mice [97]. BM transplantation (BMT) from the ApoE-/-AT1R+/+ animals to the ApoE-/-AT1R-/- mice could restore Ang II-induced aggravation of atherosclerosis and plaque destabilization, even when the recipient's vascular cells do not express AT1R [98]. The contribution of AT1R in BM cells to the pathogenesis of atherosclerosis was demonstrated in LDL-receptor-deficient mice [99]. Hypertensive hypercholesterolemic ApoE-/- mice with either normal or endogenously increased Ang II production (renovascular hypertension models) were generated in order to study the contribution of Ang II to plaque vulnerability [100]. Staging and morphology of plaques significantly differed among these groups of mice and revealed an accelerated atherosclerosis in hypertensive animals. Plaques from mice with high Ang II appeared to be vulnerable, whereas plaques from mice with unchanged Ang II levels and similar blood pressure values were stable [100]. This mouse model of vulnerable plaque induced in a mouse is important and mimics a pathophysiological state commonly found in humans.

The expression of ERK1/2 and pro-inflammatory cytokines was reduced in supernatants of human carotid atheroma explant cultures treated with ARBs [101]. Also, in the same type of atheroma ATR1 blockade led to significantly reduced Ang II, MMP-1, MMP-8 expression and soluble elastin fragments [102]. This data recognized the ability of ATR1 blockade to modify plaque stability.

There are several beneficial effects assigned to the role of AT2R in atherosclerosis. AT2R overexpression in LDLR-knockout mice reduces atherogenesis in the aorta, as well as, expression and activity of MMP-2, MMP-9 and collagen accumulation in atherosclerotic regions [103]. In the same model, the presence of AT2R modulated oxidative stress, by decreasing expression of LOX-1, endothelial NO synthase (eNOS) and heme oxygenase-1 (HO-1) [104]. Also, in mice deficient for ApoE and AT2R on a diet rich in cholesterol, the atherosclerotic changes were exaggerated [105] which was shown as increased cellularity of atherosclerotic lesions [106]. After 16 weeks on a diet high in cholesterol, ApoE (-/-)/AT2R+ mice had significantly decreased a number of macrophages, VSMCs, lipids and collagen in the plaques due to apoptosis, compared to those deficient in AT2R gene [106]. Stimulation of AT2R by exogenous Ang II reduced atherogenesis in ApoE-/-/AT1R-/- double knockout mice [107]. It is evident that AT2R exerts atheroprotective effects when AT1R is inhibited. Vascular AT2R stimulation in transgenic ApoE-/- mice (AT2R-Tg/ApoE-/-) significantly reduces atherosclerotic lesion development in an endothelial kinin/nitric oxide(NO)-dependent manner and its anti-oxidative effect is likely to be mediated by inhibition of the superoxide-producing mononuclear leukocytes accumulation [108]. In ApoE-deficient mice, direct stimulation of AT2R by agonist CGP42112 improves endothelial function and stabilizes atherosclerotic plaques [109].

Evidence suggests that AT2R and ACE2, as a part of the ACE2–Ang-(1–7)–Mas axis, play a protective role in atherogenesis. Both factors have been detected within rabbit atherosclerotic plaques, AT2R and ACE2 immunoreactivity were observed in macrophages and alpha SMC actin-positive cells [110]. ACE2 has been identified as a critical negative modulator of Ang II, counterbalancing the effects of ACE, by degrading Ang II and generating anti-atherosclerotic Ang-(1-7). Genetic ACE2 deficiency underlines vascular inflammation and atherosclerosis in the ApoE-/- mice [111]. Protective role of ACE2 and AT2R in cardiovascular pathology is supported by their decreased expression in male rat hearts on fructose-rich diet [112].

Also, ACE2 deficiency either in a whole body or in bone marrow-derived cells reduced atherosclerosis in LDLR-/- mice through regulation of Ang II/Ang-(1–7) peptides [113]. Overexpression of ACE2 in aortas of ApoE-/- mice transfected with AdACE2 (recombinant ACE2 adenovirus encoding full-length human ACE2 and co-expressing the GFP protein) led to less prominent macrophage infiltration than in aortas from control mice [114]. Also, overexpression of ACE2 enhanced plaque stability in a rabbit model of atherosclerosis [115]. Abdominal aorta segments transfected with AdACE2 showed a delayed onset of atherosclerotic lesions with fewer macrophages, less lipid deposition, more collagen contents, decreased expression of Ang II, MCP-1, LOX-1 and increased angiotensin (1–7) levels in plaque tissue [116]. In two different models of vascular disease, both hyperlipidaemia-induced atherosclerosis in ApoE-/- mice and mechanical injury-induced arterial neointimal hyperplasia in C57Bl6 mice, ACE2 deficiency resulted in significantly larger vascular lesions and neointimal hyperplasia compared with ACE2(+) controls [117]. ACE2 and exogenous Ang-(1-7) significantly inhibit early atherosclerotic lesion formation by preserving endothelial function and inhibiting of an inflammatory response in ApoE-/- mice [118, 119]. ACE2 activity and protein production were increased in atherosclerotic plaques treated with losartan *in vivo* in and *in vitro* in VSMCs [120]. Candesartan treatment restores vasoprotective and atheroprotective effects of the ACE2/Ang (1-7)/Mas receptor axis in high-cholesterol diet-fed ApoE-/- mice due to the inhibition of the pro-inflammatory-redox AT1R-mediated mechanism [121]. Increased ACE2 activation is considered to be a protective and compensatory mechanism that counterbalances ACE activity, and may play an important role in the treatment of atherosclerosis. Activation of ACE2/Ang (1-7)/Mas receptor axis by ACE2 activator (XNT) attenuates thrombus formation and reduces platelet attachment to vessels [122]. ACE2 overexpression in THP-1 (human acute monocytic leukemia cell line) *in vitro* decreases Ang II-induced MCP-1 production and this reduction is likely to be mediated by increased Ang (1-7) levels [123]. Blockage of endogenously activated Ang-(1-7) by chronic infusion of A779 attenuated late atherosclerotic plaque stability in high fat diet fed ApoE-/- mice [118]. All together ACE2 and Ang-(1–7) could be a therapeutic target for attenuation of atherosclerosis and the treatment of cardiovascular diseases.

3. Genetics of RAS in atherosclerosis

Over the past two decades, a large number of genetic investigations have been carried out to examine the association between genetic variants of RAS genes and vascular diseases, such as myocardial infarction, coronary artery disease and stroke. RAS genes were thoroughly associated with different risk factors for atherosclerosis, among which hypertension has a central role bearing in mind primary physiological role of RAS. Different cardiovascular phenotypes, such as left ventricular hypertrophy, artery stenosis, artery stiffness and vascular remodelling were studied as well.

The story started with unforgettable discovery of ACE insertion/deletion (I/D) polymorphism (rs4340) associated with increased levels of ACE [124, 125]. This was the first discovery that implicated what is now fully accepted, that naturally occurring variations in DNA sequences, or polymorphisms (SNPs, insertion/deletions, copy number variations), mostly have the modifying effect in the development of atherosclerosis and together with gene-gene and gene-environment interactions are making an important contribution to the risk.

The most widely studied polymorphism in the RAS is I/D polymorphism, a287-bp Alu repeat element in intron 16 of ACE gene. It has been considered as a functional variant, since the ACE DD genotype was associated with higher circulating [124–126] and tissue mRNA levels of ACE [127, 128]. Among 78 variations that were found by ACE gene sequencing, 17 were in absolute linkage disequilibrium with the I/D polymorphism [129]. First genetic association studies were focused on ACE D allele effect on blood pressure [130, 131] and hypertension [132–134].

In atherosclerosis, most of the studies so far have been investigating ACE I/D polymorphism in association with subclinical and intermediate atherosclerotic phenotypes, such as intima-media thickness (IMT) with conflicting results. Meta-analysis of these studies uncovered moderate positive association of ACE D allele with common carotid IMT [135]. The association of ACE I/D polymorphism studies with advanced atherosclerosis has still been rare. As different mechanisms might be dominating the different stage of atherosclerosis development, as described previously in this chapter, it is always of importance to perform a genetic association study on early non-stenotic atherosclerosis and advanced stenotic atherosclerosis. A significant independent effect of DD genotype on plaque presence in patients with high-grade carotid stenosis (>70%) was noticed only in normotensive patients [136]. Another study failed to support the hypothesis that ACE genotype is a predictor of either the prevalence or the extent of atherosclerotic plaques but only in young adults [137].

Nevertheless, its role in atherosclerotic complications was noticed in a large-scale meta-analysis where the significant associations with ischemic stroke in approximately 18,000 cases and 58,000 controls were identified for four gene polymorphisms among which was ACE I/D [138]. An astonishing discovery was made recently, 23 years after Tiret et al. [124] found that ACE I/D influence on serum ACE levels. It was observed ACE expression appears to be regulated by mitochondrial uncoupling proteins (UCPs). Serum ACE activity was influenced by allele variants in UCP2 and UCP3 genes. This was the first evidence of association of serum ACE with a genetic variant outside the ACE gene [139]. This gave a new perspective on ACE investigation, suggesting that cellular feedback regulation might exist between ACE and UCPs. Even so, genetic variations in UCPs and SIRTs were recently associated with the atherosclerotic plaque existence [140] and morphology [141].

Also, both Ang II receptor genes, AT1R and AT2R, have many SNPs in the coding and its flanking regions, but the most studied are AT1R A1166C and AT2R -1332 A/G (+G1675A).

The A1166C polymorphism (rs5186) is located in the 3′ untranslated region (UTR) of AT1R gene. Primarily, it was investigated in association with hypertension but with inconsistent findings. Association with hypertension was established in a certain subgroups of patients, e.g. only in subjects with severe, early onset, form of disease [142] and in long-term-treated subjects and/or with a family history of hypertension (HT) [143, 144] or in subjects with hypercholesterolaemia [145] or in males only [146]. A systematic review and a meta-analysis of the rs5186 variant failed to present sufficient evidence that polymorphisms in the AT1R gene are risk factors for hypertension [147].

Besides hypertension, rs5186 was associated with increased reactivity to Ang II in human arteries [148] and blood pressure response to exogenous Ang II [149]. In the context of atherosclerosis and different atherosclerotic phenotypes, previous studies addressed this polymorphism with inconsistent data. Some failed to show any significant effect for the A1166C polymorphism on mean IMT, carotid plaque formation [150] or internal carotid artery (ICA) stenosis [151]. The C-allele has been associated with a thicker carotid IMT in women [152] and increased IMT and IMT/D (common carotid artery diameter) ratio in hypertensive subjects [153]. A meta-analysis performed in 2011 suggests that the AT1R gene A1166C polymorphism is not associated with susceptibility to ischemic stroke [154]. However, the association between the AT1R 1166C allele and the presence of hypoechoic carotid plaques was recently found [155]. Confronting results could be attributed to differences in age, gender, belonging to different populations or ethnic groups, or different non-genomic and other external factors. The AT1R A1166C polymorphism is positioned in the target site for miR-155 [156, 157]. It was shown experimentally that human miR-155 downregulates expression of the 1166A allele alone [156], and that interaction between authentic miR-155 and the C allele is diminished, in a way that its ability to regulate AT1R gene expression is altered [157].

The AT2R, -1332 A/G polymorphism (rs1403543) located within the intron 1 of the gene was proposed to be functional, by affecting the mRNA alternative splicing and gene expression of AT2R. However, novel findings suggest that -1332 A/G might modulate protein expression, but not mRNA splicing [158, 159]. There are few studies that have been investigating this polymorphism in association with the presence of atherosclerotic plaques. Our study performed recently suggests that AT2R -1332 A/G polymorphism is a reliable gender-specific risk factor for carotid atherosclerotic plaque presence in females and could modify the inter-individual risk of cerebrovascular insult (CVI) among males with advanced carotid atherosclerosis [160]. It is still not clear which of the alleles, A or G, are more likely to carry a significant risk, even for hypertension and different cardiovascular phenotypes that were reproducibly investigated [161]. It was shown that a -1332 A/G polymorphism represents a risk factor for cardiovascular diseases and severe atherosclerosis by modifying systemic inflammation, especially in hypertensive males [162]. It is known that AT2R is expressed at low levels in the healthy adult vasculature. AT2R effects on cardiovascular structure and function may only become detectable under pathological conditions and/or after AT1R blockade. Expression of AT2R in human carotid atherosclerotic plaques was previously detected [163]. However, whether the stimulation of the AT2R is protective or deleterious in human atherosclerosis remains unresolved. The impact of AT2R during atherosclerosis or tissue injury should be studied by direct stimulation of AT2R to address potential therapeutic potential [164, 165].

http://dx.doi.org/10.5772/67137

4. Conclusion

Activation of RAS in the vascular wall has modulatory activities in the development of atherosclerosis by stimulating a series of cellular and molecular events. The balance between activation and repression of RAS could be decisive in the pathological remodelling, endothelial dysfunction and pathogenesis of atherosclerosis. Unfavorable and favorable effects of RAS molecules and their genetic variations, as well as consequently induced pathways, affect atherosclerosis development and following clinical events. This could have potential towards clinical application for risk stratification and therapeutics.

Acknowledgements

This work was supported by the Grants of the Ministry of Education, Science and Technological Development, Republic of Serbia: III41028 and OI 175085.

Author details

Ana Kolakovic, Maja Zivkovic and Aleksandra Stankovic*

*Address all correspondence to: alexas@vin.bg.ac.rs

Department of Health and Environment, Laboratory for Radiobiology and Molecular Genetics, VINCA Institute of Nuclear Sciences, University of Belgrade, Serbia

References

[1] Oudit GY, Crackower MA, Backx PH, Penninger JM. The role of ACE2 in cardiovascular physiology. Trends in Cardiovascular Medicine. 2003;13:93–101.

[2] Tipnis SR, Hooper NM, Hyde R, Karran E, Christie G, Turner AJ. A human homolog of angiotensin-converting enzyme. Cloning and functional expression as a captopril-insensitive carboxypeptidase. The Journal of Biological Chemistry. 2000;275:33238–43.

[3] Donoghue M, Hsieh F, Baronas E, Godbout K, Gosselin M, Stagliano N, et al. A novel angiotensin-converting enzyme-related carboxypeptidase (ACE2) converts angiotensin I to angiotensin 1–9. Circulation Research. 2000;87:E1–9.

[4] Santos RA, Ferreira AJ. Angiotensin-(1–7) and the renin-angiotensin system. Current Opinion in Nephrology and Hypertension. 2007;16:122–8.

[5] Santos RA, Simoes e Silva AC, Maric C, Silva DM, Machado RP, de Buhr I, et al. Angiotensin-(1-7) is an endogenous ligand for the G protein-coupled receptor Mas. Proceedings of the National Academy of Sciences of the United States of America. 2003;100:8258–63.

[6] Nagata S, Kato J, Sasaki K, Minamino N, Eto T, Kitamura K. Isolation and identification of proangiotensin-12, a possible component of the renin-angiotensin system. Biochemical and Biophysical Research Communications. 2006;350:1026–31.

[7] Jankowski V, Vanholder R, van der Giet M, Tolle M, Karadogan S, Gobom J, et al. Mass-spectrometric identification of a novel angiotensin peptide in human plasma. Arteriosclerosis, Thrombosis, and Vascular Biology. 2007;27:297–302.

[8] Coutinho DC, Foureaux G, Rodrigues KD, Salles RL, Moraes PL, Murca TM, et al. Cardiovascular effects of angiotensin A: a novel peptide of the renin-angiotensin system. Journal of the Renin-Angiotensin-Aldosterone System: JRAAS. 2014;15:480–6.

[9] Lautner RQ, Villela DC, Fraga-Silva RA, Silva N, Verano-Braga T, Costa-Fraga F, et al. Discovery and characterization of alamandine: a novel component of the renin-angiotensin system. Circulation Research. 2013;112:1104–11.

[10] Etelvino GM, Peluso AA, Santos RA. New components of the renin-angiotensin system: alamandine and the MAS-related G protein-coupled receptor D. Current Hypertension Reports. 2014;16:433.

[11] Bader M, Ganten D. Update on tissue renin-angiotensin systems. Journal of Molecular Medicine (Berlin, Germany). 2008;86:615–21.

[12] Campbell DJ. Clinical relevance of local Renin Angiotensin systems. Frontiers in Endocrinology. 2014;5:113.

[13] Paul M, Poyan Mehr A, Kreutz R. Physiology of local renin-angiotensin systems. Physiological Reviews. 2006;86:747–803.

[14] Speth RC, Giese MJ. Update on the Renin-Angiotensin System. J Pharmacol Clin Toxicol. 2013;1:1004.

[15] Nguyen G, Delarue F, Burckle C, Bouzhir L, Giller T, Sraer JD. Pivotal role of the renin/prorenin receptor in angiotensin II production and cellular responses to renin. The Journal of Clinical Investigation. 2002;109:1417–27.

[16] Nguyen G, Muller DN. The biology of the (pro)renin receptor. Journal of the American Society of Nephrology: JASN. 2010;21:18–23.

[17] Ahmad S, Simmons T, Varagic J, Moniwa N, Chappell MC, Ferrario CM. Chymase-dependent generation of angiotensin II from angiotensin-(1–12) in human atrial tissue. PloS One. 2011;6:e28501.

[18] Ferrario CM, Varagic J, Habibi J, Nagata S, Kato J, Chappell MC, et al. Differential regulation of angiotensin-(1–12) in plasma and cardiac tissue in response to bilateral nephrectomy. American Journal of Physiology Heart and Circulatory Physiology. 2009;296:H1184–92.

[19] Kumar R, Singh VP, Baker KM. The intracellular renin-angiotensin system: a new paradigm. Trends in Endocrinology and Metabolism: TEM. 2007;18:208–14.

[20] Simoes e Silva AC, Silveira KD, Ferreira AJ, Teixeira MM. ACE2, angiotensin-(1-7) and Mas receptor axis in inflammation and fibrosis. British Journal of Pharmacology. 2013;169:477–92.

[21] Ferrario CM. New physiological concepts of the renin-angiotensin system from the investigation of precursors and products of angiotensin I metabolism. Hypertension. 2010;55:445–52.

[22] van Kats JP, de Lannoy LM, Jan Danser AH, van Meegen JR, Verdouw PD, Schalekamp MA. Angiotensin II type 1 (AT1) receptor-mediated accumulation of angiotensin II in tissues and its intracellular half-life in vivo. Hypertension. 1997;30:42–9.

[23] Kurdi M, De Mello WC, Booz GW. Working outside the system: an update on the unconventional behavior of the renin-angiotensin system components. The International Journal of Biochemistry & Cell Biology. 2005;37:1357–67.

[24] Vargas F, Rodriguez-Gomez I, Vargas-Tendero P, Jimenez E, Montiel M. The renin-angiotensin system in thyroid disorders and its role in cardiovascular and renal manifestations. The Journal of Endocrinology. 2012;213:25–36.

[25] Kumar R, Boim MA. Diversity of pathways for intracellular angiotensin II synthesis. Current opinion in nephrology and hypertension. 2009;18:33–9.

[26] Fyhrquist F, Saijonmaa O. Renin-angiotensin system revisited. Journal of Internal Medicine. 2008;264:224–36.

[27] Filipeanu CM, Henning RH, de Zeeuw D, Nelemans A. Intracellular Angiotensin II and cell growth of vascular smooth muscle cells. British Journal of Pharmacology. 2001;132:1590–6.

[28] De Mello WC. Intracellular angiotensin II as a regulator of muscle tone in vascular resistance vessels. Pathophysiological implications. Peptides. 2016;78:87–90.

[29] Sata M, Fukuda D. Crucial role of renin-angiotensin system in the pathogenesis of atherosclerosis. The Journal of Medical Investigation: JMI. 2010;57:12–25.

[30] Daugherty A, Manning MW, Cassis LA. Angiotensin II promotes atherosclerotic lesions and aneurysms in apolipoprotein E-deficient mice. The Journal of Clinical Investigation. 2000;105:1605–12.

[31] Touyz RM. Reactive oxygen species and angiotensin II signaling in vascular cells -- implications in cardiovascular disease. Brazilian Journal of Medical and Biological Research [Revista brasileira de pesquisas medicas e biologicas/Sociedade Brasileira de Biofisica]. 2004;37:1263–73.

[32] Montezano AC, Touyz RM. Reactive oxygen species, vascular Noxs, and hypertension: focus on translational and clinical research. Antioxidants & Redox Signaling. 2014;20:164–82.

[33] Min LJ, Mogi M, Iwai M, Horiuchi M. Signaling mechanisms of angiotensin II in regulating vascular senescence. Ageing Research Reviews. 2009;8:113–21.

[34] Nickenig G, Harrison DG. The AT(1)-type angiotensin receptor in oxidative stress and atherogenesis: Part II: AT(1) receptor regulation. Circulation. 2002;105:530–6.

[35] Huang J, Hara Y, Anrather J, Speth RC, Iadecola C, Pickel VM. Angiotensin II subtype 1A (AT1A) receptors in the rat sensory vagal complex: subcellular localization and association with endogenous angiotensin. Neuroscience. 2003;122:21–36.

[36] Clausmeyer S, Reinecke A, Farrenkopf R, Unger T, Peters J. Tissue-specific expression of a rat renin transcript lacking the coding sequence for the prefragment and its stimulation by myocardial infarction. Endocrinology. 2000;141:2963–70.

[37] Peters J, Clausmeyer S. Intracellular sorting of renin: cell type specific differences and their consequences. Journal of Molecular and Cellular Cardiology. 2002;34:1561–8.

[38] Peters J, Kranzlin B, Schaeffer S, Zimmer J, Resch S, Bachmann S, et al. Presence of renin within intramitochondrial dense bodies of the rat adrenal cortex. The American Journal of Physiology. 1996;271:E439–50.

[39] Shatanawi A, Romero MJ, Iddings JA, Chandra S, Umapathy NS, Verin AD, et al. Angiotensin II-induced vascular endothelial dysfunction through RhoA/Rho kinase/p38 mitogen-activated protein kinase/arginase pathway. American Journal of Physiology Cell Physiology. 2011;300:C1181–92.

[40] Seto SW, Krishna SM, Yu H, Liu D, Khosla S, Golledge J. Impaired acetylcholine-induced endothelium-dependent aortic relaxation by caveolin-1 in angiotensin II-infused apolipoprotein-E (ApoE-/-) knockout mice. PloS One. 2013;8:e58481.

[41] Gomolak JR, Didion SP. Angiotensin II-induced endothelial dysfunction is temporally linked with increases in interleukin-6 and vascular macrophage accumulation. Frontiers in Physiology. 2014;5:396.

[42] Weiss D, Kools JJ, Taylor WR. Angiotensin II-induced hypertension accelerates the development of atherosclerosis in apoE-deficient mice. Circulation. 2001;103:448–54.

[43] Pueyo ME, Gonzalez W, Nicoletti A, Savoie F, Arnal JF, Michel JB. Angiotensin II stimulates endothelial vascular cell adhesion molecule-1 via nuclear factor-kappaB activation induced by intracellular oxidative stress. Arteriosclerosis, Thrombosis, and Vascular Biology. 2000;20:645–51.

[44] Pastore L, Tessitore A, Martinotti S, Toniato E, Alesse E, Bravi MC, et al. Angiotensin II stimulates intercellular adhesion molecule-1 (ICAM-1) expression by human vascular endothelial cells and increases soluble ICAM-1 release in vivo. Circulation. 1999;100:1646–52.

[45] Suzuki Y, Ruiz-Ortega M, Lorenzo O, Ruperez M, Esteban V, Egido J. Inflammation and angiotensin II. The International Journal of Biochemistry & Cell Biology. 2003;35:881–900.

[46] Cheng ZJ, Vapaatalo H, Mervaala E. Angiotensin II and vascular inflammation. Medical Science Monitor: International Medical Journal of Experimental and Clinical Research. 2005;11:Ra194–205.

[47] Touyz RM. Molecular and cellular mechanisms in vascular injury in hypertension: role of angiotensin II. Current Opinion in Nephrology and Hypertension. 2005;14:125–31.

[48] Dimmeler S, Rippmann V, Weiland U, Haendeler J, Zeiher AM. Angiotensin II induces apoptosis of human endothelial cells. Protective effect of nitric oxide. Circulation research. 1997;81:970–6.

[49] Song H, Gao D, Chen L, Seta K, McLaughlin JS, Wei C. Angiotensin II-mediated apoptosis on human vascular smooth muscle cells. Journal of Cardiothoracic-Renal Research. 2006;1:135–9.

[50] Keidar S, Heinrich R, Kaplan M, Hayek T, Aviram M. Angiotensin II administration to atherosclerotic mice increases macrophage uptake of oxidized ldl: a possible role for interleukin-6. Arteriosclerosis, Thrombosis, and Vascular Biology. 2001;21:1464–9.

[51] Limor R, Kaplan M, Sawamura T, Sharon O, Keidar S, Weisinger G, et al. Angiotensin II increases the expression of lectin-like oxidized low-density lipoprotein receptor-1 in human vascular smooth muscle cells via a lipoxygenase-dependent pathway. American Journal of Hypertension. 2005;18:299–307.

[52] Badimon L, Vilahur G. Thrombosis formation on atherosclerotic lesions and plaque rupture. Journal of internal medicine. 2014;276:618–32.

[53] Libby P, Nahrendorf M, Swirski FK. Monocyte heterogeneity in cardiovascular disease. Seminars in Immunopathology. 2013;35:553–62.

[54] Chistiakov DA, Bobryshev YV, Nikiforov NG, Elizova NV, Sobenin IA, Orekhov AN. Macrophage phenotypic plasticity in atherosclerosis: the associated features and the peculiarities of the expression of inflammatory genes. International Journal of Cardiology. 2015;184:436–45.

[55] Okamura A, Rakugi H, Ohishi M, Yanagitani Y, Takiuchi S, Moriguchi K, et al. Upregulation of renin-angiotensin system during differentiation of monocytes to macrophages. Journal of Hypertension. 1999;17:537–45.

[56] Jurewicz M, McDermott DH, Sechler JM, Tinckam K, Takakura A, Carpenter CB, et al. Human T and natural killer cells possess a functional renin-angiotensin system: further mechanisms of angiotensin II-induced inflammation. Journal of the American Society of Nephrology: JASN. 2007;18:1093–102.

[57] Hoch NE, Guzik TJ, Chen W, Deans T, Maalouf SA, Gratze P, et al. Regulation of T-cell function by endogenously produced angiotensin II. American Journal of Physiology Regulatory, Integrative and Comparative Physiology. 2009;296:R208–16.

[58] Chen XL, Tummala PE, Olbrych MT, Alexander RW, Medford RM. Angiotensin II induces monocyte chemoattractant protein-1 gene expression in rat vascular smooth muscle cells. Circulation Research. 1998;83:952–9.

[59] Hernandez-Presa M, Bustos C, Ortego M, Tunon J, Renedo G, Ruiz-Ortega M, et al. Angiotensin-converting enzyme inhibition prevents arterial nuclear factor-kappa B activation, monocyte chemoattractant protein-1 expression, and macrophage infiltration in a rabbit model of early accelerated atherosclerosis. Circulation. 1997;95:1532–41.

[60] Kranzhofer R, Browatzki M, Schmidt J, Kubler W. Angiotensin II activates the proinflammatory transcription factor nuclear factor-kappaB in human monocytes. Biochemical and Biophysical Research Communications. 1999;257:826–8.

[61] Kim JM, Heo HS, Ha YM, Ye BH, Lee EK, Choi YJ, et al. Mechanism of Ang II involvement in activation of NF-kappaB through phosphorylation of p65 during aging. Age (Dordrecht, Netherlands). 2012;34:11–25.

[62] Bundalo M, Zivkovic M, Culafic T, Stojiljkovic M, Koricanac G, Stankovic A. Oestradiol Treatment counteracts the effect of fructose-rich diet on matrix metalloproteinase 9 expression and NFkappaB activation. Folia Biologica. 2015;61:233–40.

[63] Esteban V, Lorenzo O, Ruperez M, Suzuki Y, Mezzano S, Blanco J, et al. Angiotensin II, via AT1 and AT2 receptors and NF-kappaB pathway, regulates the inflammatory response in unilateral ureteral obstruction. Journal of the American Society of Nephrology: JASN. 2004;15:1514–29.

[64] Bundalo M, Zivkovic M, Tepavcevic S, Culafic T, Koricanac G, Stankovic A. Fructose-rich diet-induced changes in the expression of the renin angiotensin system molecules in the heart of ovariectomized female rats could be reversed by estradiol. Hormone and Metabolic Research = Hormon- und Stoffwechselforschung = Hormones et Metabolisme. 2015;47:521–7.

[65] Tham DM, Martin-McNulty B, Wang YX, Wilson DW, Vergona R, Sullivan ME, et al. Angiotensin II is associated with activation of NF-kappaB-mediated genes and downregulation of PPARs. Physiological Genomics. 2002;11:21–30.

[66] Zhan Y, Brown C, Maynard E, Anshelevich A, Ni W, Ho IC, et al. Ets-1 is a critical regulator of Ang II-mediated vascular inflammation and remodeling. The Journal of Clinical Investigation. 2005;115:2508–16.

[67] Chen YX, Zhang M, Cai Y, Zhao Q, Dai W. The Sirt1 activator SRT1720 attenuates angiotensin II-induced atherosclerosis in apoE(-)/(-) mice through inhibiting vascular inflammatory response. Biochemical and Biophysical Research Communications. 2015;465:732–8.

[68] Koga J, Aikawa M. Crosstalk between macrophages and smooth muscle cells in atherosclerotic vascular diseases. Vascular Pharmacology. 2012;57:24–8.

[69] Touyz RM, Schiffrin EL. Signal transduction mechanisms mediating the physiological and pathophysiological actions of angiotensin II in vascular smooth muscle cells. Pharmacological Reviews. 2000;52:639–72.

[70] Zhang F, Hu Y, Xu Q, Ye S. Different effects of angiotensin II and angiotensin-(1-7) on vascular smooth muscle cell proliferation and migration. PloS One. 2010;5:e12323.

[71] Kaminska M, Mogielnicki A, Stankiewicz A, Kramkowski K, Domaniewski T, Buczko W, et al. Angiotensin II via AT1 receptor accelerates arterial thrombosis in renovascular hypertensive rats. Journal of Physiology and Pharmacology: an Official Journal of the Polish Physiological Society. 2005;56:571–85.

[72] Ishikawa M, Sekizuka E, Yamaguchi N, Nakadate H, Terao S, Granger DN, et al. Angiotensin II type 1 receptor signaling contributes to platelet-leukocyte-endothelial cell interactions in the cerebral microvasculature. American journal of Physiology Heart and Circulatory Physiology. 2007;292:H2306–15.

[73] Doller A, Gauer S, Sobkowiak E, Geiger H, Pfeilschifter J, Eberhardt W. Angiotensin II induces renal plasminogen activator inhibitor-1 and cyclooxygenase-2 expression post-transcriptionally via activation of the mRNA-stabilizing factor human-antigen R. The American Journal of Pathology. 2009;174:1252–63.

[74] Senchenkova EY, Russell J, Almeida-Paula LD, Harding JW, Granger DN. Angiotensin II-mediated microvascular thrombosis. Hypertension. 2010;56:1089–95.

[75] Nakamura S, Nakamura I, Ma L, Vaughan DE, Fogo AB. Plasminogen activator inhibitor-1 expression is regulated by the angiotensin type 1 receptor in vivo. Kidney International. 2000;58:251–9.

[76] Nishimura H, Tsuji H, Masuda H, Nakagawa K, Nakahara Y, Kitamura H, et al. Angiotensin II increases plasminogen activator inhibitor-1 and tissue factor mRNA expression without changing that of tissue type plasminogen activator or tissue factor pathway inhibitor in cultured rat aortic endothelial cells. Thrombosis and Haemostasis. 1997;77:1189–95.

[77] He M, He X, Xie Q, Chen F, He S. Angiotensin II induces the expression of tissue factor and its mechanism in human monocytes. Thrombosis Research. 2006;117:579–90.

[78] Vital SA, Terao S, Nagai M, Granger DN. Mechanisms underlying the cerebral microvascular responses to angiotensin II-induced hypertension. Microcirculation (New York, NY: 1994). 2010;17:641–9.

[79] Mogielnicki A, Chabielska E, Pawlak R, Szemraj J, Buczko W. Angiotensin II enhances thrombosis development in renovascular hypertensive rats. Thrombosis and Haemostasis. 2005;93:1069–76.

[80] Luchtefeld M, Grote K, Grothusen C, Bley S, Bandlow N, Selle T, et al. Angiotensin II induces MMP-2 in a p47phox-dependent manner. Biochemical and Biophysical Research Communications. 2005;328:183–8.

[81] Laxton RC, Hu Y, Duchene J, Zhang F, Zhang Z, Leung KY, et al. A role of matrix metalloproteinase-8 in atherosclerosis. Circulation Research. 2009;105:921–9.

[82] Djuric T, Stankovic A, Koncar I, Radak D, Davidovic L, Alavantic D, et al. Association of MMP-8 promoter gene polymorphisms with carotid atherosclerosis: preliminary study. Atherosclerosis. 2011;219:673–8.

[83] Song X, Qian X, Shen M, Jiang R, Wagner MB, Ding G, et al. Protein kinase C promotes cardiac fibrosis and heart failure by modulating galectin-3 expression. Biochimica et Biophysica Acta. 2015;1853:513–21.

[84] Dumic J, Dabelic S, Flogel M. Galectin-3: an open-ended story. Biochimica et Biophysica Acta. 2006;1760:616–35.

[85] Djordjevic A, Zivkovic M, Stankovic A, Zivotic I, Koncar I, Davidovic L, et al. Genetic Variants in the Vicinity of LGALS-3 Gene and LGALS-3 mRNA Expression in Advanced Carotid Atherosclerosis: An Exploratory Study. Journal of clinical laboratory analysis. 2016;30:1150–7.

[86] de Boer RA, Verweij N, van Veldhuisen DJ, Westra HJ, Bakker SJ, Gansevoort RT, et al. A genome-wide association study of circulating galectin-3. PloS One. 2012;7:e47385.

[87] Raitoharju E, Lyytikainen LP, Levula M, Oksala N, Mennander A, Tarkka M, et al. miR-21, miR-210, miR-34a, and miR-146a/b are up-regulated in human atherosclerotic plaques in the Tampere Vascular Study. Atherosclerosis. 2011;219:211–7.

[88] Levula M, Oksala N, Airla N, Zeitlin R, Salenius JP, Jarvinen O, et al. Genes involved in systemic and arterial bed dependent atherosclerosis--Tampere Vascular study. PloS One. 2012;7:e33787.

[89] Jovanovic I, Zivkovic M, Jovanovic J, Djuric T, Stankovic A. The co-inertia approach in identification of specific microRNA in early and advanced atherosclerosis plaque. Medical Hypotheses. 2014;83:11–5.

[90] Zhu N, Zhang D, Chen S, Liu X, Lin L, Huang X, et al. Endothelial enriched microRNAs regulate angiotensin II-induced endothelial inflammation and migration. Atherosclerosis. 2011;215:286–93.

[91] Cheng W, Liu T, Jiang F, Liu C, Zhao X, Gao Y, et al. microRNA-155 regulates angiotensin II type 1 receptor expression in umbilical vein endothelial cells from severely pre-eclamptic pregnant women. International Journal of Molecular Medicine. 2011;27:393–9.

[92] Wassmann S, Czech T, van Eickels M, Fleming I, Bohm M, Nickenig G. Inhibition of diet-induced atherosclerosis and endothelial dysfunction in apolipoprotein E/angiotensin II type 1A receptor double-knockout mice. Circulation. 2004;110:3062–7.

[93] Daugherty A, Rateri DL, Lu H, Inagami T, Cassis LA. Hypercholesterolemia stimulates angiotensin peptide synthesis and contributes to atherosclerosis through the AT1A receptor. Circulation. 2004;110:3849–57.

[94] Caligiuri G, Paulsson G, Nicoletti A, Maseri A, Hansson GK. Evidence for antigen-driven T-cell response in unstable angina. Circulation. 2000;102:1114–9.

[95] Li Z, Iwai M, Wu L, Liu HW, Chen R, Jinno T, et al. Fluvastatin enhances the inhibitory effects of a selective AT1 receptor blocker, valsartan, on atherosclerosis. Hypertension. 2004;44:758–63.

[96] Fukuda D, Enomoto S, Hirata Y, Nagai R, Sata M. The angiotensin receptor blocker, telmisartan, reduces and stabilizes atherosclerosis in ApoE and AT1aR double deficient mice. Biomedicine & Pharmacotherapy = Biomedecine & Pharmacotherapie. 2010;64:712–7.

[97] Fukuda D, Sata M, Ishizaka N, Nagai R. Critical role of bone marrow angiotensin II type 1 receptor in the pathogenesis of atherosclerosis in apolipoprotein E deficient mice. Arteriosclerosis, Thrombosis, and Vascular Biology. 2008;28:90–6.

[98] Fukuda D, Sata M. Role of bone marrow renin-angiotensin system in the pathogenesis of atherosclerosis. Pharmacology & Therapeutics. 2008;118:268–76.

[99] Cassis LA, Rateri DL, Lu H, Daugherty A. Bone marrow transplantation reveals that recipient AT1a receptors are required to initiate angiotensin II-induced atherosclerosis and aneurysms. Arteriosclerosis, Thrombosis, and Vascular Biology. 2007;27:380–6.

[100] Mazzolai L, Duchosal MA, Korber M, Bouzourene K, Aubert JF, Hao H, et al. Endogenous angiotensin II induces atherosclerotic plaque vulnerability and elicits a Th1 response in ApoE-/- mice. Hypertension. 2004;44:277–82.

[101] Clancy P, Koblar SA, Golledge J. Angiotensin receptor 1 blockade reduces secretion of inflammation associated cytokines from cultured human carotid atheroma and vascular cells in association with reduced extracellular signal regulated kinase expression and activation. Atherosclerosis. 2014;236:108–15.

[102] Clancy P, Seto SW, Koblar SA, Golledge J. Role of the angiotensin converting enzyme 1/angiotensin II/angiotensin receptor 1 axis in interstitial collagenase expression in human carotid atheroma. Atherosclerosis. 2013;229:331–7.

[103] Dandapat A, Hu CP, Chen J, Liu Y, Khan JA, Remeo F, et al. Over-expression of angiotensin II type 2 receptor (agtr2) decreases collagen accumulation in atherosclerotic plaque. Biochemical and Biophysical Research Communications. 2008;366: 871–7.

[104] Hu C, Dandapat A, Chen J, Liu Y, Hermonat PL, Carey RM, et al. Over-expression of angiotensin II type 2 receptor (agtr2) reduces atherogenesis and modulates LOX-1, endothelial nitric oxide synthase and heme-oxygenase-1 expression. Atherosclerosis. 2008;199:288–94.

[105] Iwai M, Chen R, Li Z, Shiuchi T, Suzuki J, Ide A, et al. Deletion of angiotensin II type 2 receptor exaggerated atherosclerosis in apolipoprotein E-null mice. Circulation. 2005;112:1636–43.

[106] Sales VL, Sukhova GK, Lopez-Ilasaca MA, Libby P, Dzau VJ, Pratt RE. Angiotensin type 2 receptor is expressed in murine atherosclerotic lesions and modulates lesion evolution. Circulation. 2005;112:3328–36.

[107] Tiyerili V, Mueller CF, Becher UM, Czech T, van Eickels M, Daiber A, et al. Stimulation of the AT2 receptor reduced atherogenesis in ApoE(-/-)/AT1A(-/-) double knock out mice. Journal of Molecular and Cellular Cardiology. 2012;52:630–7.

[108] Takata H, Yamada H, Kawahito H, Kishida S, Irie D, Kato T, et al. Vascular angiotensin II type 2 receptor attenuates atherosclerosis via a kinin/NO-dependent mechanism. Journal of the Renin-Angiotensin-Aldosterone System: JRAAS. 2015;16:311–20.

[109] Kljajic ST, Widdop RE, Vinh A, Welungoda I, Bosnyak S, Jones ES, et al. Direct AT(2) receptor stimulation is athero-protective and stabilizes plaque in apolipoprotein E-deficient mice. International Journal of Cardiology. 2013;169:281–7.

[110] Zulli A, Burrell LM, Widdop RE, Black MJ, Buxton BF, Hare DL. Immunolocalization of ACE2 and AT2 receptors in rabbit atherosclerotic plaques. The journal of Histochemistry and Cytochemistry: Official Journal of the Histochemistry Society. 2006;54:147–50.

[111] Thomas MC, Pickering RJ, Tsorotes D, Koitka A, Sheehy K, Bernardi S, et al. Genetic Ace2 deficiency accentuates vascular inflammation and atherosclerosis in the ApoE knockout mouse. Circulation Research. 2010;107:888–97.

[112] Bundalo MM, Zivkovic MD, Romic S, Tepavcevic SN, Koricanac GB, Djuric TM, et al. Fructose-rich diet induces gender-specific changes in expression of the renin-angiotensin system in rat heart and upregulates the ACE/AT1R axis in the male rat aorta. Journal of the Renin-Angiotensin-Aldosterone System: JRAAS. 2016;17:1470320316642915.

[113] Thatcher SE, Zhang X, Howatt DA, Lu H, Gurley SB, Daugherty A, et al. Angiotensin-converting enzyme 2 deficiency in whole body or bone marrow-derived cells increases atherosclerosis in low-density lipoprotein receptor-/- mice. Arteriosclerosis, Thrombosis, and Vascular Biology. 2011;31:758–65.

[114] Lovren F, Pan Y, Quan A, Teoh H, Wang G, Shukla PC, et al. Angiotensin converting enzyme-2 confers endothelial protection and attenuates atherosclerosis. American Journal of Physiology Heart and Circulatory Physiology. 2008;295:H1377–84.

[115] Dong B, Zhang C, Feng JB, Zhao YX, Li SY, Yang YP, et al. Overexpression of ACE2 enhances plaque stability in a rabbit model of atherosclerosis. Arteriosclerosis, Thrombosis, and Vascular Biology. 2008;28:1270–6.

[116] Zhang C, Zhao YX, Zhang YH, Zhu L, Deng BP, Zhou ZL, et al. Angiotensin-converting enzyme 2 attenuates atherosclerotic lesions by targeting vascular cells. Proceedings of the National Academy of Sciences of the United States of America. 2010;107:15886–91.

[117] Sahara M, Ikutomi M, Morita T, Minami Y, Nakajima T, Hirata Y, et al. Deletion of angiotensin-converting enzyme 2 promotes the development of atherosclerosis and arterial neointima formation. Cardiovascular Research. 2014;101:236–46.

[118] Yang J, Yang X, Meng X, Dong M, Guo T, Kong J, et al. Endogenous activated angiotensin-(1-7) plays a protective effect against atherosclerotic plaques unstability in high fat diet fed ApoE knockout mice. International Journal of Cardiology. 2015;184:645–52.

[119] Tesanovic S, Vinh A, Gaspari TA, Casley D, Widdop RE. Vasoprotective and atheroprotective effects of angiotensin (1-7) in apolipoprotein E-deficient mice. Arteriosclerosis, Thrombosis, and Vascular Biology. 2010;30:1606–13.

[120] Zhang YH, Hao QQ, Wang XY, Chen X, Wang N, Zhu L, et al. ACE2 activity was increased in atherosclerotic plaque by losartan: possible relation to anti-atherosclerosis. Journal of the Renin-Angiotensin-Aldosterone System: JRAAS. 2015;16:292–300.

[121] Pernomian L, do Prado AF, Gomes MS, Pernomian L, da Silva CH, Gerlach RF, et al. MAS receptors mediate vasoprotective and atheroprotective effects of candesartan upon

the recovery of vascular angiotensin-converting enzyme 2-angiotensin-(1-7)-MAS axis functionality. European Journal of Pharmacology. 2015;764:173–88.

[122] Fraga-Silva RA, Sorg BS, Wankhede M, Dedeugd C, Jun JY, Baker MB, et al. ACE2 activation promotes antithrombotic activity. Molecular Medicine (Cambridge, Mass). 2010;16:210–5.

[123] Guo YJ, Li WH, Wu R, Xie Q, Cui LQ. ACE2 overexpression inhibits angiotensin II-induced monocyte chemoattractant protein-1 expression in macrophages. Archives of Medical Research. 2008;39:149–54.

[124] Tiret L, Rigat B, Visvikis S, Breda C, Corvol P, Cambien F, et al. Evidence, from combined segregation and linkage analysis, that a variant of the angiotensin I-converting enzyme (ACE) gene controls plasma ACE levels. American Journal of Human Genetics. 1992;51:197–205.

[125] Rigat B, Hubert C, Alhenc-Gelas F, Cambien F, Corvol P, Soubrier F. An insertion/deletion polymorphism in the angiotensin I-converting enzyme gene accounting for half the variance of serum enzyme levels. The Journal of Clinical Investigation. 1990;86:1343–6.

[126] Ay C, Bencur P, Vormittag R, Sailer T, Jungbauer C, Vukovich T, et al. The angiotensin-converting enzyme insertion/deletion polymorphism and serum levels of angiotensin-converting enzyme in venous thromboembolism. Data from a case control study. Thrombosis and Haemostasis. 2007;98:777–82.

[127] Mizuiri S, Hemmi H, Kumanomidou H, Iwamoto M, Miyagi M, Sakai K, et al. Angiotensin-converting enzyme (ACE) I/D genotype and renal ACE gene expression. Kidney International. 2001;60:1124–30.

[128] Suehiro T, Morita T, Inoue M, Kumon Y, Ikeda Y, Hashimoto K. Increased amount of the angiotensin-converting enzyme (ACE) mRNA originating from the ACE allele with deletion. Human Genetics. 2004;115:91–6.

[129] Rieder MJ, Taylor SL, Clark AG, Nickerson DA. Sequence variation in the human angiotensin converting enzyme. Nature Genetics. 1999;22:59–62.

[130] Schunkert H, Hense HW, Muscholl M, Luchner A, Riegger GA. Association of angiotensin converting enzyme activity and arterial blood pressure in a population-based sample. Journal of Hypertension. 1996;14:571–5.

[131] Stankovic A, Ilic N, Zunic Z, Glisic S, Alavantic D. Association of the insertion/deletion polymorphism at the angiotensin I-converting enzyme locus with arterial blood pressure: population-based study. Yugoslav Medical Biochemistry. 1999;18:141–7.

[132] O'Donnell CJ, Lindpaintner K, Larson MG, Rao VS, Ordovas JM, Schaefer EJ, et al. Evidence for association and genetic linkage of the angiotensin-converting enzyme locus with hypertension and blood pressure in men but not women in the Framingham heart study. Circulation. 1998;97:1766–72.

[133] Morris BJ, Zee RY, Schrader AP. Different frequencies of angiotensin-converting enzyme genotypes in older hypertensive individuals. The Journal of Clinical Investigation. 1994;94:1085–9.

[134] Stankovic A, Zivkovic M, Alavantic D. Angiotensin I-converting enzyme gene polymorphism in a Serbian population: a gender-specific association with hypertension. Scandinavian Journal of Clinical and Laboratory Investigation. 2002;62:469–75.

[135] Sayed-Tabatabaei FA, Houwing-Duistermaat JJ, van Duijn CM, Witteman JC. Angiotensin-converting enzyme gene polymorphism and carotid artery wall thickness: a meta-analysis. Stroke; A Journal of Cerebral Circulation. 2003;34:1634–9.

[136] Kolakovic A, Zivkovic M, Radak D, Djuric T, Koncar I, Davidovic L, et al. The association of ACE I/D gene polymorphism with severe carotid atherosclerosis in patients undergoing carotid endarterectomy. Journal of the Renin-Angiotensin-Aldosterone System: JRAAS. 2012;13:141–7.

[137] Scheer WD, Boudreau DA, Hixson JE, McGill HC, Newman WP, 3rd, Tracy RE, et al. ACE insert/delete polymorphism and atherosclerosis. Atherosclerosis. 2005;178: 241–7.

[138] Casas JP, Hingorani AD, Bautista LE, Sharma P. Meta-analysis of genetic studies in ischemic stroke: thirty-two genes involving approximately 18,000 cases and 58,000 controls. Archives of Neurology. 2004;61:1652–61.

[139] Dhamrait SS, Maubaret C, Pedersen-Bjergaard U, Brull DJ, Gohlke P, Payne JR, et al. Mitochondrial uncoupling proteins regulate angiotensin-converting enzyme expression: crosstalk between cellular and endocrine metabolic regulators suggested by RNA interference and genetic studies. BioEssays: News and Reviews in Molecular, Cellular and Developmental Biology. 2016;38(Suppl. 1):S107–18.

[140] Dong C, Della-Morte D, Wang L, Cabral D, Beecham A, McClendon MS, et al. Association of the sirtuin and mitochondrial uncoupling protein genes with carotid plaque. PloS One. 2011;6:e27157.

[141] Dong C, Della-Morte D, Cabral D, Wang L, Blanton SH, Seemant C, et al. Sirtuin/uncoupling protein gene variants and carotid plaque area and morphology. International Journal of Stroke: Official Journal of the International Stroke Society. 2015;10:1247–52.

[142] Wang WY, Zee RY, Morris BJ. Association of angiotensin II type 1 receptor gene polymorphism with essential hypertension. Clinical Genetics. 1997;51:31–4.

[143] Bonnardeaux A, Davies E, Jeunemaitre X, Fery I, Charru A, Clauser E, et al. Angiotensin II type 1 receptor gene polymorphisms in human essential hypertension. Hypertension. 1994;24:63–9.

[144] Tiret L, Blanc H, Ruidavets JB, Arveiler D, Luc G, Jeunemaitre X, et al. Gene polymorphisms of the renin-angiotensin system in relation to hypertension and parental history of myocardial infarction and stroke: the PEGASE study. Projet d'Etude des Genes de

l'Hypertension Arterielle Severe a moderee Essentielle. Journal of Hypertension. 1998;16:37–44.

[145] Morisawa T, Kishimoto Y, Kitano M, Kawasaki H, Hasegawa J. Influence of angiotensin II type 1 receptor polymorphism on hypertension in patients with hypercholesterolemia. Clinica Chimica Acta; International Journal of Clinical Chemistry. 2001;304:91–7.

[146] Stankovic A, Zivkovic M, Glisic S, Alavantic D. Angiotensin II type 1 receptor gene polymorphism and essential hypertension in Serbian population. Clinica Chimica Acta; International Journal of Clinical Chemistry. 2003;327:181–5.

[147] Mottl AK, Shoham DA, North KE. Angiotensin II type 1 receptor polymorphisms and susceptibility to hypertension: a HuGE review. Genetics in Medicine: Official Journal of the American College of Medical Genetics. 2008;10:560–74.

[148] van Geel PP, Pinto YM, Voors AA, Buikema H, Oosterga M, Crijns HJ, et al. Angiotensin II type 1 receptor A1166C gene polymorphism is associated with an increased response to angiotensin II in human arteries. Hypertension. 2000;35:717–21.

[149] Lim HS, Cho JY, Oh DS, Chung JY, Hong KS, Bae KS, et al. Angiotensin II type 1 receptor 1166A/C polymorphism in association with blood pressure response to exogenous angiotensin II. European Journal of Clinical Pharmacology. 2007;63:17–26.

[150] Chapman CM, Palmer LJ, McQuillan BM, Hung J, Burley J, Hunt C, et al. Polymorphisms in the angiotensinogen gene are associated with carotid intimal-medial thickening in females from a community-based population. Atherosclerosis. 2001;159:209–17.

[151] Sticchi E, Romagnuolo I, Sofi F, Pratesi G, Pulli R, Pratesi C, et al. Association between polymorphisms of the renin angiotensin system and carotid stenosis. Journal of Vascular Surgery. 2011;54:467–73.

[152] Plat AW, Stoffers HE, de Leeuw PW, van Schayck CP, Soomers FL, Kester AD, et al. Sex-specific effect of the alpha-adducin (G460W) and AGTR1 (A1166C) polymorphism on carotid intima-media thickness. Journal of Hypertension. 2009;27:2165–73.

[153] Zhu S, Meng QH. Association of angiotensin II type 1 receptor gene polymorphism with carotid atherosclerosis. Clinical Chemistry and Laboratory Medicine. 2006;44:282–4.

[154] Zhang H, Sun M, Sun T, Zhang C, Meng X, Zhang Y, et al. Association between angiotensin II type 1 receptor gene polymorphisms and ischemic stroke: a meta-analysis. Cerebrovascular Diseases (Basel, Switzerland). 2011;32:431–8.

[155] Stankovic A, Kolakovic A, Zivkovic M, Djuric T, Bundalo M, Koncar I, et al. Angiotensin receptor type 1 polymorphism A1166C is associated with altered AT1R and miR-155 expression in carotid plaque tissue and development of hypoechoic carotid plaques. Atherosclerosis. 2016;248:132–9.

[156] Sethupathy P, Borel C, Gagnebin M, Grant GR, Deutsch S, Elton TS, et al. Human microRNA-155 on chromosome 21 differentially interacts with its polymorphic target in the AGTR1 3' untranslated region: a mechanism for functional single-nucleotide

polymorphisms related to phenotypes. American Journal of Human Genetics. 2007;81:405–13.

[157] Haas U, Sczakiel G, Laufer SD. MicroRNA-mediated regulation of gene expression is affected by disease-associated SNPs within the 3′-UTR via altered RNA structure. RNA Biology. 2012;9:924–37.

[158] Warnecke C, Mugrauer P, Surder D, Erdmann J, Schubert C, Regitz-Zagrosek V. Intronic ANG II type 2 receptor gene polymorphism 1675 G/A modulates receptor protein expression but not mRNA splicing. American Journal of Physiology Regulatory, Integrative and Comparative Physiology. 2005;289:R1729–35.

[159] Stankovic A, Zivkovic M, Kostic M, Atanackovic J, Krstic Z, Alavantic D. Expression profiling of the AT2R mRNA in affected tissue from children with CAKUT. Clinical Biochemistry. 2010;43:71–5.

[160] Kolakovic A, Stankovic A, Djuric T, Zivkovic M, Koncar I, Davidovic L, et al. Gender-specific association between angiotensin II type 2 receptor -1332 A/G gene polymorphism and advanced carotid atherosclerosis. Journal of Stroke and Cerebrovascular Diseases: the Official Journal of National Stroke Association. 2016;25:1622–30.

[161] Zivkovic M, Djuric T, Stancic O, Alavantic D, Stankovic A. X-linked angiotensin II type 2 receptor gene polymorphism -1332A/G in male patients with essential hypertension. Clinica Chimica Acta; International Journal of Clinical Chemistry. 2007;386:110–3.

[162] Tousoulis D, Koumallos N, Antoniades C, Antonopoulos AS, Bakogiannis C, Milliou A, et al. Genetic polymorphism on type 2 receptor of angiotensin II, modifies cardiovascular risk and systemic inflammation in hypertensive males. American Journal of Hypertension. 2010;23:237–42.

[163] Johansson ME, Fagerberg B, Bergstrom G. Angiotensin type 2 receptor is expressed in human atherosclerotic lesions. Journal of the Renin-Angiotensin-Aldosterone System: JRAAS. 2008;9:17–21.

[164] Namsolleck P, Recarti C, Foulquier S, Steckelings UM, Unger T. AT(2) receptor and tissue injury: therapeutic implications. Current Hypertension Reports. 2014;16:416.

[165] Matavelli LC, Siragy HM. AT2 receptor activities and pathophysiological implications. Journal of Cardiovascular Pharmacology. 2015;65:226–32.

Chapter 3

RAAS Blockade as First-Line Antihypertensive Therapy among People with CKD

Panagiotis I. Georgianos, Elias V. Balaskas and
Pantelis E. Zebekakis

Additional information is available at the end of the chapter

http://dx.doi.org/10.5772/66180

Abstract

Hypertension among people with chronic kidney disease is highly prevalent and remains often poorly controlled. To adequately control blood pressure (BP), a combination antihypertensive drug therapy is often required. The choice of the appropriate antihypertensive regimen should be individualized according to the patient clinical characteristics, the severity of chronic kidney disease (CKD), the levels at which BP should be targeted and the presence or absence of proteinuria. In proteinuric CKD, solid evidence from large-scaled randomized trials suggest that agents blocking the renin-angiotensin-aldosterone system (RAAS) should be the antihypertensive therapy of first choice, given their superiority over the other antihypertensive drug classes in reducing proteinuria and delaying nephropathy progression to end-stage-renal-disease (ESRD). In contrast, inhibition of the RAAS is shown to have no additional benefits towards renoprotection in people with non-proteinuric CKD. Combined RAAS blockade as an alternative approach to gain additive reduction in proteinuria and greater retardation of renal function decline is shown to be associated with increased risk of hypotension, serious hyperkalemia and acute kidney injury. In this chapter, we discuss the role of RAAS blockade as first-line antihypertensive therapy among people with proteinuric and non-proteinuric nephropathy, providing an overview of the evidence derived from large-scaled renal outcome trials.

Keywords: hypertension, chronic kidney disease, proteinuria, RAAS blockade, randomized controlled trials

1. Introduction

Hypertension in people with chronic kidney disease (CKD) is very common, often difficult to control and represents an independent predictor of kidney injury progression to end-stage-renal-disease (ESRD) requiring dialysis [1, 2]. Apart from achieving an adequate blood pressure (BP) control as a tool to delay nephropathy progression, the choice of the appropriate antihypertensive regimen may be another factor determining the long-term renal prognosis in people with CKD. In this regard, agents blocking the renin-angiotensin-aldosterone system (RAAS) are considered as the antihypertensive therapy of first choice in people with diabetic or nondiabetic proteinuric CKD on the basis of large-scaled outcome trials showing that these agents are superior to the other antihypertensive drug classes in retarding kidney injury progression over time [3, 4]. In contrast, RAAS blockade in people with non-proteinuric CKD is shown to confer no additional benefits toward renoprotection [4]. Furthermore, the promise that the use of combined RAAS blockade may offer additive anti-proteinuric and renoprotective effects relative to monotherapy is shown to be counteracted by an excess risk of serious hyperkalemia and acute kidney injury [5, 6].

In this chapter, we discuss the use of RAAS blockade for renoprotection in people with proteinuric and non-proteinuric CKD, summarizing the currently available evidence from large-scaled outcome trials in nephrology. We conclude with clinical practice recommendations for the choice of the appropriate antihypertensive regimen in people with CKD and provide directions for future research in this important area.

2. RAAS blockade in patients with proteinuric CKD

Accumulated evidence from large-scaled randomized controlled trials (RCTs) support the notion that inhibition of the RAAS among people with overt diabetic nephropathy confers benefits towards slower progression of kidney injury to ESRD [4]. In the Collaborate Study Group trial, 409 patients with insulin-dependent type 1 diabetes and overt nephropathy (proteinuria >500 mg/day and serum creatinine <2.5 mg/dl) were randomly assigned to receive therapy with the angiotensin-converting enzyme (ACE) inhibitor captopril or placebo for a mean follow-up of 3 years [7]. Compared with placebo, captopril treatment produced a 30% reduction in the level of proteinuria and decreased by 50% the risk of reaching the combined renal endpoint of all-cause death and need for dialysis or renal transplantation [95% confidence interval (CI) 18–70%, $p < 0.01$] [7]. The renoprotective effect of RAAS blockade among people with type 2 diabetes and overt nephropathy is supported by two landmark RCTs, the Reduction of Endpoints in NIDDM with the Angiotensin II Antagonist Losartan (RENAAL) [8] and Irbesartan Diabetic Nephropathy Trial (IDNT) [9]. The RENAAL trial enrolled 1513 patients with overt diabetic nephropathy aiming to compare the effect of the angiotensin receptor blocker (ARB) losartan (50–100 mg daily) versus placebo, both administered on top of conventional antihypertensive drug therapy, on a composite renal endpoint of doubling of serum creatinine, ESRD or death [8]. Over a mean follow-up of 3.4 years, losartan reduced by

25% the risk of doubling of serum creatinine (P = 0.006) and by 28% the risk of ESRD requiring dialysis relative to placebo (P = 0.002), but had no impact on mortality [8]. In the IDNT trial, 1715 hypertensive patients with overt diabetic nephropathy were randomized to receive irbesartan (300 mg daily), amlodipine (10 mg daily) or placebo for a mean follow-up of 2.6 years. The level of proteinuria was reduced by 33% in the irbesartan group versus 6% in the amlodipine and 10% in the placebo groups [9]. Compared with placebo, ARB treatment decreased by 20% the occurrence of the combined renal endpoint of doubling of serum creatinine, ESRD or death [relative risk (RR): 0.80; 95% CI: 0.66–0.97]; ARB therapy was also superior to the calcium channel blocker (CCB) amlodipine in improving renal outcomes (RR: 0.77; 95% CI: 0.63–0.93 for the combined renal endpoint) [9].

The renoprotective properties of ACE inhibitors and/or ARBs among patients with diabetic nephropathy are also supported by carefully conducted meta-analyses of RCTs. An earlier meta-analysis by Strippoli et al. [10] showed that compared with placebo, ACE inhibitor use was associated with a trend towards greater reduction in the risk of doubling of serum creatinine (RR: 0.60; 95% CI: 0.34–1.05) and incident ESRD (RR: 0.64; 95% CI: 0.40–1.03). ACE inhibitor use was associated with 55% reduced risk of progression from micro- to macroalbuminuria (RR: 0.45; 95% CI: 0.28–0.71) and 3.42-fold higher rate of regression from micro- to normoalbuminuria among patients with diabetic CKD (RR: 3.42; 95% CI: 1.95–5.99) [10]. Similarly to ACE inhibitors, the combined analysis of RCTs comparing the effect of ARBs versus placebo on nephropathy progression associated the use of ARBs with reduced risk of doubling of serum creatinine (RR: 0.78; 95% CI: 0.67–0.91) and ESRD incidence (RR: 0.79; 95% CI: 0.67–0.93) [10]. The favorable effect of RAAS blockade on nephropathy progression was confirmed in an updated meta-analysis of 24 RCTs showing that compared with placebo, ACE inhibitors reduced by 30% the risk of incident ESRD (RR: 0.70; 95% CI: 0.46–1.05) and by 29% the risk of doubling of serum creatinine (RR: 0.71; 95% CI: 0.56–0.91); ARB use was associated with 22% lower risk of ESRD incidence (RR: 0.78; 95% CI: 0.67–0.91) and 21% lower risk of doubling of serum creatinine (RR: 0.79; 95% CI: 0.68–0.91) [11].

In accordance with the renoprotective action of RAAS blockade among people with diabetic kidney disease, a growing body of evidence supports the notion that ACE inhibitors and ARBs are similarly effective in delaying kidney injury progression in patients with other types of proteinuric nephropathy. In the REIN-2 study (Ramipril-Efficacy-In-Nephropathy-2), 352 nondiabetic patients with CKD and proteinuria of at least 1 g/day were randomized to receive double-blind therapy with ramipril (5 mg daily) or placebo in addition to conventional antihypertensive therapy targeted at achieving a diastolic BP goal of <90 mmHg [12]. The rate of estimated glomerular filtration rate (eGFR) decline, which was the primary trial endpoint, was significantly slower over time in ramipril-treated patients than in placebo-treated patients (0.53 vs. 0.83 ml/min/1.73 m^2, P = 0.03). The proportional reduction in the level of proteinuria among ramipril-treated patients was inversely associated with the rate of eGFR decline and was an independent predictor of the risk of doubling of serum creatinine and incident ESRD during follow-up [12]. In the African American Study of Kidney Disease (AASK), 1094 African-American patients with hypertensive CKD (mean baseline eGFR: 45.6 ml/min/1.73 m^2; mean urinary protein excretion 0.6 g/day) were randomized to achieve goal mean arterial pressure

102–107 mmHg or ≤92 mmHg and to initial BP-lowering treatment with metoprolol (2.5–10 mg daily), ramipril (2.5–10 mg daily) or amlodipine (5–10 mg daily) in a 3 × 2 factorial design [13]. Compared with metoprolol and amlodipine groups, administration of the ACE inhibitor ramipril was associated with 22 and 38% reduction in the risk of reaching the composite renal outcome of decrease from baseline in eGFR by 50% or greater, incident ESRD, or death, respectively [13]. In a subsequent analysis of 224 patients with advanced stage nondiabetic CKD (baseline serum creatinine range: 3.1–5.0 mg/dl and mean proteinuria 1.6 g/day), Hou et al. [14] compared the effect of benazepril (20 mg daily) versus placebo on top of conventional antihypertensive therapy on a composite renal endpoint of doubling of serum creatinine, ESRD or death. Over a mean follow-up of 3.4 years, the risk of reaching the above combined endpoint was by 43% lower in the ACE inhibitor group than in the placebo group. Additional benefits of the ACE inhibitor therapy were an associated 52% reduction in the level of proteinuria along with a 23% slower rate of eGFR decline [14]. Additional support to the renoprotective action of ACE inhibitors is provided by an earlier meta-analysis of 11 RCTs conducted by Jafar et al. [15]. In this analysis, after adjustment for patient and trial characteristics at baseline and changes in BP and proteinuria levels during follow-up, the use of an ACE inhibitor-based antihypertensive regimen was associated with 31% greater reduction in the risk of developing ESRD (RR: 0.69; 95% CI: 0.51–0.94) and 30% decrease in the risk of doubling of serum creatinine or ESRD (RR: 0.70; 95% CI: 0.55–0.88) in comparison with antihypertensive regimens non-including ACE inhibitors [15].

Post hoc analyses of the aforementioned RCTs provided evidence that the higher the level of proteinuria at baseline the higher was the risk of nephropathy progression to ESRD [16–18]. Most importantly, achievement of an early regression of proteinuria under RAAS blockade (i.e., in the first 6 months after drug initiation) was shown to be associated with reduced long-term risk of doubling of serum creatinine, ESRD incidence or death [16–18]. The notion that drug-induced reduction in proteinuria culminates in subsequent improvement in renal outcomes is further supported by a recent meta-regression analysis of 21 RCTs involving a total of 78,342 patients and 4843 incident ESRD events [19]. The placebo-adjusted treatment effect on proteinuria significantly correlated with the treatment effect on ESRD incidence, since each 30% of drug-induced reduction in the level of proteinuria was associated with a 23.7% reduced risk of subsequent kidney injury progression to ESRD (95% CI: 11.4–34.2%, P = 0.001) [19]. Taken together, the above data support the notion that regression of proteinuria is a major target of therapy in order to delay nephropathy progression in patients with both diabetic and nondiabetic proteinuric CKD.

3. RAAS blockade in patients with non-proteinuric nephropathy

Unlike the well-documented benefits of RAAS inhibition among patients with proteinuric CKD, either diabetic or nondiabetic, it remains largely uncertain whether ACE inhibitors and/ or ARBs carry with them a similarly beneficial effect in slowing nephropathy progression among patients with non-proteinuric CKD. This issue is of major clinical relevance, given the

http://dx.doi.org/10.5772/66180

fact that high albuminuria or overt proteinuria is present only in a small proportion of the overall CKD population, whereas the vast majority of people with CKD have normoalbuminuria or microalbuminuria [20–22]. For example, the prevalence of CKD among individuals with age >70 years is estimated to be around 40%, but proteinuria is present in approximately 5% of elderly CKD patients. The prevalence of CKD in the general hypertensive population is estimated to be around 15% (ranging up to 30% in those aged >65 years), but again <5% of hypertensives with CKD exhibit macroalbuminuria [20–22]. Regardless of its high clinical significance, there are no data from properly designed RCTs to evaluate the effect of RAAS blockade on "hard" renal outcomes in patients with non-proteinuric nephropathy. The currently available evidence on this issue is derived mainly from secondary analyses of major cardiovascular outcome trials.

The first trial to evaluate the issue of renoprotection with RAAS blockade in patients with non-proteinuric CKD was the appropriate blood pressure control in diabetes (ABCD) [23]. This trial enrolled 470 patients with hypertension and type 2 diabetes, of whom only 18% had overt nephropathy (i.e., macro-albuminuria and/or impaired renal function). Study participants were randomly assigned to nisoldipine or enalapril and intensive or moderate BP control in a 2 × 2 factorial design. The rate of change in creatinine clearance over a 5.3-year-long follow-up was no different between the enalapril and nisoldipine groups [23]. However, the most definite renal endpoint of incident ESRD requiring dialysis was not evaluated in the ABCD study; accordingly, this study cannot provide direct evidence on whether the enalapril-induced reduction in the level of proteinuria would be translated into a slower kidney injury progression in a population predominantly without overt diabetic nephropathy.

The absence of additive renal benefits under RAAS blockade among patients with non-proteinuric CKD is further supported by a secondary analysis of the Antihypertensive and Lipid-Lowering Treatment to Prevent Heart Attack Trial (ALLHAT) [24]. This trial enrolled 33,000 hypertensive patients with an age of 55 years or higher and at least one additional risk factor for ischemic heart disease. The exclusion criteria included a serum creatinine >2 mg/dl and therapy with an ACE inhibitor for underlying CKD prior to the study enrolment. Although actual measurements of the level of albuminuria were not included in the protocol procedures, it is reasonable to hypothesize that participants in the ALLHAT trial were mainly hypertensives without high albuminuria. Incidence of ESRD or >50% reduction in eGFR during follow-up, which was the primary composite renal endpoint of this secondary analysis, was no different between amlodipine-treated and chlorothalidone-treated participants (RR: 1.12; 95% CI: 0.89–1.40) [24]. Similarly, the ACE inhibitor lisinopril was not superior to chlorothalidone in reducing the incidence of ESRD or >50% reduction in eGFR (RR: 1.11; 95% CI: 0.89–1.38). When the analysis was stratified according to the level of eGFR at baseline, lisinopril therapy was not associated with a reduced incidence of ESRD relative to chlorthalidone in the subgroups of patients with baseline eGFR of 60–89 ml/min/1.73 m^2 (RR: 1.34; 95% CI: 0.87–2.06) as well as in those with baseline eGFR <60 ml/min/1.73 m^2 (RR: 0.98; 95% CI: 0.73–1.31) [24]. In addition, at 4 years of follow-up, eGFR was 3–6 ml/min/1.73 m^2 higher in amlodipine-treated than in chlorothalidone-treated participants, depending on baseline eGFR stratum. The results of the ALLHAT come in sharp contrast to the clear renoprotective effect of RAAS blockade seen in trials involving patients with overt diabetic nephropathy (i.e., the aforementioned IDNT). This discrepancy is possibly explained by the different characteristics of patients included in the ALLHAT trial. It is reasonable to hypothesize that the absence of renoprotection with lisinopril therapy and the better retardation of eGFR over time in amlodipine-treated participants was possibly due to the fact that patients enrolled in the ALLHAT were more likely to suffer from ischemic rather than proteinuric nephropathy.

Additional support to for the notion that RAAS blockade is not associated with greater renoprotection in comparison to other antihypertensive drug classes among patients with non-proteinuric CKD was provided by the renal outcomes of Avoiding Cardiovascular Events through Combination Therapy in Patients Living with Systolic Hypertension (ACCOMPLISH trial) [25]. ACCOMPLISH randomized 11,506 hypertensive patients at high cardiovascular risk to receive combination therapy with benazepril plus amlodipine or benazepril plus hydrochlorothiazide. The clear benefit of the benazepril/amlodipine combination in reducing cardiovascular morbidity and mortality led to the premature termination of the ACCOMPLISH trial. Similarly to the cardiovascular benefit, the analysis of the renal outcomes showed the benazepril/amlodipine combination was associated with a slower annual rate of eGFR decline in comparison with the benazepril/hydrochlorothiazide combination (−0.88 vs. −4.22 mL/min/1.73 m^2 per year), despite the fact that proteinuria was less effectively reduced in patients receiving the ACE inhibitor/CCB combination [25]. Most importantly, compared with the benazepril/hydrochlorothiazide combination, the ACE inhibitor/CCB combination reduced by 48% the incidence of composite renal endpoint of doubling of serum creatinine or ESRD requiring dialysis [hazard ratio (HR): 0.48; 95% CI: 0.41–0.65] and by 27% the risk of doubling serum creatinine, need for dialysis or death (HR: 0.73; 95% CI: 0.64–0.84) [25]. The superiority of the ACE inhibitor/CCB combination in delaying the kidney injury progression despite its less pronounced anti-proteinuric effect could be once again explained by the characteristics of the patients participating in the ACCOMPLISH trial. ACCOMPLISH participants were predominantly older than 65 years, had preserved renal function at baseline (mean baseline eGFR of 79 mL/min/1.73 m^2) and macro-albuminuria was present in only 5% of study participants. Accordingly, it seems reasonable that patients with such clinical characteristics are less likely to benefit from a therapeutic strategy targeting on proteinuria remission; in contrast, these patients are prone to acute kidney injury due to dehydration and hypotension.

4. Dual RAAS blockade

Combining an ACE inhibitor with an ARB was suggested as an additional therapeutic tool aiming to enhance the anti-proteinuric effect of single RAAS blockade, generating the hypothesis that this manoeuvre would be translated into a more effective delay in nephropathy progression [4]. Although small RCTs showed an additive effect on proteinuria with combined RAAS blockade relative to mono-therapy [26, 27], large-scaled RCTs evaluating "hard" renal endpoints showed that the use of ACE inhibitors and ARBs in combination is associated with increased incidence of hypotension, hyperkalemia and acute kidney injury requiring support with dialysis [5, 6, 28, 29].

In the Ongoing Telmisartan Alone and in combination with Ramipril Global Endpoint Trial (ONTARGET), 25,620 patients with established cardiovascular disease or high-risk diabetes were randomly assigned to receive double-blind therapy with ramipril (10 mg daily), telmisartan (80 mg daily) or both drugs in combination for a median follow-up of 56 months [6]. Compared with mono-therapy, dual RAAS blockade was associated with a 24% higher risk of dialysis or doubling of serum creatinine [hazard ratio (HR): 1.24; 95% CI: 1.01–1.51]. Excess need for dialysis in the combination group was predominantly due to episodes of acute kidney injury, possibly attributable to the higher incidence of hypotension and hyperkalemia among patients treated aggressively with dual RAAS blockade [6]. In the Aliskiren Trial in Type 2 Diabetes Using Cardiorenal Endpoints (ALTITUDE trial), 8561 type 2 diabetic patients with CKD, cardiovascular disease or both were randomized to receive the direct renin inhibitor aliskiren (300 mg daily) or placebo on top of background therapy with an ACE inhibitor or ARB [30]. The ALTITUDE trial was prematurely terminated due to excess risk of hypotension (12.1 vs. 8.3%, $p < 0.001$) and hyperkalemia (11.2 vs. 7.2%, $p < 0.001$) in the combination group [30].

Another large-scaled RCT investigating the potential additive renoprotective effect of dual RAAS blockade was stopped early owing to safety concerns. This was the VA-NEPHRON-D (Veteran's Administration Nephron-Diabetes Trial), in which 1448 type 2 diabetic patients with overt nephropathy (i.e., urinary albumin to creatinine ratio >300 mg/g and eGFR ranging from 30 to 89.9 ml/min/1.73 m^2) already treated with the ARB losartan (100 mg daily) were randomized to receive add-on therapy with the ACE inhibitor lisinopril (10–40 mg daily) or matching placebo [5]. Once again, compared with monotherapy, combination therapy was associated with 70% excess risk of acute kidney injury (HR: 1.70; 95% CI: 1.3–2.2) and 2.8-fold elevated risk of serious hyperkalemia (HR: 2.8; 95% CI: 1.8–4.3). At the time of this interim analysis, a trend toward a benefit of dual RAAS blockade with respect to the secondary trial endpoint of first occurrence of a decline in eGFR ≥30 ml/min/1.73 m^2 or ESRD was noted (HR: 0.78; 95% CI: 0.58–1.05, P = 0.10); however, this tendency toward slower renal function decline was not sustained over time [5]. The above data suggest that even in patients with typical diabetic nephropathy and macro-albuminuria, any potential long-term renoprotective action of combined RAAS inhibition is counteracted by excess risk of serious adverse events, including hypotension, hyperkalemia and acute renal injury requiring acute dialysis.

Addition of mineralocorticoid-receptor-antagonists (MRAs) might provide renal benefits in patients with proteinuric CKD that potentially extend over and above the renoprotection provided by ACE inhibitors and/or ARBs alone [31, 32]. Add-on MRA therapy was proposed as an alternative option on the basis of data suggesting that conventional therapy with ACE inhibitors and ARBs cannot produce sustained prolonged lowering of plasma aldosterone levels, the so-called aldosterone breakthrough phenomenon. An earlier meta-analysis of 11 RCTs (including 991 patients with proteinuric CKD) showed that compared with placebo, add-on MRA therapy on top of background treatment with ACE inhibitors or ARBs was associated with a significant additive reduction in proteinuria [weighted mean difference (WMD): −0.8 g/day; 95% CI: −1.27 to −0.33 g/day]. This anti-proteinuric effect, however, was not accompanied by a slower decline in eGFR (WMD: −0.70 ml/min/1.73 m^2; 95% CI: −4.73 to 3.34 ml/min/1.73 m^2), whereas add-on MRA therapy was also associated with a significantly 3.06 times higher risk of developing hyperkalemia (pooled RR: 3.06; 95% CI: 1.26–7.41) [33]. A subsequent updated meta-analysis of 27 RCTs (including 1549 participants) confirmed in a larger frame of data that add-on MRA therapy offers an additive reduction in proteinuria [standardized mean difference (SMD): −0.61; 95% CI: −1.08 to −0.13], but MRA use aggravated the risk of hyperkalemia and gynecomastia [34]. In the albescence of properly designed RCTs evaluating the effect of add-on MRA therapy on nephropathy progression, the wide use of this therapeutic approach in people with proteinuric CKD is not recommended.

A newly introduced, selective, nonsteroidal MRA-named finerenone offers the opportunity for similarly effective anti-proteinuric action as compared with established steroidal MRAs (i.e., spironolactone and eplerenone), having also the advantage of causing less frequently clinically significant hyperkalemia [35]. The efficacy and safety of finerenone among patients with diabetic nephropathy was tested in the recent phase 2b ARTS-DN study (mineralocorticoid receptor antagonist tolerability study–diabetic nephropathy) [36], in which 821 diabetic patients with high or very high albuminuria already treated with an ACE inhibitor or an ARB were randomly assigned to double-blind therapy with finerenone (1.25 up to 20 mg once daily) or matching placebo for 3 months. Finerenone dose-dependently reduced albuminuria up to 33 and 38% in the 15 and 20 mg groups with only small increases in serum potassium (+0.17 ± 0.46 and +0.23 ± 0.37, respectively) [36]. The incidence of hyperkalemia was 4.1 and 2.6%, respectively, and not significantly different from placebo. These results suggest that finerenone may be an effective and safer approach for renoprotection in proteinuric CKD. Properly designed RCTs are warranted to fully elucidate the effect of finerenone on "hard" renal endpoints.

Recent RCTs have provided evidence that the novel oral potassium-binding resins patiromer and sodium zirconium cyclosilicate can effectively normalize elevated serum potassium and maintain in the long-term the potassium levels within the normal range in hyperkalemic patients with CKD already treated with RAAS blockers [37–39]. These emerging potassium-lowering therapies offer promise that the reduction in the risk of drug-induced hyperkalemia may facilitate the administration of RAAS blockade at adequate doses and enhance the cardiovascular and renal protection provided by these agents in people with proteinuric CKD [29].

5. Conclusion

Choice of the appropriate antihypertensive regimen in people with CKD should be individualized according to the patient clinical characteristics, with proteinuria being an important factor that needs to be taken into consideration. Among people with diabetic or nondiabetic proteinuric nephropathy, large-scaled outcome trials provided solid evidence that ACE inhibitors and/or ARBs reduce the level of proteinuria and this anti-proteinuric action is subsequently translated into slower nephropathy progression to ESRD requiring dialysis. In contrast, there is no "hard" evidence to support the use of RAAS blockers for renoprotection among elderly patients with preserved or mildly impaired renal function as well as in those with non-proteinuric CKD. The use of ACE inhibitors and ARBs in combination as an approach to achieve additive renal benefits relative to monotherapy is contraindicated in light of evidence suggesting that dual RAAS blockade is associated with increased risk of hypotension, serious hyperkalemia and acute kidney injury. Novel potassium-lowering therapies are shown to effective compensate the hyperkalemia risk associated with RAAS blockade use in people with CKD, offering promise for more adequate therapy and greater renal and cardiovascular risk protection in the future.

Conflicts of interest: The authors declare that there is no conflict of interest relevant to this work.

Financial support: This work was not supported by any source and represents an original effort of our part.

Author details

Panagiotis I. Georgianos, Elias V. Balaskas and Pantelis E. Zebekakis*

*Address all correspondence to: pzebeka@med.auth.gr

Section of Nephrology and Hypertension, 1st Department of Medicine, AHEPA Hospital, Aristotle University of Thessaloniki, Thessaloniki, Greece

References

[1] Kidney Disease Outcomes Quality Initiative (K/DOQI). K/DOQI clinical practice guidelines on hypertension and antihypertensive agents in chronic kidney disease. Am J Kidney Dis. 2004;43(5 Suppl 1):S1–290. doi:10.1053/j.ajkd.2004.03.003

[2] Mancia G, Fagard R, Narkiewicz K, et al. 2013 ESH/ESC Guidelines for the management of arterial hypertension: the Task Force for the management of arterial hypertension of the European Society of Hypertension (ESH) and of the European Society of Cardiology (ESC). J Hypertens. 2013;31:1281–357. doi:10.1097/01.hjh.0000431740.32696

[3] Sarafidis PA, Khosla N, Bakris GL. Antihypertensive therapy in the presence of proteinuria. Am J Kidney Dis. 2007;49:12–26. doi:10.1053/j.ajkd.2006.10.014

[4] Sarafidis PA, Ruilope LM. Aggressive blood pressure reduction and renin-angiotensin system blockade in chronic kidney disease: time for re-evaluation? Kidney Int. 2014;85:536–46. doi:10.1038/ki.2013.355

[5] Fried LF, Emanuele N, Zhang JH, et al. Combined angiotensin inhibition for the treatment of diabetic nephropathy. N Engl J Med. 2013;369:1892–903. doi:10.1056/NEJMoa1303154

[6] Mann JF, Schmieder RE, McQueen M, et al. Renal outcomes with telmisartan, ramipril, or both, in people at high vascular risk (the ONTARGET study): a multicentre, randomised, double-blind, controlled trial. Lancet. 2008;372:547–53.doi:10.1016/S0140-6736(08)61236-2

[7] Lewis EJ, Hunsicker LG, Bain RP, Rohde RD. The effect of angiotensin-converting-enzyme inhibition on diabetic nephropathy. The Collaborative Study Group. N Engl J Med. 1993;329:1456–62. doi:10.1056/NEJM199311113292004

[8] Brenner BM, Cooper ME, de Zeeuw D, et al. Effects of losartan on renal and cardiovascular outcomes in patients with type 2 diabetes and nephropathy. N Engl J Med. 2001;345:861–9. doi:10.1056/NEJMoa011161

[9] Lewis EJ, Hunsicker LG, Clarke WR, et al. Renoprotective effect of the angiotensin-receptor antagonist irbesartan in patients with nephropathy due to type 2 diabetes. N Engl J Med. 2001;345:851–60. doi:10.1056/NEJMoa011303

[10] Strippoli GF, Craig M, Deeks JJ, Schena FP, Craig JC. Effects of angiotensin converting enzyme inhibitors and angiotensin II receptor antagonists on mortality and renal outcomes in diabetic nephropathy: systematic review. BMJ. 2004;329:828–38. doi:10.1136/bmj.38237.585000.7C

[11] Sarafidis PA, Stafylas PC, Kanaki AI, Lasaridis AN. Effects of renin-angiotensin system blockers on renal outcomes and all-cause mortality in patients with diabetic nephropathy: an updated meta-analysis. Am J Hypertens. 2008;21:922–9. doi:10.1038/ajh.2008.206

[12] The GISEN Group (Gruppo Italiano di Studi Epidemiologici in Nefrologia). Randomised placebo-controlled trial of effect of ramipril on decline in glomerular filtration rate and risk of terminal renal failure in proteinuric, non-diabetic nephropathy.. Lancet. 1997;349:1857–63. doi:10.1016/S0140-6736(96)11445-8

[13] Wright JT, Jr., Bakris G, Greene T, et al. Effect of blood pressure lowering and antihypertensive drug class on progression of hypertensive kidney disease: results from the AASK trial. JAMA. 2002;288:2421–31. doi:10.1001/jama.288.19.2421

[14] Hou FF, Zhang X, Zhang GH, et al. Efficacy and safety of benazepril for advanced chronic renal insufficiency. N Engl J Med. 2006;354:131–40. doi:10.1056/NEJMoa053107

[15] Jafar TH, Schmid CH, Landa M et al. Angiotensin-converting enzyme inhibitors and progression of nondiabetic renal disease. A meta-analysis of patient-level data. Ann Intern Med. 2001;135:73–87. doi:10.7326/0003-4819-135-2-200107170-00007

[16] Atkins RC, Briganti EM, Lewis JB, et al. Proteinuria reduction and progression to renal failure in patients with type 2 diabetes mellitus and overt nephropathy. Am J Kidney Dis. 2005;45:281–7. doi:10.1053/j.ajkd.2004.10.019

[17] De Zeeuw D, Remuzzi G, Parving HH, et al. Proteinuria, a target for renoprotection in patients with type 2 diabetic nephropathy: lessons from RENAAL. Kidney Int. 2004;65:2309–20. doi:10.1111/j.1523-1755.2004.00653.x

[18] Lea J, Greene T, Hebert L, et al. The relationship between magnitude of proteinuria reduction and risk of end-stage renal disease: results of the African American study of kidney disease and hypertension. Arch Intern Med. 2005;165:947–53. doi:10.1001/archinte.165.8.947

[19] Heerspink HJ, Kropelin TF, Hoekman J, de Zeeuw D. Drug-induced reduction in albuminuria is associated with subsequent renoprotection: a meta-analysis. J Am Soc Nephrol. 2015;26:2055–64. doi:10.1681/ASN.2014070688

[20] Bruck K, Jager KJ, Dounousi E, et al. Methodology used in studies reporting chronic kidney disease prevalence: a systematic literature review. Nephrol Dial Transplant. 2015;30(Suppl 4):iv6–16. doi:10.1093/ndt/gfv131

[21] Coresh J, Byrd-Holt D, Astor BC, et al. Chronic kidney disease awareness, prevalence, and trends among U.S. adults, 1999 to 2000. J Am Soc Nephrol. 2005;16:180–8. doi: 10.1681/ASN.2004070539

[22] O'Hare AM, Kaufman JS, Covinsky KE, Landefeld CS, McFarland LV, Larson EB. Current guidelines for using angiotensin-converting enzyme inhibitors and angiotensin II-receptor antagonists in chronic kidney disease: is the evidence base relevant to older adults? Ann Intern Med 2009;150:717–24. doi: 10.7326/0003-4819-150-10-200905190-00010

[23] Estacio RO, Jeffers BW, Gifford N, Schrier RW. Effect of blood pressure control on diabetic microvascular complications in patients with hypertension and type 2 diabetes. Diabetes Care. 2000;23(Suppl 2):B54–B64.

[24] Rahman M, Pressel S, Davis BR, et al. Renal outcomes in high-risk hypertensive patients treated with an angiotensin-converting enzyme inhibitor or a calcium channel blocker vs a diuretic: a report from the Antihypertensive and Lipid-Lowering Treatment to Prevent Heart Attack Trial (ALLHAT). Arch Intern Med. 2005;165:936–46. doi:10.1001/archinte.165.8.936

[25] Bakris GL, Sarafidis PA, Weir MR, et al. Renal outcomes with different fixed-dose combination therapies in patients with hypertension at high risk for cardiovascular events (ACCOMPLISH): a prespecified secondary analysis of a randomised controlled trial. Lancet. 2010;375:1173–81. doi:10.1016/S0140-6736(09)62100-0

[26] Hollenberg NK, Parving HH, Viberti G, et al. Albuminuria response to very high-dose valsartan in type 2 diabetes mellitus. J Hypertens. 2007;25:1921–6. doi:10.1097/HJH.0b013e328277596e

[27] Schmieder RE, Klingbeil AU, Fleischmann EH, Veelken R, Delles C. Additional antiproteinuric effect of ultrahigh dose candesartan: a double-blind, randomized, prospective study. J Am Soc Nephrol. 2005;16:3038–45. doi:10.1681/ASN.2005020138

[28] Majewski C, Bakris GL. Has RAAS blockade reached its limits in the treatment of diabetic nephropathy? Curr Diab Rep. 2016;16:24. doi:10.1007/s11892-016-0713-y

[29] Sarafidis PA, Georgianos PI, Bakris GL. Advances in treatment of hyperkalemia in chronic kidney disease. Expert Opin Pharmacother. 2015;16:2205–15. doi: 10.1517/14656566

[30] Parving HH, Brenner BM, McMurray JJ, et al. Cardiorenal end points in a trial of aliskiren for type 2 diabetes. N Engl J Med. 2012;367:2204–13. doi:10.1056/NEJMoa1208799

[31] Chrysostomou A, Becker G. Spironolactone in addition to ACE inhibition to reduce proteinuria in patients with chronic renal disease. N Engl J Med. 2001;345:925–6. doi: 10.1056/NEJM200109203451215

[32] Rossing K, Schjoedt KJ, Smidt UM, Boomsma F, Parving HH. Beneficial effects of adding spironolactone to recommended antihypertensive treatment in diabetic nephropathy: a randomized, double-masked, cross-over study. Diabetes Care. 2005;28:2106–12.

[33] Navaneethan SD, Nigwekar SU, Sehgal AR, Strippoli GF. Aldosterone antagonists for preventing the progression of chronic kidney disease: a systematic review and meta-analysis. Clin J Am Soc Nephrol. 2009;4:542–51. doi:10.2215/CJN.04750908

[34] Bolignano D, Palmer SC, Navaneethan SD, Strippoli GF. Aldosterone antagonists for preventing the progression of chronic kidney disease. Cochrane Database Syst Rev 2014;4:CD007004. doi:10.1002/14651858.CD007004

[35] Haller H, Bertram A, Stahl K, Menne J. Finerenone: a new mineralocorticoid receptor antagonist without hyperkalemia: an opportunity in patients with CKD? Curr Hypertens Rep. 2016;18:41. doi:10.1007/s11906-016-0649-2

[36] Bakris GL, Agarwal R, Chan JC, et al. Effect of finerenone on albuminuria in patients with diabetic nephropathy: a randomized clinical trial. JAMA. 2015;314:884–94. doi: 10.1001/jama.2015.10081

[37] Bakris GL, Pitt B, Weir MR, et al. Effect of patiromer on serum potassium level in patients with hyperkalemia and diabetic kidney disease: the AMETHYST-DN randomized clinical trial. JAMA. 2015;314:151–61. doi:10.1001/jama.2015.7446

[38] Packham DK, Rasmussen HS, Lavin PT, et al. Sodium zirconium cyclosilicate in hyperkalemia. N Engl J Med. 2015;372:222–31. doi:10.1056/NEJMoa1411487

[39] Weir MR, Bakris GL, Bushinsky DA, et al. Patiromer in patients with kidney disease and hyperkalemia receiving RAAS inhibitors. N Engl J Med. 2015;372:211–21. doi: 10.1056/NEJMoa1410853

Chapter 4

Signaling Pathways of Cardiac Remodeling Related to Angiotensin II

Carolina Baraldi Araujo Restini,
Arthur F. Engracia Garcia, Henrique Melo Natalin,
Guilherme Melo Natalin and Elen Rizzi

Additional information is available at the end of the chapter

http://dx.doi.org/10.5772/66076

Abstract

Heart failure affects more than 23 million people worldwide, and its prognosis remains poor. Hypertension is one of the most prominent human health problem and places individuals at a higher risk for heart failure. Several factors interplay the development of hypertension contributing for decompensated heart hypertrophy. The renin-angiotensin system (RAS) has been shown to be the foremost regulator of blood pressure. Many evidences have pointed out the importance of RAS and its key mediator, angiotensin II (Ang II), on signaling pathways involved in cardiac remodeling. The Ang II-induced hypertrophic effects seem to be related to increased reactive oxygen species (ROS). Under oxidative stress conditions, as those observed in hypertension and heart failure, the matrix metalloproteinases (MMP) is activated. Ang II is connected with TNF-α and TGF-β by ROS-NF-κB-MMP mechanisms, which are involved in heart failure. The rationale of the present chapter is structured on the progression of heart failure related to Ang II, TNF-α and TGF-β by common signaling pathways. Pharmacotherapeutics approaches to the heart failure abound, but the mortality rates remain high. This chapter will also describe molecular mechanisms involved in heart failure highlighting that TGF-β and/or TNF-α inhibitors could contribute to treatment to this serious clinical condition.

Keywords: heart failure, renin-angiotensin system (RAS), hypertension, transforming growth factor-beta (TGF-β), tumor necrosis factor (TNF)-α, metalloproteinases (MMP)

1. Introduction

Cardiac remodeling is generally triggered due to cardiovascular diseases, such as myocardial infarction, pressure overload, idiopathic dilated cardiomyopathy or volume overload [1].

Cardiac remodeling is also the most common factor in heart failure progress, a chronic disease defined as a complex syndrome. In this sense, heart failure is associated with intensive and progressive cardiac structural and functional modifications, leading to impaired cardiac output [2, 3].

More than 23 million people worldwide are affected by heart failure. In the United States, approximately 5 million patients have heart failure and this number increases by more than half a million cases per year [4]. It is estimated that an increase in the 46% in the prevalence of heart failure from 2012 to 2030 in people with 18-year old or more [5].

There are several criteria to diagnose heart failure as revised by Roger VL [6]. These criteria are important to determine the kind of heart failure treatment and also contribute to improving the accuracy of epidemical data. Despite the progress of the heart failure treatment, mortality rates are still high. Nowadays, the available treatments for heart failure improve the survival rates but raise hospitalizations as well as hospital readmissions. Among these treatments, there are angiotensin-converting enzyme inhibitors (ACEi) and beta-adrenoceptors blockers that alleviate the symptoms in individuals with advanced heart failure and depressed ejection fraction in end-stage disease [7]. Therefore, heart failure is a growing public health problem, in which a projection from 2012 to 2030 heart failure will account more than $69 billion in health-care cost in the United States. It will be a significant increase from 127% [5].

Several risk factors are associated with heart failure, such as smoking, obesity, diabetes mellitus, coronary heart disease and hypertension among others. Hypertension—chronic elevation of blood pressure—is the most prominent human health problem, and it is the main comorbidity linking obesity, cardiovascular and metabolic diseases. According to Framingham study, hypertension is considered the major risk factor attributed to heart failure, and its prevalence in hypertension exceeds 50% [6, 8]. Hereupon, hypertension is the cause of deaths because it often coexists with heart failure and also places individuals at a higher risk for kidney failure, stroke, etc.

2. The progression of cardiac remodeling in hypertension

Hypertension-induced cardiac remodeling is an initial adaptive response of the heart in order to compensate the increased left ventricle wall stress induced by an augmented hemodynamic load. This remodeling is named adaptive hypertrophy, which is featured by growing inwards of the left ventricle and septum wall, resulting in a reduction in left ventricle chamber (**Figure 1**) [2, 3]. The structural changes may occur due to additional contractile-protein units within the cardiomyocytes leading to an expansion in the myocyte width. In parallel to the cellular growth, the cardiac extracellular matrix is also hypertrophied. An important hallmark in chronic hypertension is the intensive turnover from the extracellular matrix, resulting in a progressive collagen deposition [3]. Amount evidences have shown that the cardiac fibrosis could contribute to initial diastolic dysfunction harming the re-lengthening of myocytes during diastole [2, 8, 9]. Thus, despite being called "adaptive", this hypertrophy generates several maladaptive molecular and/or cellular mechanisms triggered in the initial remodeling.

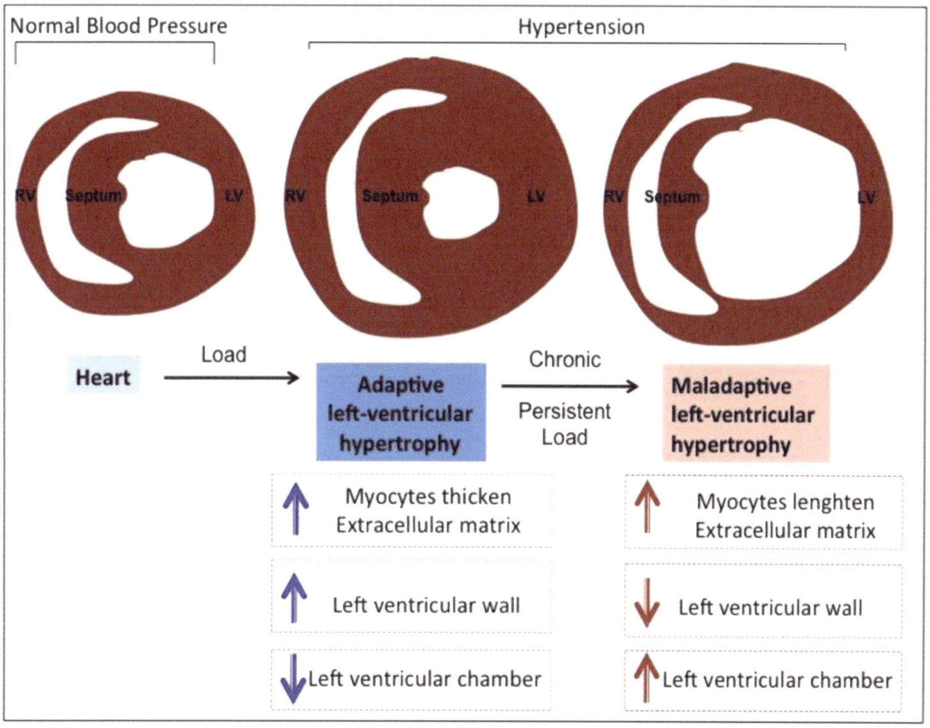

Figure 1. The hypertension induced progression from adaptive hypertrophy to maladaptive hypertrophy. Cardiac remodeling is progressive in hypertension. Initially, an adaptive hypertrophy occurs in the left ventricle that grows inwards reducing the left ventricle chamber. The cardiac remodeling may progress to maladaptive hypertrophy. The left ventricular chamber is dilated and left ventricle and septum wall are thinned. The strength of cardiac contraction may be reduced mainly due the loss of contractile proteins. The heart is therefore considered decompensated, which may result in heart failure. Both, adaptive and maladaptive hypertrophies are characterized by increased heart size and weight. RV: right ventricle and LV: left ventricle.

Hypertensive patients may progress from adaptive to maladaptive hypertrophy, which is characterized by increased left ventricle chamber accompanied by thinning of a left ventricle and septum wall (**Figure 1**). The myocytes are still hypertrophied, but the length is increased [1–3, 9]. The mechanisms involved in the transitions from adaptive to maladaptive hypertrophy are poorly understood. Nonetheless, some studies point out to the excessive matrix extracellular degradation during maladaptive hypertrophy disrupting the cellular organization [2], which could contribute to myocytes lengthening and left ventricular chamber dilatation. It has been also accepted that cell death is associated with this alteration in myocytes [2, 10].

Pathogenic cellular and interstitial changes in hypertension-induced cardiac remodeling are orchestrated by several molecular mechanisms that may be transduced from mechanical force into myocardial growth. In this regard, renin-angiotensin system (RAS) is activated in hypertension and may be involved in cardiac hypertrophy and failure. Clinical and experimental studies have shown significant benefit conferred by pharmacological blockade of RAS [7, 11–13] arousing interest by mechanisms underlying the action of angiotensin II (Ang II).

3. Angiotensin II and cardiac remodeling

Ang II is the primary effector peptide of the RAS. The hypertrophic effects of this peptide on the heart are associated with its vasoconstrictor and hypertensive properties. However, it is currently known that independently of its blood pressure effects, Ang II is a powerful hypertrophic agent. *In vitro* studies show that Ang II activates different hypertrophic signaling pathways in cardiac myocytes [11]. In addition, the crucial components to initiate synthetic route to Ang II production are present in the heart. Thus, Ang II is also locally synthesized at the myocardium, acting as an autocrine factor [11]. Increased cardiac Ang II synthesis is mediated, *in vitro*, by cardiomyocyte under stretch conditions [14]. Similarly, the rise in cardiac Ang II was also observed in hypertrophied heart from animals after overload pressure as well as in patients from end-stage heart failure, which suggests the hypertrophy have resulted from local RAS activation [11, 15].

The Ang II hypertrophic effects are mediated by the activation of specific receptor AT1 that plays a crucial role in heart failure pathophysiology, but both AT1 and AT2 receptor are present in the cardiac tissue [16–19]. The AT1 receptor is 7-transmembrane domain coupled to Gq protein (GPCR). Ang II is able to perform the signaling transduction to adaptive and maladaptive remodeling pathway [2]. AT1 receptor stimulated by Ang II leads to the protein kinase C activation [17], which in turn activates the mitogen-activated protein kinase (MAPK). The intracellular signaling cascade generated from MAPK is constituted by a phosphorylation-based amplification network and results in hypertrophic signals to cardiac adaptive or maladaptive remodeling [2, 10]. Three MAPKs, such as p38 kinases, c-Jun-terminal kinases (JNK) and ERK 1/2 have been described as signaling pathways in cardiac myocytes or extracellular matrix changes along the heart failure progression [10].

In the compensatory response to overload pressure, ERK 1/2 activation has been related to adaptive changes and increased width of the myocytes [20]. Further, some studies have suggested that JNK could contribute to maladaptive remodeling due to its pivotal role in cell death [2, 10, 21]. The MAPK signaling from cardiomyocyte cytoplasm drives to nuclei where transcriptional factors such as factor nuclear kappa B (NF-kB), activating protein-1 (AP-1) and Smad are intracellular proteins to transduce extracellular signals from transforming growth factor beta ligands to the nucleus where they activate downstream gene transcription, rising the transcription of key proteins and developing essential function to the cardiac remodeling progression [22–25].

The NF-kB is an oxidative-sensitive transcriptional factor [26]. Likewise, multiple signal transduction pathways are activated in response to reactive oxygen species (ROS) [27]. In this regard, emergent evidences have shown that Ang II-mediated hypertrophic response may be dependent of increased ROS production, particularly during hypertension [25, 28–30].

Several studies have confirmed the key role of ROS in the genesis and progression of cardiac remodeling [28, 31, 32]. Low levels of ROS are important to many downstream regulators in a physiological condition such as ion channel, receptors, kinases, phosphatases and transcriptional factor. However, increased ROS production characterizes oxidative stress, disrupts redox signaling within the cells and the interstice, promoting activation of calcium/calmodulin-dependent protein kinase I (CaMKI), increased NF-kB, AP-1 and other transcriptional factors signaling [33, 34]. Oxidative stress also elicits post-transductional pathways that result in activation of some proteins, e.g., matrix metaloproteinases (MMP) [35]. Consequently, oxidative stress has been associated with cardiac contraction dysfunction, increased collagen deposition and myocytes hypertrophy that contribute to cardiac dysfunction, myocyte hypertrophy and cell death [27, 35].

Considering the relevance of ROS to cardiac diseases, a substantial body of studies has investigated which enzyme could be more important to ROS synthesis. Along the progression of cardiac remodeling, a family of complex enzymes termed nicotinamide adenine dinucleotide phosphate-oxidase (NADPH oxidase) seems to play a central position to ROS production [27, 29]. Increased expression and activity of NADPH oxidase have been persistently observed in both preclinical and clinical studies of heart failure [27, 36]. There are seven Nox family isoforms (Nox1-5 and DUOX1 and 2), and the main cardiac enzymes are Nox2 and Nox4 [37].

Nox4 contribute to myocyte hypertrophy and cardiac fibrosis induced by AngII [38]. However, the role of Nox4 to cardiac hypertrophy is not yet fully comprehended [39].

Amount evidences show Nox2 associated with detrimental effects in the heart [27, 39]. The low-level activity of Nox2 is continuously present in the presence of nanomolar ROS levels but may be increased at the Ang II, endothelin, transforming growth factor (TGF)-β, tumor necrosis factor (TNF)-α presence as well as due to mechanical force [27]. Interestingly, Ang II-induced cardiac hypertrophy and fibrosis were reduced in knockout mice for Nox2 when compared to the wild type [38]. Currently, the contribution of Nox2 to Ang II hypertrophic effects appears to involve ERK1/2, Akt and NF-kB signaling [27, 41, 43]. In addition, increased Ang II-induced MMP activation and expression seem to be dependent of ROS [30, 42, 44] resulting in cardiac adaptive remodeling and fibrosis [43, 44]. **Figure 2** summarizes relationship between Ang II-induced cardiac remodeling and Nox2.

The important signaling in Ang II-induced fibrosis predominantly requires the differentiation from fibroblast into myofibroblast cells [3]. This phenotypic transformation from fibroblast is characterized by α-smooth muscle actin (α-SMA) expression and increased production of extracellular matrix, which is a key event in connective tissue remodeling involved in the heart failure progression [3, 45]. Rossi [9] has shown an intensive and progressive accumulation of collagen, accompanied by increased heart weight in hypertensive subjects. In addition, the study revealed an association among connective matrix, cardiac systolic and diastolic dysfunction in

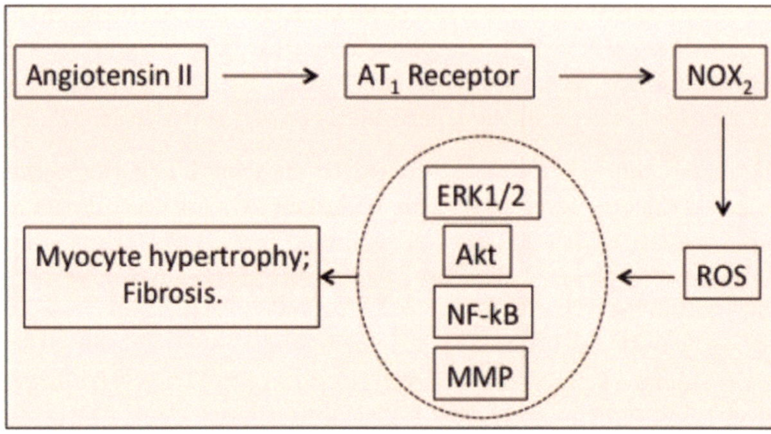

Figure 2. Main pathways concerning Ang II-induced cardiac remodeling. Nox2 is activated by Ang II via AT1 receptor, triggering ROS formation, which activates intracellular pathways related to the cardiac hypertrophy. Nox2: NADPH oxidase isoform 2; ROS: reactive oxygen species; Akt: serine/threonine-specific protein kinase; ERK1/2: extracellular.

hypertension suggesting that collagen deposition could contribute to decreased myocardial compliance and disrupted heart electrical properties [9]. Currently, it is well known the relevance of fibrosis not only to the structure of the cardiac hypertrophy but also to the heart dysfunction [46]. Collagen is the main component of the extracellular matrix in the myocardium, which is synthesized by fibroblasts. However, its deposition in the heart during hypertension also depends of its degradation [3]. Thus, a large body of studies has shown the contribution of the MMP, which is the main proteases to collagen degradation, strongly contributing to the cardiac remodeling after pressure overload or infarct [28, 47]. The imbalances between MMP and endogenous tissue inhibitor (TIMP) are key mechanisms to control the collagen formation and deposition [2, 3, 48]. Indeed, some transcriptional factors such as AP-1 and NF-kB may modulate the MMP activity increasing its MMP expression and also TIMP expression [28, 47]. Posttranslational mechanisms such as oxidative stress, particularly peroxynitrite and hydrogen peroxide, may activate MMP and inhibit TIMP activity [35, 49, 50], suggesting a possible mechanism to ROS-induced fibrosis in hypertensive rats [51]. Thus, MMP activity is regulated at three levels: (i) transcriptional level, (ii) endogenous inhibitors and (iii) factor activators (ROS). Interestingly, Ang II may increase MMP activity involving redox-sensitive signaling in fibroblast, thus triggering NF-kB and AP-1 transcriptional factor activation [52]. In fact, antioxidant therapy reverses Ang II-induced cardiac hypertrophy and MMP activity in left ventricle from hypertensive rats [30]. Taken together, Ang II promotes myocyte on the heart and matrix extracellular hypertrophy by similar mechanisms involving redox signaling, which not only activates the RNA expression of proteins in the myocytes or fibroblasts, but also rises the activity of enzymes already present in the heart, such as MMP.

Furthermore, it must be recognized that Ang II induces inflammation by triggering cardiac remodeling. The proinflammatory effects of Ang II have been described since 1970 by Finn Olsen [53]. Thenceforward, several studies have supported the contribution of the inflammatory processes associated with Ang II to cardiovascular disorders, including hypertension and heart remodeling [23, 25, 54]. Since inflammation contributes to this important clinical condition, numerous evidences have reported the connection between Ang II and two pivotal mediators for heart remodeling, the cytokines transforming growth factor (TGF)-β [23] and the tumoral necrosis factor (TNF)-α [25].

4. Angiotensin II and TGF-β in cardiac remodeling

Increased expression of TGF-β was found in the myocardium during cardiac hypertrophy and heart failure [55]. Classically, TGF-β is a multifunctional cytokine recognized as a powerful profibrotic factor. Three isoforms of the TGF-β family have been identified in mammals [56], but TGF-β1 has been constantly associated with several cardiovascular diseases, particularly during the transition from adaptive cardiac hypertrophy into heart failure [56–59]. The overexpression of TGF-β1 induced fibrosis and myocyte hypertrophy in transgenic mice after they were 8 weeks old [58]. Upregulated TGF-β1 mRNA is found in the pressure-overloaded human heart [60], as well as in the dilated cardiomyopathy [57]. The latent form of TGF-β1 is composed of 390-amino acid complexed with the signal peptide and the large amino-terminal prodomains (known as latency-associated proteins, LAPs) which are required for correct folding and dimerization of the carboxyl terminal domain of the growth factor (the mature peptide) [61]. TGF-β1 can be released and activated by the proteolytic cleavage, which disrupts its non-covalent attachment with LAP [62]. The intracellular signaling induced by TGF-β underlies the activation of serine/threonine kinases receptor resulting in Smad phosphorylation, which is responsible to activate target genes [61]. TGF-β may also promote the regulation of the transcription by TGF-β-activated kinase-1 (TAK1) triggering p38 MAPK phosphorylation and activating transcriptional factor (ATF)-2 [56].

Myriad experimental studies reported Ang II-mediated TGF-beta induction, particularly of its expression [63–65]. AT1 receptor seems to be involved with TGF-β upregulation expression at the transcriptional level in as much as losartan treatment inhibited the rise of this cytokine in animals after Ang II infusion [63].

Since AT1 activation produces ROS via NADPH oxidase, Wenzel et al. [63] demonstrated that the induction of TGF-β in cardiomyocytes was diminished in the presence of NADPH oxidase inhibitors. Consistently, antioxidant treatments have shown decreased cardiac TGF-β expression in the experimental model of RAS activation [23, 30]. The redox signaling involved in Ang II-induced TGF-β upregulation seems to be dependent on p38 MAPK and AP-1 pathway, such was observed in ventricular cardiac myocytes [23, 63]. In this regard, the first direct evidence about the causal relation between two important factors for cardiac hypertrophy (Ang II e TGF-β) was observed in TGF-β1-deficient mice. The marked cardiac hypertrophy and the impaired cardiac function induced by chronic suppressor doses of Ang II were not observed in TGF-β1-deficient mice [66]. Thus, cardiac TGF-β is required to hypertrophy signaling induced by Ang II, which in turn activates its AT1 receptor upregulating this cytokine expression.

TGF-β and Ang II are involved in fibroblast differentiation and MMP activity control [3]. In this regard, an imbalance between MMP/TIMP is possibly another common signaling consequently involved in the heart hypertrophy. Ang II-induced increased MMP transcriptional expression has been reported by several studies [30, 42, 44]. Despite AP-1 contribution to the transcription of MMP-2 [47], the NF-kB inhibition attenuated MMP-2 upregulation in both heart and aorta from 2-kidney and 1-clip (2K1C) hypertensive rats [44]. Transgenic mice overexpressing cardiac MMP-2 presented marked decompensated hypertrophy, including not only collagen deposition but also significant systolic dysfunction [67]. MMP-2 seems to degrade some contractile proteins from heart sarcomeres, such as myosin and troponin [35], which have constantly been associated with impaired heart capacity to contract in experimental models of heart disease [68]. In this regard, several findings have stated that MMP-2 inhibition ameliorates remodeling and cardiac dysfunction [35, 47, 69]. In addition, Ang II-induced MMP activation may be associated with adaptive remodeling and cardiac dysfunction in 2K1C rats [69]. The Ang II activates MMP-2 by mechanisms involving NADPH oxidase activation and ROS formation [30, 42]. In this sense, TGF-β could increase MMP-2 activation since this cytokine also increases ROS formation. Indeed, some studies have shown increased TGF-β levels and MMP-2 activity in the left ventricle from hypertensive rats [3, 30]. Hence, the TGF-β-dependent mechanisms to Ang II-induced cardiac remodeling may involve MMP-2 activation by redox signaling. However, future studies are necessary to support the causal relation between MMP-2 activation and TGF-β in Ang II hypertrophy.

5. Angiotensin II and TNF-α in cardiac remodeling

The proinflammatory cytokine TNF-α was first defined as an antimutagenic. Nowadays, amount findings revealed a wide range of pleitropic TNF-α effects including cell proliferation, apoptosis and production of other proinflammatory cytokines [2].

Growing body of evidences evaluated the role of TNF-α in many diseases, particularly in cardiovascular disease. TNF-α has been found upregulated in myocardial from humans and animals with heart failure [70]. A wide variety of cells including macrophages, fibroblast and endothelial cells produce TNF-α. It has been described that cardiomyocytes themselves are capable of synthesizing TNF-α [71]. Bryant et al. [72] have shown that TNF-α synthesized by cardiomyocytes was sufficient to cause severe cardiac remodeling suggesting maladaptive hypertrophy, which may also occur in human heart failure.

The TNF-α is secreted as a cell surface protein (homotrimeric type II transmembrane protein) containing 233-amino-acid, which is activated by proteolytic cleavage to a 76-amino-acid signal peptide [73, 74]. The TNF-α released as a mature protein, which acts as a soluble cytokine through its two receptors: TNF receptor 1 (TNFR1) and TNFR2 [75, 76]. Despite the homology between TNFR1 and TNFR2 in extracellular domains, both intracellular domains of TNFR1 and TNFR2 are different. Once activated, TNFR1 leads to recruitment of a protein TRADD (TNFR1 associated death domain protein), which subsequently interacts with three other intracellular proteins forming a complex. When activated, TNFR2 directly recruits TRAF2 and TRAF1 (TNF receptor-associated factor). These differences in TNFR-induced intracellular signaling suggest each receptor has distinct cellular functions. In this sense, dual effects of TNF-α have been suggested during the progress of cardiac disease. Low concentration of TNF-α has been associated with the protective effects while its high concentrations present deleterious effects [77]. This study did not evaluate the TNF-α receptors contribution. However, other evidences have been shown that the effects of the two receptors on heart failure were opposite, TNFR1 showed proapoptotic and prohypertrophic while TNFR2 developed antiapoptotic and antihypertrophic effects [78]. In addition, other findings have suggested that TNFR1 is responsible for the major deleterious effects produced by TNF-α in hypertrophic signaling [79, 80]. Moreover, soluble TNFR1 is a predictor of mortality and heart failure in patients with acute myocardial infarct [81]. Preclinical studies demonstrated that TNFR1 plays an important role in Ang II-induced fibrosis in rats while TNFR2 did not affect the increased collagen deposition in response to Ang II infusion [80].

TNF-α-induced intracellular signaling involves canonical NF-kB activation. The complex of intracellular protein is formed when TNFR1 is activated, specific mitogen-activated protein kinase kinases (MAPKKs) are phosphorylated consequently activating c-Jun N terminal kinase (JNK), AP1 and p38 MAPK signaling pathways. Taken together, TNF-α-induced intracellular signaling controls the expression of inflammatory proteins and antiapoptotic genes. Another signaling complex is triggered as a response to the TNFR1 activation resulting in stimulation of the effective caspases, which in turn lead to apoptosis [82].

TNF-α has induced increased ROS formation in endothelial cells by a mechanism dependent of NADPH oxidase subunit: p47 phox subunit [83]. Indeed, cardiomyocytes hypertrophy was induced by recombinant human TNF-α at least in part due to ROS generation [84]. Through experimental models of heart failure, TNF-α inhibition decreased oxidative stress and apoptosis improving cardiac remodeling and dysfunction [85]. Thus, ROS seems to foster a key function in the cardiac hypertrophy induced by TNF-α.

As described above, it is possible to observe common signaling pathways between TNF-α and Ang II. Since Ang II notably has increased TNF-α *in vivo* [86] and *in vitro* studies [87], some evidences have reported a potential role of TNF-α in Ang II-induced cardiac hypertrophy [25, 88–90]. In this context, chronic Ang II infusion promotes cardiac hypertrophy, which was attenuated in TNF-α knockout mice [89]. These findings were further confirmed by the pharmacological inhibition by etanercept, an inhibitor of TNF-α, which blunted cardiac hypertrophy in mice under Ang II infusion [25]. Indeed, the authors showed the involvement of TNF-α in the intracellular signaling in Ang II-induced hypertrophy. Both TNF-α and Ang II induced activation of NF-kB, p38 MAPK and JNK. Accordingly, heart TNF-α knockout mice attenuated the activation of NF-kB, p38 MAPK and JNK signaling in Ang II infusion, suggesting TNF-α is required to induce Ang II cardiac hypertrophy by intracellular signaling pathways [25]. It was observed that the TNFR1 deficient mice did not develop fibrosis under Ang II stimulation, while TNFR2 deficient mice showed increased collagen accumulation in the heart under Ang II infusion [88], which may indicate a promising role of TNF-α in activating TNFR1 as crucial signaling to Ang II inducing cardiac remodeling.

Ang II and TNF-α are involved in increased production of ROS, which in turn activate NF-kB. In this regard, Sriramula et al. [25] also suggest that redox signaling induced by Ang II may be dependent of TNF-α. The authors have found that the increased mRNA, 2 expression and also the expression of other NADPH oxidase isoforms were blunted in TNF-α knockout mice, which have resulted in lower levels of ROS. Collectively, all findings point out to a causal relation between hypertrophic signaling of Ang II and TNF-α that involve redox pathways on NF-kB, JNK and p38 activation.

6. Conclusion

Ang II and these cytokines (TGF-β and TNF-α) activate some intracellular pathways involved in hypertrophy, including increased ROS production through NADPH oxidase. Ang II activates NF-κB, which is a possible mechanism to Ang II-induced increased levels TNF-α and other proinflammatory cytokines. NF-κB and ROS pathway seems to be also involved TGF-β-increased MMP activity. In addition, cytokines, TNF-α and TGF-β, and Ang II are closely related with a MAPK, which is a known key pathway involved in cardiac hypertrophy and MMP regulation. Taken together, Ang II is associated to the TNF-α and TGF-β by mechanisms involving ROS-NF-κB-MMP then contributing to the heart failure.

Author details

Carolina Baraldi Araujo Restini[1,2*], Arthur F. Engracia Garcia[1], Henrique Melo Natalin[1], Guilherme Melo Natalin[1] and Elen Rizzi[2]

*Address all correspondence to: carolbaraldi@hotmail.com

1 Medical School, University of Ribeirao Preto, SP-UNAERP, São Paulo, Brazil

2 Department of Biotechnology, University of Ribeirao Preto, SP-UNAERP, São Paulo, Brazil

References

[1] Rossi MA, Carillo SV. Cardiac hypertrophy due to pressure and volume overload: distinctly different biological phenomena? Int J Cardiol 1991;31:133–41. DOI: 10.1016/0167-5273(91)90207-6.

[2] Opie LH, Commerford PJ, Gersh BJ, Pfeffer MA. Controversies in ventricular remodelling. Lancet 2006;367:356–67. DOI: 1016/S0140-6736(06)68074-4.

[3] Berk BC, Fujiwara K, Lehoux S. ECM remodeling in hypertensive heart disease. J Clin Invest 2007;117:568–75. DOI: 10.1172/JCI31044.

[4] Hunt SA. ACC/AHA 2005 guideline update for the diagnosis and management of chronic heart failure in the adult: a report of the American College of Cardiology/

American Heart Association Task Force on Practice Guidelines (Writing Committee to Update the 2001 Guidelines for the Evaluation and Management of Heart Failure). J Am Coll Cardiol 2005;46:e1-82. DOI: 10.1016/j.jacc.2005.08.022.

[5] Heidenreich PA, Albert NM, Allen LA, Bluemke DA, Butler J, Fonarow GC, et al. Forecasting the impact of heart failure in the United States: a policy statement from the American Heart Association. Circ Heart Fail 2013;6:606–19 DOI: 10.1161/HHF. 0b013e318291329a.

[6] Roger VL. Epidemiology of heart failure. Circ Res 2013;113:646–59 DOI: 10.1161/ CIRCRESAHA.113.300268.

[7] Dusing R. Mega clinical trials which have shaped the RAS intervention clinical practice. Ther Adv Cardiovasc Dis 2016;10:133–501. DOI: 10.1177/1753944716644131.

[8] Levy D, Larson MG, Vasan RS, Kannel WB, Ho KK. The progression from hypertension to congestive heart failure. JAMA 1996;275:1557–62. DOI: 10.1001/jama. 1996.03530440037034

[9] Rossi MA. Pathologic fibrosis and connective tissue matrix in left ventricular hypertrophy due to chronic arterial hypertension in humans. J Hypertens 1998;16:1031–41. PMID:9794745

[10] Opie LH. Cellular basis for therapeutic choices in heart failure. Circulation 2004;110:2559–61. DOI: 10.1161/01.CIR.0000146803.14063.F7.

[11] Wollert KC, Drexler H. The renin-angiotensin system and experimental heart failure. Cardiovasc Res 1999;43:838–49. DOI: 10.1016/S0008-6363(99)00145-5.

[12] Tamargo J, Lopez-Sendon J. Novel therapeutic targets for the treatment of heart failure. Nat Rev Drug Discov 2011;10:536–55. DOI:10.1038/nrd3431.

[13] Martins-Oliveira A, Castro MM, Oliveira DM, Rizzi E, Ceron CS, Guimaraes D, et al. Contrasting effects of aliskiren versus losartan on hypertensive vascular remodeling. Int J Cardiol 2013;167:1199–20. DOI: 10.1016/j.ijcard.2012.03.137.

[14] Leri A, Claudio PP, Li Q, Wang X, Reiss K, Wang S, et al. Stretch-mediated release of angiotensin II induces myocyte apoptosis by activating p53 that enhances the local renin-angiotensin system and decreases the Bcl-2-to-Bax protein ratio in the cell. J Clin Invest 1998;101:1326–42. DOI: 10.1172/JCI316.

[15] De Mello WC, Danser AH. Angiotensin II and the heart: on the intracrine renin-angiotensin system. Hypertension 2000;35:1183-8. DOI: 10.1161/01.HYP.35.6.1183.

[16] Sechi LA, Griffin CA, Grady EF, Kalinyak JE, Schambelan M. Characterization of angiotensin II receptor subtypes in rat heart. Circ Res 1992;71:1482-9. DOI: 10.1161/01.RES.71.6.1482

[17] Sadoshima J, Izumo S. Signal transduction pathways of angiotensin II-induced c-fos gene expression in cardiac myocytes in vitro. Roles of phospholipid-derived second messengers. Circ Res 1993;73:424–38.DOI: 10.1161/01.RES.73.3.424

[18] Suzuki J, Matsubara H, Urakami M, Inada M. Rat angiotensin II (type 1A) receptor mRNA regulation and subtype expression in myocardial growth and hypertrophy. Circ Res 1993;73:439–47. DOI:10.1161/01.RES.73.3.439

[19] Lopez JJ, Lorell BH, Ingelfinger JR, Weinberg EO, Schunkert H, Diamant D, et al. Distribution and function of cardiac angiotensin AT1- and AT2-receptor subtypes in hypertrophied rat hearts. Am J Physiol 1994;267:H844–52. PMID:8067441

[20] Bueno OF, De Windt LJ, Tymitz KM, Witt SA, Kimball TR, Klevitsky R, et al. The MEK1-ERK1/2 signaling pathway promotes compensated cardiac hypertrophy in transgenic mice. EMBO J 2000;19:6341–50 DOI: 10.1093/emboj/19.23.6341.

[21] Rose BA, Force T, Wang Y. Mitogen-activated protein kinase signaling in the heart: angels versus demons in a heart-breaking tale. Physiol Rev 2010;90:1507–46. DOI: 10.1152/physrev.00054.2009 [doi].

[22] Brasier AR, Jamaluddin M, Han Y, Patterson C, Runge MS. Angiotensin II induces gene transcription through cell-type-dependent effects on the nuclear factor-kappaB (NF-kappaB) transcription factor. Mol Cell Biochem 2000;212:155–69. PMID:11108147

[23] Rosenkranz S. TGF-beta1 and angiotensin networking in cardiac remodeling. Cardiovasc Res 2004;63:423–32. DOI: 10.1016/j.cardiores.2004.04.030.

[24] Lim H, Zhu YZ. Role of transforming growth factor-beta in the progression of heart failure. Cell Mol Life Sci 2006;63:2584–96. DOI:10.1007/s00018-006-6085-8.

[25] Sriramula S, Francis J. Tumor necrosis factor-alpha is essential for angiotensin II-induced ventricular remodeling: role for oxidative stress. PLoS One 2015;10:e0138372. DOI:10.1371/journal.pone.0138372.

[26] Ushio-Fukai M. Redox signaling in angiogenesis: role of NADPH oxidase. Cardiovasc Res 2006;71:226–35. DOI:10.1016/j.cardiores.2006.04.015.

[27] Sag CM, Santos CX, Shah AM. Redox regulation of cardiac hypertrophy. J Mol Cell Cardiol 2014;73:103–11. DOI:10.1016/j.yjmcc.2014.02.002.

[28] Deschamps AM, Spinale FG. Pathways of matrix metalloproteinase induction in heart failure: bioactive molecules and transcriptional regulation. Cardiovasc Res 2006;69:666–76. DOI:10.1016/j.cardiores.2005.10.004.

[29] Briones AM, Touyz RM. Oxidative stress and hypertension: current concepts. Curr Hypertens Rep 2010;12:135–42. DOI:10.1007/s11906-010-0100-z.

[30] Rizzi E, Castro MM, Ceron CS, Neto-Neves EM, Prado CM, Rossi MA, et al. Tempol inhibits TGF-beta and MMPs upregulation and prevents cardiac hypertensive changes. Int J Cardiol 2013;165:165–73. DOI: 10.1016/j.ijcard.2011.08.060.

[31] Murdoch CE, Zhang M, Cave AC, Shah AM. NADPH oxidase-dependent redox signalling in cardiac hypertrophy, remodelling and failure. Cardiovasc Res 2006;71:208–15. DOI: 10.1016/j.cardiores.2006.03.016.

[32] Zhang M, Perino A, Ghigo A, Hirsch E, Shah AM. NADPH oxidases in heart failure: poachers or gamekeepers? Antioxid Redox Signal 2013;18:1024–41. DOI: 10.1089/ars.2012.4550.

[33] Siwik DA, Colucci WS. Regulation of matrix metalloproteinases by cytokines and reactive oxygen/nitrogen species in the myocardium. Heart Fail Rev 2004;9:43–51. DOI: 10.1023/B:HREV.0000011393.40674.13.

[34] Burgoyne JR, Mongue-Din H, Eaton P, Shah AM. Redox signaling in cardiac physiology and pathology. Circ Res 2012;111:1091–106. DOI: 10.1161/CIRCRESAHA.111.255216.

[35] Schulz R. Intracellular targets of matrix metalloproteinase-2 in cardiac disease: rationale and therapeutic approaches. Annu Rev Pharmacol Toxicol 2007;47:211–42. DOI:10.1146/annurev.pharmtox.47.120505.105230.

[36] Heymes C, Bendall JK, Ratajczak P, Cave AC, Samuel JL, Hasenfuss G, et al. Increased myocardial NADPH oxidase activity in human heart failure. J Am Coll Cardiol 2003;41:2164–71. DOI: :10.1016/S0735-1097(03)00471-6.

[37] Lassegue B, San Martin A, Griendling KK. Biochemistry, physiology, and pathophysiology of NADPH oxidases in the cardiovascular system. Circ Res 2012;110:1364–90. DOI: 10.1161/CIRCRESAHA.111.243972.

[38] Zhao QD, Viswanadhapalli S, Williams P, Shi Q, Tan C, Yi X, et al. NADPH oxidase 4 induces cardiac fibrosis and hypertrophy through activating Akt/mTOR and NFkappaB signaling pathways. Circulation 2015;131:643–55. DOI: 10.1161/CIRCULATIONAHA.114.011079.

[39] Shah AM. Parsing the role of NADPH oxidase enzymes and reactive oxygen species in heart failure. Circulation 2015;131:602-4. DOI: 10.1161/CIRCULATIONAHA.115.014906.

[40] Bendall JK, Cave AC, Heymes C, Gall N, Shah AM. Pivotal role of a gp91(phox)-containing NADPH oxidase in angiotensin II-induced cardiac hypertrophy in mice. Circulation 2002;105:293-6. DOI: 10.1161/hc0302.103712.

[41] Sarman B, Skoumal R, Leskinen H, Rysa J, Ilves M, Soini Y, et al. Nuclear factor-kappaB signaling contributes to severe, but not moderate, angiotensin II-induced left ventricular remodeling. J Hypertens 2007;25:1927–39. DOI: 10.1097/HJH.0b013e3281e66653.

[42] Luchtefeld M, Grote K, Grothusen C, Bley S, Bandlow N, Selle T, et al. Angiotensin II induces MMP-2 in a p47phox-dependent manner. Biochem Biophys Res Commun 2005;328:183-8.DOI: 10.1016/j.bbrc.2004.12.152.

[43] Belo VA, Guimaraes DA, Castro MM. Matrix metalloproteinase 2 as a potential mediator of vascular smooth muscle cell migration and chronic vascular remodeling in hypertension. J Vasc Res 2015;52:221–31. DOI: 10.1159/000441621.

[44] Cau SB, Guimaraes DA, Rizzi E, Ceron CS, Gerlach RF, Tanus-Santos JE. The nuclear factor kappaB inhibitor pyrrolidine dithiocarbamate prevents cardiac remodelling and matrix metalloproteinase-2 up-regulation in renovascular hypertension. Basic Clin Pharmacol Toxicol 2015;117:234–41. DOI: 10.1111/bcpt.12400.

[45] Gonzalez A, Lopez B, Querejeta R, Diez J. Regulation of myocardial fibrillar collagen by angiotensin II. A role in hypertensive heart disease? J Mol Cell Cardiol 2002;34:1585–93. DOI: 10.1006/jmcc.2002.2081.

[46] Weber KT, Sun Y, Tyagi SC, Cleutjens JP. Collagen network of the myocardium: function, structural remodeling and regulatory mechanisms. J Mol Cell Cardiol 1994;26:279–92. DOI: 10.1006/jmcc.1994.1036.

[47] Spinale FG. Myocardial matrix remodeling and the matrix metalloproteinases: influence on cardiac form and function. Physiol Rev 2007;87:1285–342. DOI: 10.1152/physrev.00012.2007.

[48] Brew K, Nagase H. The tissue inhibitors of metalloproteinases (TIMPs): an ancient family with structural and functional diversity. Biochim Biophys Acta 2010;1803:55–71. DOI: 10.1016/j.bbamcr.2010.01.003.

[49] Donnini S, Monti M, Roncone R, Morbidelli L, Rocchigiani M, Oliviero S, et al. Peroxynitrite inactivates human-tissue inhibitor of metalloproteinase-4. FEBS Lett 2008;582:1135–40. DOI: 10.1016/j.febslet.2008.02.080.

[50] Kandasamy AD, Chow AK, Ali MA, Schulz R. Matrix metalloproteinase-2 and myocardial oxidative stress injury: beyond the matrix. Cardiovasc Res 2010;85:413–23. DOI: 10.1093/cvr/cvp268 [doi].

[51] Rizzi E, Ceron CS, Guimaraes DA, Prado CM, Rossi MA, Gerlach RF, et al. Temporal changes in cardiac matrix metalloproteinase activity, oxidative stress, and TGF-beta in renovascular hypertension-induced cardiac hypertrophy. Exp Mol Pathol 2013;94:1-9. DOI: 10.1016/j.yexmp.2012.10.010.

[52] Chen J, Mehta JL. Angiotensin II-mediated oxidative stress and procollagen-1 expression in cardiac fibroblasts: blockade by pravastatin and pioglitazone. Am J Physiol Heart Circ Physiol 2006;291:H1738–45. DOI: 10.1152/ajpheart.00341.2006.

[53] Olsen F. Type and course of the inflammatory cellular reaction in acute angiotensin-hypertensive vascular disease in rats. Acta Pathol Microbiol Scand A 1970;78:143–50. DOI: 10.1111/j.1699-0463.1970.tb00249.x.

[54] McMaster WG, Kirabo A, Madhur MS, Harrison DG. Inflammation, immunity, and hypertensive end-organ damage. Circ Res 2015;116:1022–33. DOI: 10.1161/CIRCRESAHA.116.303697.

[55] Bujak M, Frangogiannis NG. The role of TGF-beta signaling in myocardial infarction and cardiac remodeling. Cardiovasc Res 2007;74:184–95. DOI: 10.1016/j.cardiores. 2006.10.002.

[56] Poniatowski LA, Wojdasiewicz P, Gasik R, Szukiewicz D. Transforming growth factor Beta family: insight into the role of growth factors in regulation of fracture healing biology and potential clinical applications. Mediators Inflamm 2015;2015:137823–40 DOI: 10.1155/2015/137823.

[57] Pauschinger M, Knopf D, Petschauer S, Doerner A, Poller W, Schwimmbeck PL, et al. Dilated cardiomyopathy is associated with significant changes in collagen type I/III ratio. Circulation 1999;99:2750-6. DOI: 10.1161/01.CIR.99.21.2750.

[58] Rosenkranz S, Flesch M, Amann K, Haeuseler C, Kilter H, Seeland U, et al. Alterations of beta-adrenergic signaling and cardiac hypertrophy in transgenic mice overexpressing TGF-beta(1). Am J Physiol Heart Circ Physiol 2002;283:H1253–62. DOI 10.1152/ajpheart.00578.2001.

[59] Creemers EE, Pinto YM. Molecular mechanisms that control interstitial fibrosis in the pressure-overloaded heart. Cardiovasc Res 2011;89:265–72. DOI: 10.1093/cvr/cvq308.

[60] Villar AV, Llano M, Cobo M, Exposito V, Merino R, Martin-Duran R, et al. Gender differences of echocardiographic and gene expression patterns in human pressure overload left ventricular hypertrophy. J Mol Cell Cardiol 2009;46:526–35 DOI:10.1016/j.yjmcc.2008.12.024.

[61] Massague J, Seoane J, Wotton D. Smad transcription factors. Genes Dev 2005;19:2783–810. DOI: 10.1101/gad.1350705.

[62] Lyons RM, Keski-Oja J, Moses HL. Proteolytic activation of latent transforming growth factor-beta from fibroblast-conditioned medium. J Cell Biol 1988;106:1659–65.PMCID: PMC2115066.

[63] Wenzel S, Taimor G, Piper HM, Schluter KD. Redox-sensitive intermediates mediate angiotensin II-induced p38 MAP kinase activation, AP-1 binding activity, and TGF-beta expression in adult ventricular cardiomyocytes. FASEB J 2001;15:2291–310. DOI: 1096/fj.00-0827fje.

[64] Sun Y, Zhang J, Zhang JQ, Ramires FJ. Local angiotensin II and transforming growth factor-beta1 in renal fibrosis of rats. Hypertension 2000;35:1078–84. DOI: 10.1161/01.HYP.35.5.1078.

[65] Wheeler JB, Ikonomidis JS, Jones JA. Connective tissue disorders and cardiovascular complications: the indomitable role of transforming growth factor-beta signaling. Adv Exp Med Biol 2014;802:107–27. DOI: 10.1007/978-94-007-7893-1_8.

[66] Schultz Jel J, Witt SA, Glascock BJ, Nieman ML, Reiser PJ, Nix SL, et al. TGF-beta1 mediates the hypertrophic cardiomyocyte growth induced by angiotensin II. J Clin Invest 2002;109:787–96. DOI: 10.1172/JCI14190.

[67] Bergman MR, Teerlink JR, Mahimkar R, Li L, Zhu BQ, Nguyen A, et al. Cardiac matrix metalloproteinase-2 expression independently induces marked ventricular remodeling and systolic dysfunction. Am J Physiol Heart Circ Physiol 2007;292:H1847–60. DOI: 10.1152/ajpheart.00434.2006.

[68] Hughes BG, Schulz R. Targeting MMP-2 to treat ischemic heart injury. Basic Res Cardiol 2014;109:424. DOI: 10.1007/s00395-014-0424-y.

[69] Rizzi E, Castro MM, Prado CM, Silva CA, Fazan R, Jr., Rossi MA, et al. Matrix metalloproteinase inhibition improves cardiac dysfunction and remodeling in 2-kidney, 1-clip hypertension. J Card Fail 2010;16:599–608. DOI: 10.1016/j.cardfail.2010.02.005.

[70] Torre-Amione G, Vooletich MT, Farmer JA. Role of tumour necrosis factor-alpha in the progression of heart failure: therapeutic implications. Drugs 2000;59:745–51. DOI: 10.2165/00003495-200059040-00002.

[71] Kapadia SR, Oral H, Lee J, Nakano M, Taffet GE, Mann DL. Hemodynamic regulation of tumor necrosis factor-alpha gene and protein expression in adult feline myocardium. Circ Res 1997;81:187–95. DOI: 10.1161/01.RES.81.2.187.

[72] Bryant D, Becker L, Richardson J, Shelton J, Franco F, Peshock R, et al. Cardiac failure in transgenic mice with myocardial expression of tumor necrosis factor-alpha. Circulation 1998;97:1375–81. DOI: 10.1161/01.CIRC.97.14.1375.

[73] Camussi G, Albano E, Tetta C, Bussolino F. The molecular action of tumor necrosis factor-alpha. Eur J Biochem 1991;202:3-14. DOI: 10.1111/j.1432-1033.1991.tb16337.x.

[74] Amour A, Slocombe PM, Webster A, Butler M, Knight CG, Smith BJ, et al. TNF-alpha converting enzyme (TACE) is inhibited by TIMP-3. FEBS Lett 1998;435:39–44. DOI: 10.1016/S0014-5793(98)01031-X.

[75] Tartaglia LA, Goeddel DV. Two TNF receptors. Immunol Today 1992;13:151–301. DOI: 10.1016/0167-5699(92)90116-O.

[76] Winsauer C, Kruglov AA, Chashchina AA, Drutskaya MS, Nedospasov SA. Cellular sources of pathogenic and protective TNF and experimental strategies based on utilization of TNF humanized mice. Cytokine Growth Factor Rev 2014;25:115–23. DOI: 10.1016/j.cytogfr.2013.12.005 [doi].

[77] Mann DL. Stress-activated cytokines and the heart: from adaptation to maladaptation. Annu Rev Physiol 2003;65:81–101. DOI: 10.1146/annurev.physiol.65.092101.142249.

[78] Hamid T, Gu Y, Ortines RV, Bhattacharya C, Wang G, Xuan YT, et al. Divergent tumor necrosis factor receptor-related remodeling responses in heart failure: role of nuclear factor-kappaB and inflammatory activation. Circulation 2009;119:1386–97. DOI: 10.1161/CIRCULATIONAHA.108.802918.

[79] von Haehling S, Jankowska EA, Anker SD. Tumour necrosis factor-alpha and the failing heart--pathophysiology and therapeutic implications. Basic Res Cardiol 2004;99:18–28. DOI: 10.1007/s00395-003-0433-8.

[80] Duerrschmid C, Crawford JR, Reineke E, Taffet GE, Trial J, Entman ML, et al. TNF receptor 1 signaling is critically involved in mediating angiotensin-II-induced cardiac fibrosis. J Mol Cell Cardiol 2013;57:59–67. DOI: 10.1016/j.yjmcc.2013.01.006.

[81] Valgimigli M, Ceconi C, Malagutti P, Merli E, Soukhomovskaia O, Francolini G, et al. Tumor necrosis factor-alpha receptor 1 is a major predictor of mortality and new-onset heart failure in patients with acute myocardial infarction: the Cytokine-Activation and Long-Term Prognosis in Myocardial Infarction (C-ALPHA) study. Circulation 2005;111:863–70. DOI: 10.1161/01.CIR.0000155614.35441.69.

[82] Borghi A, Verstrepen L, Beyaert R. TRAF2 multitasking in TNF receptor-induced signaling to NF-kappaB, MAP kinases and cell death. Biochem Pharmacol 2012; 116 (15): 1–10. DOI:10.1016/j.bcp.2016.03.009.

[83] Li JM, Mullen AM, Yun S, Wientjes F, Brouns GY, Thrasher AJ, et al. Essential role of the NADPH oxidase subunit p47(phox) in endothelial cell superoxide production in response to phorbol ester and tumor necrosis factor-alpha. Circ Res 2002;90:143–50. DOI: 10.1161/hh0202.103615.

[84] Nakamura K, Fushimi K, Kouchi H, Mihara K, Miyazaki M, Ohe T, et al. Inhibitory effects of antioxidants on neonatal rat cardiac myocyte hypertrophy induced by tumor necrosis factor-alpha and angiotensin II. Circulation 1998;98:794-9. DOI: 10.1161/01.CIRC.98.8.794.

[85] Moe GW, Marin-Garcia J, Konig A, Goldenthal M, Lu X, Feng Q. In vivo TNF-alpha inhibition ameliorates cardiac mitochondrial dysfunction, oxidative stress, and apoptosis in experimental heart failure. Am J Physiol Heart Circ Physiol 2004;287:H1813–20. DOI: 10.1152/ajpheart.00036.2004.

[86] Haudek SB, Cheng J, Du J, Wang Y, Hermosillo-Rodriguez J, Trial J, et al. Monocytic fibroblast precursors mediate fibrosis in angiotensin-II-induced cardiac hypertrophy. J Mol Cell Cardiol 2010;49:499–507. DOI: 10.1016/j.yjmcc.2010.05.005.

[87] Pellieux C, Montessuit C, Papageorgiou I, Lerch R. Angiotensin II downregulates the fatty acid oxidation pathway in adult rat cardiomyocytes via release of tumour necrosis factor-alpha. Cardiovasc Res 2009;82:341–50. DOI:10.1093/cvr/cvp004 [doi].

[88] Duerrschmid C, Trial J, Wang Y, Entman ML, Haudek SB. Tumor necrosis factor: a mechanistic link between angiotensin-II-induced cardiac inflammation and fibrosis. Circ Heart Fail 2015;8:352–61. DOI: 10.1161/CIRCHEARTFAILURE.114.001893.

[89] Sriramula S, Haque M, Majid DS, Francis J. Involvement of tumor necrosis factor-alpha in angiotensin II-mediated effects on salt appetite, hypertension, and cardiac hyper-

trophy. Hypertension 2008;51:1345–51. DOI: 10.1161/HYPERTENSIONAHA . 107.102152.

[90] Sriramula S, Cardinale JP, Francis J. Inhibition of TNF in the brain reverses alterations in RAS components and attenuates angiotensin II-induced hypertension. PLoS One 2013;8:e63847–56. DOI: 10.1371/journal.pone.0063847.

Section 3

RAS and Reproduction

Chapter 5

Renin-Angiotensin System on Reproductive Biology

Anthony C.S. Castilho, Patrícia K. Fontes,
Fernanda F. Franchi, Priscila H. Santos and
Eduardo M. Razza

Additional information is available at the end of the chapter

http://dx.doi.org/10.5772/66997

Abstract

In the female reproductive system, angiotensin II (ANG II) is a potential signaling molecule involved in ovarian follicle development, which acts through two transmembrane receptors. Within the ovarian follicle, there appear to be species differences in the precise pattern of localization of AGTR2 protein and it has an important role in in vitro maturation of oocytes in mammals. The infusion of ANG II induced ovulation in rabbits and the use of ANG II antagonists inhibited ovulation in rabbits, rats, and cattle. In fetal ovaries, AGTR2 protein was detected in ovigerous cords and preantral follicles throughout porcine and bovine gestation. In the oviduct, ANG II is responsible for the orchestration of the transport of gametes. In the male reproductive system, there is considerable evidence for the local synthesis of components of renin-angiotensin system (RAS) in male reproductive tissues. The roles of RAS in local processes at these sites are still uncertain, although there is evidence for involvement in tubular contractility, spermatogenesis, sperm maturation, capacitation, acrosomal exocytosis, and fertilization.

Keywords: oviduct, ovary, bovine, reproduction, testis

1. Introduction

Many peptides are responsible for the coordination of functions in reproductive tissues, including angiotensin II (ANG II). In the oviduct, ANG II induces morphological and physiological alterations in the infundibulum, ampulla, and isthmus to provide an ideal microenvironment for oocyte transport and maturation, sperm capacitation and transport, and fertilization and early embryonic development.

In the ovary, the AT2 receptor is important for ovulation in many species (cattle, rats, and rabbits) and follicle stimulating hormone (FSH) is an important regulator in bovine granulosa cells *in vivo* and *in vitro*. Moreover, the presence of this system in bovine, caprine and procine fetal ovaries ovaries suggests a role in preantral follicle development. In addition, in female germ cells, ANG II plays a key role in the oocytes during in vitro maturation in porcine and Cattle. In male reproduction as an important role in spermatogenesis to guarantee fertilization.

Aiming to clarify the localization, role, and practical implications of the renin-angiotensin system (RAS) in male and female reproductive biology, this chapter highlights the roles of RAS in mammalian reproductive physiology, specifically, in the ovaries, testes, oviducts, and other reproductive tissues.

2. Role in follicular microenvironment and ovulatory capacity

Oocyte and follicle development start during the fetal stage. Initially, the primordial germ cells migrate from the endoderm of the embryonic yolk sac to the gonadal ridge, where during migration the cells undergo mitotic divisions. In the gonadal ridge, cells are internalized and cease mitotic division. After being enclosed in ovigerous cords, the cells become referred to as oogonia. The oogonia present the onset of meiosis but are interrupted in prophase I, the moment that the chromosomes are decondensed and contained in the germinal vesicle. One layer of flattened epithelial cells (pre-granulosa cells) is formed around the oogonia, becoming a primordial follicle, and when the pre-granulosa cells become cuboidal granulosa cells (primary follicle), follicular growth begins, with the proliferation of granulosa cells turning into a secondary follicle (two to six layers), and later an antral follicle (more than six layers) (reviewed for [1, 2]).

The presence of prorenin, renin, angiotensinogen, angiotensin-converting enzyme, and ANG II and ANG II receptors (AT1 and AT2 receptors) in the ovary is suggestive of a functional ovarian RAS. In cattle, the expression of ANG II is greatest in large follicles, suggesting that it is important during follicular growth and maturation [9]. Within the ovarian follicle, there appear to be species differences in the precise pattern of localization of AGTR2 protein. Infusion of ANG II induced ovulation in rabbits and the use of ANG II antagonists inhibited ovulation in rabbits, rats, and cattle [3–7].

ANG II acts through two distinct transmembrane receptors, namely AT1 (encoded by the AGTR1 gene) and AT2 (encoded by the AGTR2 gene [8]). In rabbits, the receptors are mostly AT2 receptors and are expressed in the granulosa cells of preovulatory follicles, consistent with the role of ANG II in ovulation. A similar role has been suggested in cattle by [7], who observed that AGTR2 mRNA in bovine granulosa cells was more abundant in healthy compared with atretic follicles.

Regarding the effects on oocyte maturation, Giometti et al. [9] investigated the role of ANG II in bovine oocyte nuclear maturation and suggested a role of ANG II in blocking the inhibitory effect of theca cells on nuclear maturation of bovine oocytes. Moreover, Barreta et al. [10] found strong evidence that ANG II mediates the resumption of meiosis induced by a luteinizing hormone (LH) surge in bovine oocytes, probably through the effects of prostaglandins produced by follicular cells. Recently, Siqueira et al. [11, 12] suggested that progesterone is also involved in oocyte meiotic resumption induced by the gonadotropin surge in cattle.

Furthermore, some reproductive biotechnologies, such as ovarian hyperstimulation, seem to affect ANG II in the ovaries. Numerous treatment protocols to induce multiple ovulations in cattle, using different gonadotropins, doses, routes of administration, and various hormone combinations and schedules, have been proposed in an attempt to improve embryo yield [13–16]. Recently, Barros et al. [17] showed higher levels of AGTR2 mRNA in cows submitted to ovarian hyperstimulation using FSH. These findings substantiate those of [7], who observed increases in AT2 receptor mRNA and protein levels after adding FSH to granulosa cell culture.

Although the focus of RAS is on antral follicle development and oocyte competence, RAS has also been detected in fetal ovaries; however, not much is known about the regulation of development of pre-antral follicles. ANG II could be one of the factors that activate oogonia and oocytes. Embryologically, ovarian development in mammals originates from the nephrogenic ridge, as well as fetal kidney [18], where ANG II plays a role in kidney development [19]. Renin was identified in pig and mouse mesonephros [18]. It is believed that mesonephric cells are the precursors of granulosa cells (reviewed for [1]).

ANG II is produced in fetal porcine ovaries, as well as other components of RAS (prorenin, angiotensin, AT1, and AT2 receptors) required for the production and action of ANG II. These components are present at about 45 days of gestation. The abundance of mRNA prorenin increases until day 90 and then stabilizes [20].

In early gestation in porcines, there is the presence of AT2 mRNA but the abundance decreases with the progress of gestation, unlike AT1 mRNA that remains stable during gestation. In addition, the protein of the receptors appears alternately; AT1 receptor is present throughout gestation but the amount decreases during evolution while AT2 appears steadily [20].

Still in porcines, proteins of the receptors are present in the epithelial surface with a predominance of AT1 receptors, in primordial germ cells [20, 21], granulosa cells of primordial, primary, and secondary follicles, and also in oocytes (except for oocytes of secondary follicles). However, proteins of the receptors are not present in theca or stroma cells [20].

In cattle, there is only one study confirming the presence of AT2 in fetal ovaries. Protein was detected in the cytoplasm of oogonia up to 60 days of gestation, becoming weak and unstable from day 75 of gestation. The AT2 protein appears again from day 210 in granulosa cells of primary and secondary follicles, and granulosa and theca cells of antral follicles. The mRNA AT2 abundance does not change throughout gestation [22].

The difference in the expression pattern of the protein and AT2 mRNA mentioned above is easily explained by the differences in follicular development between the species. The primary follicles appear earlier in bovines than in porcines, but in bovines the gestation is approximately three times longer than in porcines [22]. In caprine pre-antral ovaries, a high expression of AT1 and AT2 has been demonstrated in primordial follicles. It was also expressed in secondary follicles, but at a lower level [23].

Despite the presence of RAS components in fetal ovaries, the function of the system is not well understood. In pre-antral follicles, ANG II is associated with conserving follicular viability through binding to its receptors [23], and seems to be related to cellular atresia by binding to AT2 [20]. Furthermore, when porcine pre-antral follicles are cultured in a long-term culture system with the addition of ANG II, it seems to stimulate the division of granulosa cells and steroid synthesis [24].

3. Role in oviductal function

In the oviduct, endocrine and paracrine factors induce morphological, biochemical, and physiological alterations in the infundibulum, ampulla, and isthmus to provide an ideal microenvironment for oocyte transport and maturation, sperm capacitation and transport, and fertilization and early embryonic development. Thus, the temporal and spatial organization of each of these events is fundamental to reproductive efficiency [6, 25]. It is known that some peptides are responsible for the orchestration of these processes, including angiotensin II (ANG II) [26, 27].

ANG II is the major bioactive peptide of the renin-angiotensin system. This vasoactive peptide is derived from angiotensinogen in a two-step process that first involves the renin-dependent conversion of angiotensinogen to angiotensin I (ANG I), followed by ANG I conversion to ANG II via angiotensin-converting enzyme I (ACE-I). The fact that ANG II has a reproductive role in the female mammal is demonstrated by the presence of ANG II receptors in reproductive tissues in several species. There are two types of ANG II receptors: type 1 (ANGR1) and type 2 (ANGR2) [28].

The oviductal cells are capable of producing ANG II [29]. It has been reported that the ACE-1 mRNA abundance is higher during the postovulatory phase and that ANG II released by oviductal tissues is greater in the follicular and postovulatory phases than the luteal phase of the bovine estrous cycle [29]. In women, ANG II concentration in the fallopian tubes is higher in the secretory phase of the menstrual cycle [30].

Both receptors are present in the oviduct. In the human fallopian tube, ANGR1 receptor is in the epithelial cells of the mucosa; there are higher levels in the ampulla than in the fimbria and isthmus [31, 32], and ANGR1 receptor concentration is higher in the proliferative phase than in the secretory phase. In the bovine oviduct, the presence of ANGR2 has been demonstrated in all oviducts during the pre-ovulatory period [33].

ANG II is involved in the ciliary beat frequency (CBF) of oviductal ciliary cells. ANG II stimulates the increase in CBF in the mucosa of human fallopian tubes acting on the ANGR1 [31, 32]. Additionally, elevated ANG II interacts with other contraction-release substances to activate oviductal smooth muscle contractions [29].The combination of the action of ANG II to activate CBF and muscle contraction during the peri-ovulatory phase suggests the important function of ANG II in the rapid transport of gametes to the fertilization site [29].

In addition, ANG II is involved in sperm survival. In the bovine oviduct, ANG II participates in the local immunological response of the oviduct against allogeneic sperm, modulating the phagocytic activity of neutrophils [34].

4. Role in male reproduction

The renin-angiotensin system (RAS) appears to be quite important for fertility in the male reproductive system. This system is isolated from the plasmatic RAS by the blood testicular barrier, which protects fertility from AT1 blockers and angiotensin-converting enzyme (ACE) inhibitors. Many researchers have found strong evidence of renin activity in mouse, rat, and human testicular tissue. The Leydig cells have continuously been considered as the most likely origin of renin in this tissue. Other key players of the RAS, for example, ACE, ANG I, ANG II, and ANG III, have also been extensively detected in many cell types including Leydig cells [35].

As learned from mice, testicular ACE is highly tissue-specific and, although Leydig cells were once suggested as being the origin of ACE in the testis, it was later confirmed that germinal cells are the actual source of ACE activity in the testes. During spermiogenesis, ACE is highly expressed by germ cells and the administration of ANG II can decrease ACE expression in the testis [36, 37].

Although present in the prostate, until now there has been no evidence of renin in the epididymis [38]. One interesting observation was that if the spermatozoa access to the epididymis is blocked by efferent duct legation, for instance, the ACE activity is greatly reduced in the epididymis, suggesting an important but still unclear role of the RAS in this process [39, 40].

ACE is very active in the seminal vesicle and its levels in the testis are very high; therefore, potential ACE secretion in the seminal fluid is strongly suggested [41–43]. Also, both isoenzymes of ACE have been detected in rat epididymis [41, 44]. In human seminal plasma, the ACE is highly active and probably originates from the epididymal tubules of the vas deferens. Known to be highly expressed in germ cells, testicular ACE seems to be dependent on sexual maturation, since it exists in mature sperm and in spermatocytes with mature spermatids, and also in spermatids of sexually mature mammals [43, 44].

ACE activity is low in the prostate under normal conditions; however, prostatic hyperplasia can increase ACE activity [41, 43, 45, 46]. Likewise, ANG II AT1 receptors are predominant in the prostate, but their binding is reduced during hyperplasia, suggesting an effect of prostatic hyperstimulation [47]. ACE isoforms are strongly present in the vas deferens, but with low activity [44, 48]. Low ACE activity has also been identified in seminal vesicles [48].

The activity of the ACE enzyme is low in immature mammals and increases with the onset of sexual maturity [42, 49]. Sexual stimulation was shown to enhance ACE activity in semen [50, 51] but remains basal in oligospermic males [50]. The ACE enzyme may play a role in fertilization, since its levels increase during sperm capacitation [52–55].

The action of ACE in male fertility has been investigated by the use of knockout mice [56, 57], where males lacking ACE are indeed infertile; however, their sperm content, motility, viability, capacitation, and induction of acrosome reaction were completely normal. Although these knockout sperms present normal functionality, barely any of them reach the uterine tube, and even if they do, they seem incompetent at zona pellucida binding to the potentially present oocyte in the ampulla region of the oviduct. The probable reason for this is that ACE may provide sperm with the capacity to detach from the oviduct epithelium in the female reproductive tract. It is important to highlight that these genetically modified male mice, such as those resulting from the insertion of a modified ACE allele through homologous recombination [58], present distinctly low blood pressure, deeply impaired kidneys, and a high infertility index. In addition, ANG II can increase sperm motility and AT1 receptor antagonists can inhibit this action [59].

Additionally, angiotensinogen is present in testicular tissue in the majority of mammals, excluding rats [37, 60–66]. Molecular investigations have found that AT1A is the predominantly expressed receptor in mouse testis [67] and ANG II receptor was also found to be acting on Leydig cells of mammals [59, 68]. Likewise, ANG I and ANG II are also present in rat epididymis and the level of ANG II in the epididymis can be clearly reduced after efferent duct ligation [38, 40, 69]. ANG receptors AT1 and AT2 have been detected in rat epididymis [70], where the presence of AT1 receptors is higher than AT2 receptors, and both receptors are much more numerous in fully mature rat epididymis than in younger stages. AT1 receptors were also found in primary spermatogonia and spermatid tails [59].

There is evidence of linked RAS regulation between the circulatory system and testes, as hypophysectomy decreases renin levels in the testes while slightly increasing plasma renin [71]. Estrogen and other gonadotrophin hyperstimulation treatments can deplete renin signalization in Leydig cells [72, 73]. On the other hand, renin activity, as well as ANG production, can be increased in Leydig cells in vitro by human chorionic gonadotropin (hCG) or bovine luteinizing hormone administration [74]. There is also evidence that renin levels in plasma are also increased by hCG [75].

In 1998, Hirai et al. [76] verified that AT1 and AT2 expression in rat testes depends on the pituitary action, since after hypophysectomy the gene expression of both receptors was significantly increased. In addition, chorionic gonadotropin has been shown to reduce AT1 and AT2 gene expression. Furthermore, the AT2 expression in rat testes is variable according to the developmental stage of the male. For instance, as the aging process progresses the expression of both AT1 and AT2 substantially decreases [77]. Similarly, we can observe plenty of ANG II receptors in non-differentiated mesenchymal cells of the interstitium in immature testes, but ANG II binding systematically decreases throughout development [68].

ANG is one of the peptide hormones in the epididymis responsible for stimulating the secretion of anion and fluid [39]. Some evidence suggests that the majority of its action is attributed to ANG II action on the apical surface of the epididymal epithelium, in which it may exert an effect through interaction with the AT1 receptor [70, 78].

In summary, the variability of the RAS in the testes or epididymis is gradually affected as development progresses, with a decrease in concentrations of AT1 and AT2 receptors and also a reduction in ANG II receptor binding (predominantly AT2 receptor) in the testes. By adulthood, the testes contain almost exclusively AT1 receptors [77].

Acknowledgments

Funding for studies was provided by the São Paulo Research Foundation (FAPESP; grant #2011/50593-2 and #2013/11480-3).

Author details

Anthony C.S. Castilho[1]*, Patrícia K. Fontes[2], Fernanda F. Franchi[2], Priscila H. Santos[2] and Eduardo M. Razza[2]

*Address all correspondence to: castilho.anthony@gmail.com

1 University of Western Sao Paulo, Presidente Prudente, Sao Paulo, Brazil

2 University of Sao Paulo State, Botucatu, Sao Paulo, Brazil

References

[1] Fair, T., Follicular oocyte growth and acquisition of developmental competence. Anim Reprod Sci, 2003. **78**(3-4): pp. 203-16.

[2] Adams, G.P., et al., Progress in understanding ovarian follicular dynamics in cattle. Theriogenology, 2008. **69**(1): p. 72-80.

[3] Pellicer, A., et al., Blockage of ovulation by an angiotensin antagonist. Science, 1988. **240**(4859): p. 1660-1.

[4] Yoshimura, Y., et al., Locally produced angiotensin II induces ovulation by stimulating prostaglandin production in in vitro perfused rabbit ovaries. Endocrinology, 1993. **133**(4): p. 1609-16.

[5] Kuji, N., et al., Involvement of angiotensin II in the process of gonadotropin-induced ovulation in rabbits. Biol Reprod, 1996. **55**(5): p. 984-91.

[6] Ferreira, R., et al., The role of angiotensin II in the early stages of bovine ovulation. Reproduction, 2007. **134**(5): p. 713-9.

[7] Portela, V.M., et al., Regulation of angiotensin type 2 receptor in bovine granulosa cells. Endocrinology, 2008. **149**(10): p. 5004-11.

[8] Paul, M., Poyan Mehr, A., and Kreutz, R. Physiology of local renin-angiotensin systems. Physiol Rev, 2006. **86**(3): p. 747-803.

[9] Giometti, I.C., et al., Angiotensin II reverses the inhibitory action produced by theca cells on bovine oocyte nuclear maturation. Theriogenology, 2005. **63**(4): p. 1014-25.

[10] Barreta, M.H., et al., Evidence that the effect of angiotensin II on bovine oocyte nuclear maturation is mediated by prostaglandins E2 and F2alpha. Reproduction, 2008. **136**(6): p. 733-40.

[11] Siqueira, L.C., et al., Angiotensin II, progesterone, and prostaglandins are sequential steps in the pathway to bovine oocyte nuclear maturation. Theriogenology, 2012. **77**(9): p. 1779-87.

[12] Siqueira, L.C., et al., Preovulatory changes in the angiotensin II system in bovine follicles. Reprod Fertil Dev, 2013. **25**(3): p. 539-46.

[13] Barros, C.M. and Nogueira, M.F. Embryo transfer in Bos indicus cattle. Theriogenology, 2001. **56**(9): p. 1483-96.

[14] Barros, C.M., et al., Use of knowledge regarding LH receptors to improve superstimulatory treatments in cattle. Reprod Fertil Dev, 2010. **22**(1): p. 132-7.

[15] Baruselli, P.S., et al., Superovulation and embryo transfer in Bos indicus cattle. Theriogenology, 2006. **65**(1): p. 77-88.

[16] Bo, G.A., et al., The timing of ovulation and insemination schedules in superstimulated cattle. Theriogenology, 2006. **65**(1): p. 89-101.

[17] Barros, C.M., et al., Effect of superstimulatory treatments on the expression of genes related to ovulatory capacity, oocyte competence and embryo development in cattle. Reprod Fertil Dev, 2012. **25**(1): p. 17-25.

[18] Kon, Y., et al., An immunohistochemical study on the embryonic development of renin-containing cells in the mouse and pig. Anat Histol Embryol, 1989. **18**(1): p. 14-26.

[19] Chen, Y., Lasaitiene, D., and Friberg, P. The renin-angiotensin system in kidney development. Acta Physiol Scand, 2004. **181**(4): p. 529-35.

[20] Pountain, S.J., Pipkin, F.B., and Hunter, M.G. The ontogeny of components of the renin-angiotensin system in the porcine fetal ovary. Anim Reprod Sci, 2010. **117**(1-2): p. 119-26.

[21] Shuttleworth, G., et al., Immunocytochemical localization of angiotensin II receptor subtypes 1 and 2 in the porcine fetal, prepubertal and postpubertal ovary. J Anat, 2002. **201**(3): p. 267-74.

[22] Portela, V.M., et al., Localization of angiotensin receptor type 2 in fetal bovine ovaries. Anim Reprod Sci, 2016. **168**: p. 34-9.

[23] Bruno, J.B., et al., Expression of angiotensin II receptors in the caprine ovary and improvement of follicular viability in vitro. Zygote, 2016. **24**(4): p. 568-77.

[24] Shuttleworth, G., Broughton Pipkin, F., and Hunter, M.G. In vitro development of pig preantral follicles cultured in a serum-free medium and the effect of angiotensin II. Reproduction, 2002. **123**(6): p. 807-18.

[25] Rodrigues, D.B., et al., In situ detection of inflammatory cytokines and apoptosis in pemphigus foliaceus patients. Arch Pathol Lab Med, 2009. **133**(1): p. 97-100.

[26] Machado, G.M., et al., Effect of Percoll volume, duration and force of centrifugation, on in vitro production and sex ratio of bovine embryos. Theriogenology, 2009. **71**(8): p. 1289-97.

[27] Iwanczyk, J.S., et al., Mercuric iodide polycrystalline films. Penetrating Radiation Systems and Applications III, Proc.SPIE, 2001. **4508**: p. 28-40.

[28] Regitz-Zagrosek, V., et al., Molecular biology of angiotensin receptors and their role in human cardiovascular disease. J Mol Med (Berl), 1996. **74**(5): p. 233-51.

[29] Wijayagunawardane, M.P., et al., Angiotensin II secretion by the bovine oviduct is stimulated by luteinizing hormone and ovarian steroids. J Reprod Dev, 2009. **55**(5): p. 570-5.

[30] Johnson, M.C., et al., Presence of angiotensin II and expression of angiotensin II type-2 receptor in human fallopian tube. Fertil Steril, 1998. **70**(4): p. 740-6.

[31] Saridogan, E., et al., Angiotensin II receptors and angiotensin II stimulation of ciliary activity in human fallopian tube. J Clin Endocrinol Metab, 1996. **81**(7): p. 2719-25.

[32] Saridogan, E., et al., Type 1 angiotensin II receptors in human endometrium. Mol Hum Reprod, 1996. **2**(9): p. 659-64.

[33] Fontes, P.K., et al., Prostaglandin receptors (EP2 and EP4) and angiotensin receptor (AGTR2) mRNA expression increases in the oviducts of Nelore cows submitted to ovarian superstimulation. Anim Reprod Sci, 2014. **151**(3-4): p. 112-8.

[34] Marey, M.A., et al., Angiotensin II increases sperm phagocytosis by neutrophils in vitro: A possible physiological role in the bovine oviduct. Mol Reprod Dev, 2016. **83**(7): p. 630-9.

[35] Watson, A.J. and Barcroft, L.C. Regulation of blastocyst formation. Front Biosci, 2001. **6**: p. D708-30.

[36] Schunkert, H., et al., Feedback regulation of angiotensin converting enzyme activity and mRNA levels by angiotensin II. Circ Res, 1993. **72**(2): p. 312-8.

[37] Pandey, K.N., Misono, K.S., and Inagami, T. Evidence for intracellular formation of angiotensins: coexistence of renin and angiotensin-converting enzyme in Leydig cells of rat testis. Biochem Biophys Res Commun, 1984. **122**(3): p. 1337-43.

[38] Leung, P.S., Wong, T.P., and Sernia, C. Angiotensinogen expression by rat epididymis: evidence for an intrinsic, angiotensin-generating system. Mol Cell Endocrinol, 1999. **155**(1-2): p. 115-22.

[39] Wong, P.Y., et al., Effect of angiotensins on electrogenic anion transport in monolayer cultures of rat epididymis. J Endocrinol, 1990. **125**(3): p. 449-56.

[40] Wong, P.Y. and Uchendu, C.N. The role of angiotensin-converting enzyme in the rat epididymis. J Endocrinol, 1990. **125**(3): p. 457-65.

[41] Hohlbrugger, G., Schweisfurth, H., and Dahlheim, H. Angiotensin I converting enzyme in rat testis, epididymis and vas deferens under different conditions. J Reprod Fertil, 1982. **65**(1): p. 97-103.

[42] Cushman, D.W. and Cheung, H.S. Concentrations of angiotensin-converting enzyme in tissues of the rat. Biochim Biophys Acta, 1971. **250**(1): p. 261-5.

[43] van Sande, M., et al., Tripeptidyl carboxypeptidase activity of angiotensin-converting enzyme in human tissues of the urogenital tract. Urol Int, 1985. **40**(2): p. 100-2.

[44] Berg, T., et al., Immunohistochemical localization of two angiotensin I-converting isoenzymes in the reproductive tract of the male rabbit. J Histochem Cytochem, 1986. **34**(6): p. 753-60.

[45] Yokoyama, M., et al., Angiotensin-converting enzyme in human prostate. Clin Chim Acta, 1980. **100**(3): p. 253-8.

[46] Naruse, K., et al., Immunohistological evidence for renin in human endocrine tissues. J Clin Endocrinol Metab, 1985. **61**(1): p. 172-7.

[47] Dinh, D.T., et al., Angiotensin AT(4) receptors in the normal human prostate and benign prostatic hyperplasia. Mol Cell Endocrinol, 2001. **184**(1-2): p. 187-92.

[48] Vanha-Perttula, T., et al., Localization of the angiotensin-converting enzyme activity in testis and epididymis. Biol Reprod, 1985. **33**(4): p. 870-7.

[49] Jaiswal, A.K., et al., Age related development of angiotensin converting enzyme in testes and epididymis of rat. Andrologia, 1983. **15**(4): p. 347-9.

[50] Hohlbrugger, G., Pschorr, J., and Dahlheim, H. Angiotensin I converting enzyme in the ejaculate of fertile and infertile men. Fertil Steril, 1984. **41**(2): p. 324-5.

[51] Jaiswal, A., et al., Angiotensin converting enzyme in the testis and epididymis of mammals. Andrologia, 1984. **16**(5): p. 410-6.

[52] Foresta, C., et al., Angiotensin-converting enzyme content of human spermatozoa and its release during capacitation. Fertil Steril, 1987. **47**(6): p. 1000-3.

[53] Foresta, C., et al., Evidence for the involvement of sperm angiotensin converting enzyme in fertilization. Int J Androl, 1991. **14**(5): p. 333-9.

[54] Köhn, F.M., Miska, W., and Schill, W.B. Release of angiotensin-converting enzyme (ACE) from human spermatozoa during capacitation and acrosome reaction. J Androl, 1995. **16**(3): p. 259-65.

[55] Singh, U.S., Kumar, M.V., and Panda, J.N. Angiotensin converting enzyme in semen and its possible role in capacitation. Andrologia, 1985. **17**(5): p. 472-5.

[56] Krege, J.H., et al., Male-female differences in fertility and blood pressure in ACE-deficient mice. Nature, 1995. **375**(6527): p. 146-8.

[57] Hagaman, J.R., et al., Angiotensin-converting enzyme and male fertility. Proc Natl Acad Sci U S A, 1998. **95**(5): p. 2552-7.

[58] Esther, C.R., et al., Mice lacking angiotensin-converting enzyme have low blood pressure, renal pathology, and reduced male fertility. Lab Invest, 1996. **74**(5): p. 953-65.

[59] Vinson, G.P., et al., Type 1 angiotensin II receptors in rat and human sperm. J Endocrinol, 1995. **144**(2): p. 369-78.

[60] Dzau, V.J., et al., A comparative study of the distributions of renin and angiotensinogen messenger ribonucleic acids in rat and mouse tissues. Endocrinology, 1987. **120**(6): p. 2334-8.

[61] Campbell, D.J. and Habener, J.F. Angiotensinogen gene is expressed and differentially regulated in multiple tissues of the rat. J Clin Invest, 1986. **78**(1): p. 31-9.

[62] Ekker, M., Tronik, D., and Rougeon, F. Extra-renal transcription of the renin 6genes in multiple tissues of mice and rats. Proc Natl Acad Sci U S A, 1989. **86**(13): p. 5155-8.

[63] Poisner, A.M., et al., Renin and inactive renin in human amnion at term pregnancy. Proc Soc Exp Biol Med, 1982. **169**(1): p. 4-6.

[64] Paul, M., et al., Quantification of renin mRNA in various mouse tissues by a novel solution hybridization assay. J Hypertens, 1988. **6**(3): p. 247-52.

[65] Miller, C.C., et al., Differential extra-renal expression of the mouse renin genes. Nucleic Acids Res, 1989. **17**(8): p. 3117-28.

[66] Deschepper, C.F., et al., Analysis by immunocytochemistry and in situ hybridization of renin and its mRNA in kidney, testis, adrenal, and pituitary of the rat. Proc Natl Acad Sci U S A, 1986. **83**(19): p. 7552-6.

[67] Kitami, Y., et al., Differential gene expression and regulation of type-1 angiotensin II receptor subtypes in the rat. Biochem Biophys Res Commun, 1992. **188**(1): p. 446-52.

[68] Aguilera, G., Millan, M.A., and Harwood, J.P. Angiotensin II receptors in the gonads. Am J Hypertens, 1989. **2**(5 Pt 1): p. 395-402.

[69] Zhao, W., et al., Localization and distribution of angiotensin II in the rat epididymis. J Endocrinol, 1996. **149**(2): p. 217-22.

[70] Leung, P.S., et al., Angiotensin II receptors: localization of type I and type II in rat epididymis of different developmental stages. J Membr Biol, 1997. **157**(1): p. 97-103.

[71] Naruse, M., et al., Gonadotropin-dependent renin in the rat testes. Proc Soc Exp Biol Med, 1984. **177**(2): p. 337-42.

[72] Pandey, K.N., Ascoli, M., and Inagami, T. Induction of renin activity by gonadotropic hormones in cultured Leydig tumor cells. Endocrinology, 1985. **117**(5): p. 2120-6.

[73] Parmentier, M., et al., Pituitary-dependent renin-like immunoreactivity in the rat testis. Endocrinology, 1983. **112**(4): p. 1318-23.

[74] Pandey, K.N. and Inagami, T. Regulation of renin angiotensins by gonadotropic hormones in cultured murine Leydig tumor cells. Release of angiotensin but not renin. J Biol Chem, 1986. **261**(9): p. 3934-8.

[75] Okuyama, A., et al., Demonstration of gonadotropin-induced plasma renin activity in human internal spermatic vein. Acta Endocrinol (Copenh), 1988. **117**(2): p. 268-72.

[76] Hirai, K., et al., Pituitary-dependent expression of the testicular angiotensin II receptor and its subtypes in rats. Int J Androl, 1998. **21**(4): p. 177-85.

[77] Kanehara, H., et al., Involvement of angiotensin II receptor subtypes during testicular development in rats. Int J Androl, 1998. **21**(4): p. 186-95.

[78] Leung, P.S., et al., Angiotensin II receptors, AT1 and AT2 in the rat epididymis. Immunocytochemical and electrophysiological studies. Biochim Biophys Acta, 1997. **1357**(1): p. 65-72.

Chapter 6

Role of the Renin-Angiotensin System in Healthy and Pathological Pregnancies

Émilie Pepin, Shahin Shabanipour Dehboneh,
Nozha Raguema, Maedeh Talebi Esfandarani and
Julie L. Lavoie

Additional information is available at the end of the chapter

http://dx.doi.org/10.5772/66748

Abstract

Introduction: Pregnancy is a physiological process that necessitates many cardiovascular and hemodynamic adaptations to ensure the survival of the foetus and well-being of the mother. The renin-angiotensin system (RAS) has been suggested as key player in many of these changes as it is critical for blood pressure control as well as fluid and salt homeostasis in the non-pregnant state.

Body: Normal pregnancy is characterized by an increase in the circulating levels of prorenin, renin, angiotensinogen and angiotensin-II. However, this is coupled to a diminished endothelial sensitivity to angiotensin-II, which may explain the lack of increase in blood pressure in pregnancy. Conversely, an increase in circulating levels of aldosterone and anti-diuretic hormone during pregnancy can be observed and could contribute to the enhanced renal sodium and water reabsorption, respectively. Moreover, dysregulation of the RAS has been implicated in the development of gestational hypertensive disorders such as preeclampsia.

Conclusion: The difference in the RAS effects observed during normal pregnancy may be attributable to local modifications of the RAS as well as to non-classic RAS such as the angiotensin-(1-7) axis. These adaptations may be dysregulated during preeclampsia and may contribute to the development of the disease.

Keywords: gestation, reproductive system, cardiovascular adaptations to gestation, preeclampsia, exercise training

1. Menstrual cycle, implantation and pregnancy

The female reproductive system includes the ovaries, fallopian tubes, uterus, cervix and vagina. It is involved in the production and transportation of gametes, the production of sex hormones and development of embryo. The oviducts extend from the uterus to the ovaries. The egg bursts from the ovary and moves through the oviduct towards the uterus. In humans, an egg lives approximately 6–24 hours, unless fertilization occurs, which results in zygote formation. A developing embryo normally reaches the uterus after several days, and then implantation occurs. During implantation, the embryo embeds in the uterine lining, which has been prepared to receive it. The lining of the uterus, called the endometrium, participates in the formation of the placenta, which has a main role in supplying nutrients needed for embryonic and foetal development [1]. At menarche (first menstrual period), females undergo monthly reproductive cycles regulated by the hypothalamus, pituitary gland and ovaries. This so-called menstrual cycle prepares the reproductive system for pregnancy. As shown in **Figure 1**, each menstrual cycle is composed of an ovarian and an uterine cycle based on processes taking place in the ovary and uterus, respectively [1, 2].

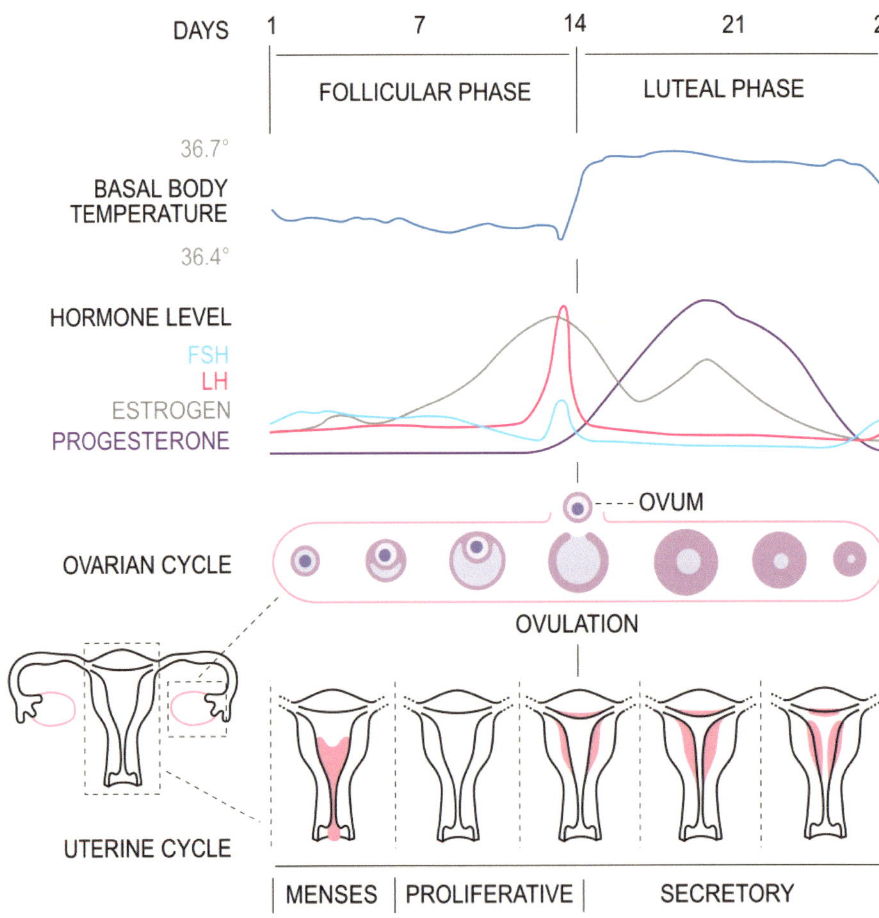

Figure 1. Human ovarian and menstrual cycles. Diagram of the menstrual cycle (based on several different sources) by Isometrik through Wikimedia Commons licensed under CC BY-SA 3.0.

The ovarian cycle begins with the menstrual phase from day 1 and lasts, on average, for 5 days. The menstrual phase is followed by the follicular phase, which ends at ovulation at approximately day 14. The third phase is called the luteal phase which lasts from day 14 to 28 and ends with the beginning of menstruations and the start of a new cycle (**Figure 1**) [3]. During the ovarian cycle, there are two hormones released from the anterior pituitary by the stimulatory action of the gonadotropin-releasing hormone (GnRH): the follicle-stimulating hormone (FSH), which stimulates the development of ovarian follicles and production of estrogen by the follicular cells, and the luteinizing hormone (LH), which serves as the trigger for ovulation and stimulates the follicular cells and corpus luteum to produce progesterone [2]. The cyclic changes in the ovaries with hormonal stimulation of FSH and LH allow follicle maturation and oogenesis, and lead to the release of the secondary oocyte into the oviduct during a process called ovulation (**Figure 1**) [1].

Estrogen and progesterone produced by the ovarian follicles and corpus luteum during the ovarian cycle cause cyclic changes in the endometrium of the uterus, also known as the uterine cycle. Both ovarian and uterine cycles last on average 28 days. Menstruation, characterized by the endometrium's breaking down, is the first phase of the uterine cycle and lasts from day 1 to day 5. It also spans part of the follicular phase of the ovarian cycle. Menstruation is followed by the proliferative phase, characterized by estrogen secretion from the primary follicles and lasts for almost 9 days. This phase, which coincides with the growth of the ovarian follicles in the ovarian cycle, leads to increasing thickness of the endometrium. At the very end of the proliferative phase on day 14, the ovulation occurs. After that, the uterine secretory phase begins. This phase lasts for 13 days and coincides with the formation, function and growth of the corpus luteum in the ovarian cycle [1, 2]. During days 15–28, increased production of progesterone by the corpus luteum in the ovary causes the endometrium of the uterus to double or triple in thickness [1]. This phenomenon prepares the endometrium for receiving the developing embryo in the short period of receptivity known as the window of implantation [4]. If fertilization does not occur, the corpus luteum degenerates and the concomitant decrease in progesterone level causes timely destruction of the fully developed endometrium, leading to menstruation. However, if fertilization occurs, the zygote cleavage (increase in cell number without increase in mass) takes place. Following blastocyst formation, the embryo implantation occurs, typically on the sixth day of the luteal phase. This leads to the secretion of the human chorionic gonadotropin (hCG) by the syncytiotrophoblasts of the developing placenta, which acts on the ovaries to maintain the secretion of estrogen and progesterone and prevent the degradation of the corpus luteum. As a result, the luteal phase is prolonged, which prevents the start of the menstrual cycle, and the endometrium continues to grow and undergoes further morphological and molecular changes to provide sufficient support for the growing embryo during the pregnancy [2].

Although it was once thought to be a systemic entity, the presence of local tissue-specific renin-angiotensin systems (RASs) has been recently demonstrated. Indeed, different tissues have been found to express all the functional components of the RAS [5, 6]. The reproductive system and placental RAS play a key role in ovulation, implantation, placentation and development of the uteroplacental and umbilicoplacental circulations [7]. Additionally, this local RAS contributes to the activity of circulating maternal renin-angiotensin-aldosterone system (RAAS), and as such, influences maternal cardiovascular and renal function [8]. Moreover, the reproductive system RAS has been shown to be implicated in different aspects of reproduction, from fertility to embryo implantation and later through pregnancy [9, 10]. Important modulations of the RAS are observed from the very beginning of pregnancy and aberrant changes in RAS component expression can cause gestational problems such as preeclampsia [11–13]. The implication of the RAS in both normal and pathological pregnancy will be discussed in this book chapter.

2. RAS in the reproductive system

2.1. RAS and ovary and follicular development

Prorenin is produced by the ovarian follicular cells at different stages in oocyte maturation. As the ovarian follicle undergoes maturation, the prorenin concentration increases and remains elevated until the end of the luteal phase, near the start of menstruation, where it falls in parallel with progesterone levels [14]. Prorenin secretion in the ovary is regulated by gonadotropins, and thus, the rise in plasma-luteinizing hormone (LH) levels shortly precedes the elevation of plasma prorenin, secreted into circulation mainly by the ovary [15, 16]. Of note, concentrations of prorenin, the inactive precursor of renin, are typically higher in the reproductive system than those of renin and it was originally postulated that it was locally activated by an unknown process. As such, studies demonstrating the expression of cathepsin B, a potential activator of prorenin, in the maturating oocyte suggest that the increase in prorenin expression in the ovary can contribute to the rise in renin levels in the follicular fluid. Moreover, prorenin can activate the prorenin/renin receptor ((P)RR) and thus become active as well as stimulate Ang-II-independent pathways, which are associated to this receptor [17]. For instance, binding of prorenin to the (P)RR can promote cell growth and oocyte maturation [18]. More specifically, the (P)RR has recently been suggested to induce resumption of meiosis in oocytes [19].

Similarly to prorenin, local ovarian renin activity has been shown to be increased following the LH surge in rats, rabbits and human [20–22]. Moreover, increased renin mRNA expression has been measured in rat and primate following follicle-stimulating hormone (FSH), estradiol or human chorionic gonadotropin (hCG) stimulation [23], suggesting that prorenin could be activated locally in the ovary and could contribute to the stimulation of the local RAS [15].

The ovarian expression of angiotensinogen (Agt) has been studied in rats and humans and has been shown to vary between species. In rat, Agt expression is found in ovaries, more specifically during the mid- and late-maturation of follicles (not during maturation of early-primary or primary follicles) [24]. The timing of Agt expression in maturing follicles matches the expression of gonadotropins. As such, given that Agt expression has been shown to be stimulated by estradiol in rat liver, it has been suggested that Agt expression in maturating follicles could be driven by gonadotropin-stimulated-estradiol local production. In humans, Agt has been measured in the follicular fluid and its levels are comparable or lower to circulating Agt [7]. However, there is no evidence of local ovarian Agt mRNA expression, suggesting that local ovarian Agt protein levels are derived from the circulation [15].

In contrast to the other RAS components mentioned above, the angiotensin-converting enzyme (ACE) expression in the ovary does not follow gonadotropin-stimulated cyclic expression pattern during the oestrous cycle since high ACE levels are found in the early stages of follicle maturation and in atretic follicles with very low levels in preovulatory follicles. This suggests that ACE has a role in early maturation of the follicles as well as their atresia [15].

Angiotensin II (Ang II) has been found to be produced and secreted by rabbit and rat ovaries in response to hCG elevation [21]. Since renin activity is stimulated by gonadotropins during preovulation, this increased renin activity probably drives the production of local Ang II. Similar observations have been made in women with natural or gonadotropin-stimulated cycles [25].

Ang II mediates its actions in the ovary through both AT1R and AT2R. However, each receptor has different functions within the reproductive system. Indeed, AT1R has been reported to be mainly involved in the maintenance of ovarian vasculature which supplies nutrients to the developing follicles [26], whereas AT2R would be implicated in both the follicular development as well as in the regression of the luteal vasculature towards the end of the ovarian cycle. However, the timing of AT2R expression during oocyte maturation is uncertain and varies between species. Indeed, a study using autoradiography and gene expression measurements reported the expression of AT2R in granulosa cells of rat atretic follicles while it is almost absent in healthy follicles [27]. In contrast, studies in bovine ovaries demonstrate that AT2R expression is increased during follicular growth and maturation [15]. As such, it is very difficult to conclude on a clear role of the ATRs in the ovary. In addition, the signalling pathways involved in AT2R modulation of follicular growth and maturation have not yet been studied. However, neuronal studies of AT2R signalling demonstrate that the MAPK pathway and activation of nitric oxide promotes cell differentiation and could be putative pathways involved in follicular maturation in the ovary [28]. On the other hand, studies in rabbits have shown that ovarian RAS activation leads to estradiol production through AT2R stimulation. Based on the fact that gonadotropins stimulate the expression of many components of the RAS cascade, an intra-ovarian paracrine or autocrine loop would exist between Ang II and estradiol [15]. However, the mechanisms responsible for the control of the autocrine loop are not well understood and more data are needed to confirm its activity in other species such as rodents and humans.

2.2. RAS during ovulation

The process of ovulation depends on different signalling cascades involving cAMP release, steroids, prostaglandins and other chemical mediators [29, 30]. Several *in vitro* and *in vivo* studies have demonstrated that the RAS, especially through AT2R stimulation, has a role to play in ovulation. In particular, studies using *in vitro* perfused ovaries have demonstrated a dose-dependent effect of Ang II on estradiol and prostaglandin secretion, correlating with the initiation of ovulation [31]. Therefore, the use of ACE inhibitors (which would lead to a decrease in Ang II production) for the treatment of hypertension in women who want to become pregnant may not be recommended. Of note, insulin-like growth factor 1 (IGF-1), through the activation of the plasminogen activator (PA), has been proposed to increase Ang

II production, leading to the production of prostaglandins necessary for the rupture of the follicular wall and ovulation [32]. Hence, this could be a mechanism by which the IGF-1 produces its important effects on ovarian physiology and follicle development [33].

Studies on human follicular fluid samples collected from *in vitro* fertilization samples suggest that RAS activity correlates with follicular development. In particular, prorenin activity in follicular fluid is associated with the development, maturity and viability of the oocytes [18]. Indeed, low levels of follicular prorenin are associated with immature follicles while high prorenin levels are correlated with atretic follicles, the latter being characterized by high levels of testosterone and low levels of estradiol. Intermediate levels of prorenin would therefore be necessary for normal ovulation to proceed. Interestingly, in our recently characterized model of preeclampsia superimposed on chronic hypertension, mice that overexpress both human renin and angiotensinogen (R^+A^+), we observed that these mice have reduced litter size [34]. Given that this is not associated with increased foetal or neonatal mortality, this suggests that hypertension or the overexpression of the RAS in the reproductive system may decrease fertility by modulating ovulation or embryo implantation.

2.3. Corpus luteum

Following ovulation, the remaining follicular cells undergo rapid remodelling and capillary invasion. Studies have shown that microvascular endothelial (MVE) cells in the corpus luteum express ACE and can convert Ang I to Ang II [26]. Both AT1R and AT2R have been detected in MVE cells with different levels of expression throughout the ovarian cycle: AT1R expression levels seem unchanged, whereas AT2R expression is lowest during the mid-luteal phase and highest during the late luteal phase [26]. The regulation of angiogenic processes is a crucial step to ensure the constant flow of growth, maturation and demise of the corpus luteum. This angiogenic step requires the secretion of angiogenic factors such as the basic fibroblast growth factor (bFGF). Ang II would be one of the drivers of this rapid capillary invasion through AT1R-dependent stimulation of bFGF expression. Hence, in luteal cells, the surge in LH that precedes ovulation would lead to increased Ang II production and enhanced AT1R stimulation which would drive the expression of bFGF. This would then promote angiogenesis and appropriate maintenance of the corpus luteum [35]. In contrast, the regression of the luteal vasculature would be attributed to the Ang II-AT2R axis of the RAS [36].

2.4. Atresia

At the beginning of each ovarian cycle, several primordial (immature) follicles undergo maturation. Due to the inefficient nature of folliculogenesis, most of those primordial follicles will not reach the final stage of maturation, and in humans, only one follicle will undergo ovulation. The remaining follicles degenerate through a process known as atresia. Atretic follicles are characterized by abnormally high prorenin levels associated with a low estradiol/progesterone ratio [37]. These follicles have a thin layer of degenerated granulosa cells and the remaining active theca cells secrete prorenin [38]. In atretic granulosa cells, the Ang II receptor isoform that is most expressed is AT2R, which has been shown to drive apoptosis

[27]. In follicles, FSH acts as a mild repressor of AT2R expression, so apoptosis cannot be triggered during the maturation phase of follicular development. However, in the luteal phase, FSH levels are reduced which relieves the inhibition on AT2R expression. As such, given the high Ang II level, AT2 stimulation increases granulosa cells apoptosis, promoting the atresia of immature follicles.

2.5. RAS and the placenta

The placenta is an organ that provides nutrients and oxygen to the developing foetus and removes toxic waste products from the foetal circulation [39]. The formation of the placenta starts with the implantation of the embryo (at this developmental stage, the blastocyst) in the endometrium (known as the decidua during pregnancy). The blastocyst is composed of an inner cell mass (which will give rise to the foetus and the amniotic cavity) and the trophoblastic cells (a 'sticky' layer of cells forming the outer layer of the blastocyst). Implantation is initiated when the trophoblastic cells adhere to the surface of the decidua. This stimulates the proliferation of the trophoblastic cells, which divide into two cell types: the syncytial trophoblasts and cellular trophoblasts (also known as the chorion). The syncytial trophoblastic cells are multinucleated cells which are highly invasive. They secrete proteolytic enzymes that are responsible for the destruction of the decidua which creates cavities (known as endometrial lacunae). Simultaneously, the proliferating trophoblastic cells form protrusions, known as the chorionic villi, which become highly branched as well as vascularised by ramifications of the umbilical vein and artery. The endometrial lacunae will then be invaded by the branching chorionic villi, allowing the blastocyst to penetrate into the decidua and establishing the interface between the maternal and foetal blood where nutrients, blood gas and wastes will be exchanged. By the end of the first trimester, the uteroplacental circulation is fully established [40]. Maintaining optimal placental blood osmotic pressure and flow is crucial for the production of a viable offspring. Placental RAS is a key player in the regulation of maternal-foetal blood flow during pregnancy [41]. Since many components of the RAS have been shown to be expressed in whole human placental extracts, human placental cell lines (human umbilical venous endothelial cells (HUVEC)), and in isolated primary placental cell fractions (primary trophoblastic cells fraction, primary macrophage-rich fraction and primary villous endothelial cells) [42–44], the RAS is believed to have a considerable influence in this organ [11, 45–48]. However, functional data of the placental RAS are very rare. RAS proteins have different level of expression in various areas of the placenta. Agt, renin, Ang I, Ang II, ACE, AT1R, and AT2R have been localized to the human and rat maternal decidua [49, 50], whereas Ang II and ACE have also been found in pericytes of endometrial spiral arteries. RAS components such as Agt and renin have also been detected in foetal capillaries [51] and AT1R has been found in cytotrophoblastic and syncytiotrophoblastic cells as well as in foetal capillaries. Many studies have suggested the implication of the placental RAS in promoting trophoblastic cell migration, proliferation of the foetal vascular endothelium and vasodilation of the maternal vasculature [52, 53]. Hence, changes in placental RAS potentially contribute to alterations in uteroplacental perfusion, which are associated with gestational complications such as preeclampsia [54].

2.6. RAS and the uterus/endometrium

Most components of the RAS can be found in both myometrium and endometrium of the uterus. However, the role of the RAS in the non-pregnant uterus is still unknown [55]. Elevated expression and secretion of prorenin in stromal cells have been associated with decidualisation of the endometrium in early to mid-proliferative phase [56]. Activation of the (P)RR by prorenin has been shown to promote vascular endothelial growth factor (VEGF) expression and could thus increase vascularity of the decidua to ensure an adequate blood flow to the placenta [56]. In addition, Ang II as well as AT1R and AT2R show a cyclical pattern of expression depending on the phase of the uterine cycle. First, AT2R is expressed at higher levels compared to AT1R, although both receptors show a similar expression pattern. Their expression gradually increases during the proliferative phase, reaching a maximum in late proliferative and early secretory phases, followed by a gradual decrease in expression through the rest of the secretory phase [57]. In comparison, plasma Ang II levels gradually increase through the menstrual cycle, reaching a peak in the late secretory phase [58]. Moreover, in the early to mid-proliferative phase, endometrial Ang II levels and ATRs expression are mostly localized to the glandular and stromal cells of the endometrium, which could highlight a role for the RAS in modulating decidualisation and neovascularisation of the endometrium. Alternatively, in late secretory phase, they are localized mostly around blood vessels, where Ang II could contribute to the vasoconstriction of spiral arterioles which is necessary for the induction of menstruation [57]. In addition, angiotensin-(1-7) (Ang-(1-7), a heptapeptide generated from Ang II cleavage by the enzyme ACE 2) and its receptor MAS (MAS-R) have been shown to be expressed in the endometrium. While MAS-R expression is localized to the epithelial and stromal cells and does not change throughout the menstrual cycle, Ang-(1-7) concentrations are highest in the glandular epithelium and in the stroma of the endometrium in mid- to late-secretory phase [59]. Although the function of the Ang-(1-7)—Mas-R axis is not well understood in the endometrium, by its vasodilatory, antiangiogenic and antimitotic properties, Ang-(1-7) could counterbalance Ang II actions and, possibly regulate endometrial regenerating processes according to homeostatic needs.

3. Pregnancy and RAS

Pregnancy is characterized by an elevation in the levels of maternal circulating estrogen. Consequently, maternal circulating prorenin and renin are also increased during pregnancy. Prorenin reaches a peak within 20 days after conception and remains high until parturition while plasma-renin activity rises during the first few weeks of pregnancy [60]. ACE is the only RAS component that decreases during pregnancy [61] while plasma Agt and Ang II levels are particularly elevated during the last trimester of normal gestation [62]. The elevated Ang II levels could be attributed in part to the stimulatory effect of estrogen on Agt expression but also to the elevated renin levels [63]. In addition, increased urinary and plasma aldosterone levels are observed during pregnancy which produces the increased plasma volume required for the growing placenta and foetus [64].

The increase in RAS in pregnant women should normally be associated with an increase in blood pressure. However, elevated blood pressure in not typically observed during normal

http://dx.doi.org/10.5772/66748

pregnancy. On the contrary, due to the vasodilating effect of progesterone, a decrease in blood pressure is typically seen in the first and second trimesters, returning to baseline by delivery [65]. Indeed, although Ang II levels are increased during pregnancy, normotensive pregnant women are actually refractory to its vasopressor effects. Studies have reported a twofold increase in plasma Ang II levels concomitantly with a twofold decrease in the sensitivity to Ang II vasoconstrictive effects [66, 67]. Moreover, studies in pregnant women and animals have demonstrated that the elevation of plasma Ang-(1-7) would contribute to the reduction in blood pressure during pregnancy by counterbalancing the vasoconstrictor actions of elevated Ang II [68–70]. It was also demonstrated in rats, that arteries were more responsive to the vasodilatory effects of Ang-(1-7) during pregnancy [71]. The capacity of Ang-(1-7) to stimulate the release of the vasodilatory molecules prostaglandins would potentiate its own vasodilatory actions and would oppose Ang II effects [72]. A balance of the two biologically active peptides of the RAS, Ang II, a vasoconstrictor and angiogenic molecule, and Ang-(1-7), a vasodilator and anti-angiogenic molecule, may therefore be essential for the maintenance of normal pregnancy [11, 73].

Trophoblasts are rich in AT1Rs and are thus responsive to the changes in Ang II concentrations that occur during pregnancy [74]. Recent studies demonstrate that multiple genes are regulated by AT1R signalling and include those encoding secreted proteins associated with trophoblast invasion (e.g., plasminogen activator inhibitor-1, PAI-I) and angiogenesis (soluble fms-like tyrosine receptor-1, sFlt-1) which could promote endometrium decidualisation. Ang II signalling also activates NF-kappa B and stimulates NADPH-oxidase synthesis by trophoblasts which would promote trophoblastic proliferation and invasiveness [75].

4. RAS and gestational pathophysiological conditions

Since the RAS has a wide array of important functions in the body, any dysfunction in this system may lead to complications [41]. Studies have shown that the RAS is involved in reproductive conditions such as preeclampsia, polycystic ovary (PCOS) [76]. Moreover, it has a role in tumour progression in gynaecological cancers, highlighting the implication of the RAS in on tumour cell proliferation, vascular function and angiogenesis [54]. The following sections will describe the implication of RAS in the development of gestational pathologies, with the main emphasis being put on preeclampsia.

4.1. Polycystic ovary syndrome

Polycystic ovary syndrome (PCOS) is the leading cause of anovulatory infertility in women of reproductive age. Evidence of enhanced systemic RAS activity (increased plasma renin, Ang II and aldosterone) has been demonstrated to be responsible for the development of this disease [76, 77]. In PCOS patients, the maturation and oocyte quality are both affected by the increased intra-follicular renin level [54]. Moreover, there is evidence indicating that a polymorphism in ACE gene is associated to insulin resistance (IR) in women with PCOS [76, 78, 77]. Thus, treatment with ACE inhibitors aiming at increasing insulin sensitivity could result in an increased fertility in PCOS patients, but since RAS inhibitors are known to be teratogenic, further studies and much care would be needed to validate this therapeutic approach.

4.2. Ovarian cancer

Ovarian cancer is the most lethal gynaecological malignancy in women worldwide [79]. Ovarian cancer cells express Ang II and AT1R [80]. Elevated AT1R levels have been measured in borderline lesions and in invasive epithelial ovarian cancers [81]. Moreover, prognosis is worse for patients with tumours expressing high AT1R levels compared to patients with AT1R-negative tumours. The Ang II—AT1R pathway stimulates cell proliferation while the simultaneous increase in VEGF expression and Ang II levels promotes angiogenesis [54]. Therefore, targeting the Ang II-AT1R pathway could be part of a future treatment strategy for invasive epithelial ovarian cancer.

4.3. Endometrial cancer

Endometrial cancer (EC) is the most common gynaecological malignancy. Moreover, since obesity is a major risk factor, its incidence could increase in the future in parallel with the growing metabolic syndrome pandemic [82]. The endometrial RAS, like other tissue RASs, has been implicated in angiogenesis, neovascularisation and cell proliferation, which are processes involved in tumour growth and metastasis. Increased expression of Ang II, AT1R, AT2R, VEGF and estrogen receptor alpha (NR3A1) has been identified in EC tissues [83]. Moreover, a strong positive correlation has been detected between the levels of Ang II and AT1R/AT2R expression in endometrial tumours with advancing stage of the tumour [54, 83]. Overactivation of the RAS can often be attributed to single nucleotide polymorphisms (SNPs) in a RAS gene [84]. In a study by Freitas-Silva et al., an ACE polymorphism was described to be associated with early onset of EC. In summary, high activity of the local RAS in endometrial cancer is associated with higher incidence, earlier onset and increased rates of angiogenesis [54].

4.4. Preeclampsia

4.4.1. Definition of the pathology

Preeclampsia is a gestational complication that affects 2–5% of women in North America [85]. Preeclampsia risk factors include primiparity, multiparity as well as pre-existing conditions such as type 2 diabetes mellitus, obesity, hypertension and thrombophilia [86]. Moreover, women with preeclampsia are more likely to develop cardiovascular diseases later in life [87]. Clinical diagnostic is determined by the presence of new onset of hypertension (systolic pressure ≥140 mmHg or diastolic pressure ≥90 mmHg) and proteinuria (≥300 mg in 24h) after 20 weeks of gestation. Other potential clinical manifestations are placental alterations, cerebral ischemia, liver abnormalities, cardiac hypertrophy and impaired vascular reactivity, although they are not seen in all preeclamptic women [88]. Patients with severe preeclampsia can also develop pulmonary oedema, haemolysis, elevated liver enzymes and low platelets syndrome, severe central nervous system symptoms, renal failure and intrauterine growth restriction [89].

Several factors have been involved in the development of preeclampsia, such as placental abnormalities, oxidative stress, endothelial dysfunction, inflammation and immunity, but none have been clearly proven [86]. Preventive therapies such as antioxidants have not demonstrated any beneficial effects while calcium supplementation only helps patients with calcium depletion [90, 91]. Therefore, physicians usually try to control the progression of the disease using antihypertensive therapies, such as methyldopa (an α-adrenergic agonist), labetalol (an α- and β-blocker) and nifedipine (a calcium channel antagonist), which are considered relatively safe for the foetus. On the contrary, other drugs, such as RAS inhibitors, which are teratogenic and diuretic, are not compatible with regards to the hypovolemic state associated with preeclampsia. As such, they are not recommended for the treatment of this disease [92]. Ultimately, premature delivery of the foetus is the only effective treatment available, which can be problematic if the development of the foetus, has not sufficiently progressed.

4.4.2. Preeclampsia and RAS

Dysregulation of the RAS has been observed in preeclampsia compared to women with healthy pregnancies [6, 93, 94]. In particular, contrarily to normal pregnancy, preeclamptic women suffer from a hypovolemic hypertension (as mentioned above) characterized by a reduction in plasma renin, Ang I, and Ang II levels [70]. However, PE is characterized by a heightened sensitivity to vasoconstrictors when compared to normal pregnancy [6] partly due to an upregulation of the Ang II type 1 receptors [93], which would contribute to the increased blood pressure associated with this condition. Moreover, recent human studies revealed that both plasma Ang-(1-7) and Ang II are increased in normal pregnancy but decreased in preeclampsia [70]. However, the analysis of the Ang-(1-7)/Ang II ratio demonstrates that there is a greater decrease in Ang-(1-7) relatively to Ang II levels in preeclamptic [70], tipping the vasopressive balance towards increased vasoconstriction in pathological pregnancies. In addition, many epidemiological studies have suggested a relation between alleles of the RAS and PE [95]. For instance, women carrying specific polymorphisms of ACE [96] or Ang [97–99] genes have been reported to have an increased PE risk. Interestingly, these alleles are associated with an increase in systemic RAS [100].

In contrast, patients with preeclampsia have also been reported to have an increased Ang II content and AT1R expression in maternal decidua and in the placenta itself. Brosnihan's group also found in placental chorionic villi from human preeclamptic pregnancies an increase in Ang II and AT1R while Ang-(1-7) was not elevated and the Mas-R was significantly decreased [44]. They proposed that this increased Ang II effect in the chorionic villi could produce a decrease in foetal blood flow, and thus contribute to a reduction in foetal oxygen and nutrients as well as to the development of the intra-uterine growth restriction observed in these pregnancies. The same group showed that the placental increase in Ang-(1-7) content observed during normal pregnancy was reduced in a rat model of PE (the reduced uterine perfusion pressure model), although this was not accompanied by a concomitant decrease in ACE2 [101]. Moreover, we have demonstrated that R^+A^+ mice, an animal model of preeclampsia, have increased AT1Rand decreased Mas-R protein in both placenta and aorta, a condition expected to decrease angiotensin-(1-7) effects in favour of angiotensin II effects [102]. The importance of different RAS components in the development of preeclampsia will be further discussed below.

4.4.3. *Prorenin and prorenin receptor ((P)RR) and preeclampsia*

Expression of the (P)RR has been shown to be localized to the syncytiotrophoblasts both in normotensive and preeclamptic pregnant women [103]. Placental prorenin and (P)RR levels as well as the circulating soluble form of (P)RR (s(P)RR) were shown to be significantly higher in preeclamptic compared to normotensive pregnant women [104]. Moreover, placental (P)RR expression positively correlates with systolic blood pressure only in preeclamptic women. The concomitant modulations of prorenin and (P)RR in preeclamptic women reinforce the idea that an increase in RAS local activation could promote the elevation of blood pressure in this pathology. However, the implication of an increase in s(P)RR in the development of preeclampsia is still misunderstood.

4.4.4. *AT1 receptors autoantibodies in preeclampsia*

In recent years, a wealth of evidence has emerged supporting a role for AT1R autoantibodies (AT1-AA) in the development of preeclampsia. Studies have shown that these autoantibodies are elevated in patients with preeclampsia compared to normal pregnancies and have been shown to specifically stimulate Ang II type 1 receptors, suggesting that these autoantibodies may be involved in the development of preeclampsia [93, 105]. Studies in animal models of preeclampsia have shown that the hypoxia used to induce the disease (caused by the reduction in placental perfusion in pregnant rats) strongly stimulated AT1-AA production [106]. Moreover, infusion of AT1-AA from preeclamptic patients in normal pregnant animal was able to trigger hypertension through an increase in endothelin-1 expression, a potent vasoconstrictor [107]. *In vitro* and *in vivo* studies have demonstrated the binding of those autoantibodies to AT1R on different cell types [108]. In particular, AT1-AA binding at the surface of human trophoblastic cells cause an activation of NADPH oxidase, contributing to the rise in oxidative stress putatively involved in the development of preeclampsia [109]. In addition, activation of AT1R in this cell-type stimulates the release of PAI-1, resulting in decreased trophoblastic invasiveness causing a defect in placentation [110]. It was also observed that AT1-AA stimulates the release of sFlt-1 and s-Eng by the placenta which stimulates endothelial dysfunction [111, 112]. Overall, these results indicate that the vasoconstrictor angiotensin receptor signalling is a key pathway involved in the development of PE.

4.4.5. *RAS and angiogenic factors in preeclampsia*

A molecular hallmark of preeclampsia is a decrease in plasmatic angiogenic markers, free VEGF and placental growth factor (PlGF), along with an increase in the circulating levels of anti-angiogenic markers, soluble fms-like tyrosine-1 (sFlt-1, a soluble variant of the VEGF receptor) and soluble endoglin (sEng), compared to normal pregnancies [113–115]. The decrease in VEGF and PlGF would lead to the improper spiral artery remodelling which is associated with preeclampsia [116]. Moreover, hypoxia, through an increased expression of hypoxia-inducible factor 1 α (HIF-1α), stimulates the expression of sFlt-1, and therefore amplifies the hypoxic placental microenvironment [117, 118]. HIF-1α has also been shown to upregulate the expression of both endothelin-1 and endoglin, a membrane-bound precursor of sEng [119, 120]. In addition, increased secretion of sEng has been measured from both chorionic villi from preeclamptic placenta and hypoxic trophoblastic cells [121]. The increase in endothelin-1 would promote the increase in blood pressure associated with preeclampsia, while the increase in sEng levels would prevent trophoblastic differentiation and invasion.

4.4.6. Beneficial effects of exercise training on preeclampsia could be through modulation of the RAS

While exercise training is well known for its health benefits in the general population, it has also been shown to improve pregnancy outcome during normal human gestation [122]. Moreover, there are data demonstrating that it can also reduce the prevalence of human pregnancy disorders such as gestational diabetes. There is also a significant body of evidence supporting the exercise training-induced reduction in risk of developing PE by 35% to 78% [123]. We have recently demonstrated that exercise training (mouse voluntary wheel running) before and during gestation significantly prevents the development of preeclampsia superimposed on chronic hypertension phenotypes in our mouse model of that disease [102]. We noted that the pregnant mice naturally reduce the duration and intensity of their exercise training throughout pregnancy and cease exercising 2–3 days prior to delivery, a phenomenon we call the graded intensity or GI-exercise training program. Indeed, this GI-exercise training program normalized the mouse preeclampsia phenotypes, and: (1) prevented the increase in blood pressure; (2) reduced the development of the proteinuria; (3) abolished the increase in placental mRNA and circulating levels of sFlt-1; and (4) prevented the development of the placental pathology characteristic of preeclampsia, and thus also prevented the associated foetal intra-uterine growth restriction phenotype. In support of this beneficial effect of the GI-exercise training program, we also observed similar benefits in a mouse model of preeclampsia (*hAGT*hREN model*; normotensive female mice which overexpress human angiotensinogen, bred with males that overexpress human renin) [124]. Interestingly, we found that these beneficial effects of exercise training in R^+A^+ mice were associated to a normalisation of AT1R and MasR in the placenta as well as an increase Mas receptor content in the aorta [102]. Hence, this could contribute to the prevention of the increase in blood pressure and the normalisation of placental development observed in this animal model.

5. Conclusion

In conclusion, the reproductive system's local RAS has been clearly shown to be implicated in fertility, reproduction and pregnancy. Moreover, dysregulation of the RAS has been associated with gestational pathologies, although more work is needed to clearly identify the molecular mechanisms involved. As such, the development of new therapies aiming at amplifying the vasodilating arm of the RAS could help in improving both maternal and foetal outcomes although caution needs to be taken given that RAS inhibitors have been shown to be teratogenic.

Author details

Émilie Pepin[1], Shahin Shabanipour Dehboneh[1,2], Nozha Raguema[1,3], Maedeh Talebi Esfandarani[1,4] and Julie L. Lavoie[1,2]*

*Address all correspondence to: julie.lavoie.3@umontreal.ca

1 CRCHUM, Université de Montréal, Montreal, Canada

2 Department of Kinesiology, Université de Montréal, Montreal, Canada

3 University of Carthage, Human Genome and Multifactorial Disease Laboratory, Faculty of Pharmacy at Monastir, Tunisia

4 Department of Biochemistry, Université de Montréal, Montreal, Canada

References

[1] Mader SS, Windelspecht M, Preston L. Essentials of Biology. Boston: McGraw-Hill Higher Education; 2007.

[2] Moore KL, Persaud TVN, Torchia MG. Before We Are Born: Essentials of Embryology and Birth Defects with Student Consult Online Access. Philadelphia: Elsevier Health Sciences; 2015.

[3] Jones RE, Lopez KH. Human Reproductive Biology. Waltman: Elsevier Science; 2013.

[4] Cakmak H, Taylor HS. Implantation failure: molecular mechanisms and clinical treatment. Human Reproduction Update. 2011;**17**(2):242-253.

[5] Paul M, Poyan MA, Kreutz R. Physiology of local renin-angiotensin systems. Physiological Reviews. 2006;**86**(3):747-803. DOI: 10.1152/physrev.00036.2005

[6] Irani RA, Xia Y. The functional role of the renin-angiotensin system in pregnancy and preeclampsia. Placenta. 2008;**29**(9):763-771. DOI: 10.1016/j.placenta.2008.06.011

[7] Vinson GP, Saridogan E, Puddefoot JR, Djahanbakhch O. Tissue renin-angiotensin systems and reproduction. Human Reproduction. 1997;**12**(4):651-662. DOI: 10.1093/humrep/12.4.651

[8] Lumbers ER, Pringle KG. Roles of the circulating renin-angiotensin-aldosterone system in human pregnancy. American Journal of Physiology-Regulatory, Integrative and Comparative Physiology. 2014;**306**(2):R91–R101.

[9] Tufro-McReddie A, Romano LM, Harris JM, Ferder L, Gomez RA. Angiotensin II regulates nephrogenesis and renal vascular development. American Journal of Physiology. 1995;**269**(1 Pt 2):F110–F115.

[10] Lumbers ER. Functions of the renin-angiotensin system during development. Clinical and Experimental Pharmacology and Physiology. 1995;**22**(8):499-505. DOI: 10.1111/j.1440-1681.1995.tb02057.x

[11] Anton L, Brosnihan KB. Systemic and uteroplacental renin--angiotensin system in normal and pre-eclamptic pregnancies. Therapeutic Advances in Cardiovascular Disease. 2008;**2**(5):349-362. DOI: 10.1177/1753944708094529

[12] Laskowska M, Vinson GP, Szumilo J, Laskowska K, Leszczynska-Gorzelak B, Oleszczuk J. Comparative analysis of the angiotensin-II receptor in placental vascular endothelial cells in preeclamptic and normotensive patients. Gynecologic Obstetric Investestigation. 2003;**56**(1):55-60. DOI: 72704

[13] Anton L, Merrill DC, Neves LA, Diz DI, Corthorn J, Valdes G, et al. The uterine placental bed Renin-Angiotensin system in normal and preeclamptic pregnancy. Endocrinology. 2009;**150**(9):4316-4325. DOI: 10.1210/en.2009-0076

[14] Sealey JE, Atlas SA, Glorioso N, Manapat H, Laragh JH. Cyclical secretion of prorenin during the menstrual cycle: Synchronization with luteinizing hormone and progesterone. Proceedings of National Academy of Sciences U S A. 1985;**82**(24):8705-8709.

[15] Yoshimura Y. The ovarian renin-angiotensin system in reproductive physiology. Frontiers in Neuroendocrinology. 1997;**18**(3):247-291. DOI: 10.1006/frne.1997.0152

[16] Itskovitz J, Sealey JE, Glorioso N, Rosenwaks Z. Plasma prorenin response to human chorionic gonadotropin in ovarian-hyperstimulated women: Correlation with the number of ovarian follicles and steroid hormone concentrations. Proceedings of National Academy of Sciences U S A. 1987;**84**(20):7285-7289.

[17] Oksjoki S, Soderstrom M, Vuorio E, Anttila L. Differential expression patterns of cathepsins B, H, K, L and S in the mouse ovary. Molecular Human Reproduction. 2001;**7**(1):27-34. DOI: 10.1093/molehr/7.1.27

[18] Itskovitz J, Rubattu S, Rosenwaks Z, Liu HC, Sealey JE. Relationship of follicular fluid prorenin to oocyte maturation, steroid levels, and outcome of in vitro fertilization. Journal of Clininical Endocrinology and Metabolism. 1991;**72**(1):165-171. DOI: 10.1210/jcem-72-1-165

[19] Dau AM, da Silva EP, da Rosa PR, Bastiani FT, Gutierrez K, Ilha GF, et al. Bovine ovarian cells have (pro)renin receptors and prorenin induces resumption of meiosis in vitro. Peptides. 2016;**81**:1-8. DOI: 10.1016/j.peptides.2016.03.010

[20] Fernandez LA, Tarlatzis BC, Rzasa PJ, Caride VJ, Laufer N, Negro-Vilar AF, et al. Renin-like activity in ovarian follicular fluid. Fertility and Sterility. 1985;**44**(2):219-223.

[21] Yoshimura Y, Koyama N, Karube M, Oda T, Akiba M, Yoshinaga A, et al. Gonadotropin stimulates ovarian renin-angiotensin system in the rabbit. Journal of Clinical Investigation. 1994;**93**(1):180-187. DOI: 10.1172/JCI116943

[22] Lightman A, Deschepper CF, Mellon SH, Ganong WG, Naftolin F. In situ hybridization identifies renin mRNA in the rat corpus luteum. Gynecological Endocrinology. 1987;**1**:227-233.

[23] Itskovitz J, Bruneval P, Soubrier F, Thaler I, Corvol P, Sealey JE. Localization of renin gene expression to monkey ovarian theca cells by in situ hybridization. Journal of Clinical Endocrinology and Metabolism. 1992;**75**(5):1374-1380. DOI: 10.1210/jcem.75.5.1430100

[24] Thomas WG, Sernia C. The immunocytochemical localization of angiotensinogen in the rat ovary. Cell Tissue Resistance. 1990;**261**(2):367-373.

[25] Lightman A, Tarlatzis BC, Rzasa PJ, Culler MD, Caride VJ, Negro-Vilar AF, et al. The ovarian renin-angiotensin system: Renin-like activity and angiotensin II/III immunoreactivity in gonadotropin-stimulated and unstimulated human follicular fluid. American Journal of Obstetrics and Gynecology. 1987;**156**(4):808-816. DOI: 10.1016/0002-9378(87)90336-X

[26] Hayashi K, Miyamoto A, Berisha B, Kosmann MR, Okuda K, Schams D. Regulation of angiotensin II production and angiotensin receptors in microvascular endothelial cells from bovine corpus luteum. Biological of Reproduction. 2000;**62**(1):162-167. DOI: 10.1095/?biolreprod62.1.162

[27] Kotani E, Sugimoto M, Kamata H, Fujii N, Saitoh M, Usuki S, et al. Biological roles of angiotensin II via its type 2 receptor during rat follicle atresia. American Journal of Physiology. 1999;**276**(1 Pt 1):E25–E33.

[28] Gendron L, Payet MD, Gallo-Payet N. The angiotensin type 2 receptor of angiotensin II and neuronal differentiation: From observations to mechanisms. Journal of Molecular Endocrinology. 2003;**31**(3):359-372. DOI: 10.1677/jme.0.0310359

[29] Marsh JM. The role of cyclic AMP in gonadal steroidogenesis. Biological Reproduction. 1976;**14**(1):30-53. DOI: 10.1095/?biolreprod14.1.30

[30] Craig GM. Prostaglandins in reproductive physiology. Postgradraduate Medical Journal. 1975;**51**(592):74-84.

[31] Yoshimura Y, Karube M, Oda T, Koyama N, Shiokawa S, Akiba M, et al. Locally produced angiotensin II induces ovulation by stimulating prostaglandin production in *in vitro* perfused rabbit ovaries. Endocrinology. 1993;**133**(4):1609-1616. DOI: 10.1210/endo.133.4.8404601

[32] Yoshimura Y, Aoki N, Sueoka K, Miyazaki T, Kuji N, Tanaka M, et al. Interactions between insulin-like growth factor-I (IGF-I) and the renin-angiotensin system in follicular growth and ovulation. Journal of Clinical Investestigation. 1996;**98**(2):308-316. DOI: 10.1172/JCI118794

[33] Richards JS, Russell DL, Ochsner S, Hsieh M, Doyle KH, Falender AE, et al. Novel signalling pathways that control ovarian follicular development, ovulation, and luteinization. Recent Progress in Hormone Research. 2002;**57**:195-220.

[34] Falcao S, Stoyanova E, Cloutier G, Maurice RL, Gutkowska J, Lavoie JL. Mice overexpressing both human angiotensinogen and human renin as a model of superimposed preeclampsia on chronic hypertension. Hypertension. 2009;**54**(6):1401-1407. DOI: 10.1161/HYPERTENSIONAHA.109.137356

[35] Stirling D, Magness RR, Stone R, Waterman MR, Simpson ER. Angiotensin II inhibits lutenizing hormone stimulated cholesterol side chain cleavage expression and stimulates basic fibroblast growth factor expression in bovine luteal cells in primary culture. Journal of Biological Chemistry. 1990;**265**:5-8.

[36] Schams D, Berisha B, Neuvians T, Amselgruber W, Kraetzl WD. Real-time changes of the local vasoactive peptide systems (angiotensin, endothelin) in the bovine corpus luteum after induced luteal regression. Molecular Reproduction and Development. 2003;**65**(1):57-66. DOI: 10.1002/mrd.10257

[37] Mukhopadhyay AK, Holstein K, Szkudlinski M, Brunswig-Spickenheier B, Leidenberger FA. The relationship between prorenin levels in follicular fluid and follicular Atresia in bovine ovaries. Endocrinology. 1991;**129**(5):2367-75. DOI: 10.1210/endo-129-5-2367

[38] Barnes CD, Johnston C. Brain-gut Peptides and Reproductive Function. Bota Raton: CRC Press; 1991.

[39] Kay HN DM, Wang Y. The placenta: from development to disease. Chichester: Wiley-Blackwell; 2011 April 2011. p. 360 DOI: 10.1002/9781444393927

[40] Wang Y, Zhao S. Cell Types of the Placenta. Vascular Biology of the Placenta. Integrated Systems Physiology: From Molecules to Function to Disease. Williston: Morgan & Claypool; 2010. DOI: 10.4199/C00016ED1V01Y201008ISP009

[41] Vaswani K, Chan H-W, Verma P, Nitert MD, Peiris HN, Wood-Bradley RJ, et al. The rat placental renin-angiotensin system-a gestational gene expression study. Reproductive Biology and Endocrinology. 2015;**13**(1):1.

[42] Pan N, Frome WL, Dart RA, Tewksbury D, Luo J. Expression of the renin-angiotensin system in a human placental cell line. Clinical and Medical Research. 2013;**11**(1):1-6. DOI: 10.3121/cmr.2012.1094

[43] Ito M, Itakura A, Ohno Y, Nomura M, Senga T, Nagasaka T, et al. Possible activation of the renin-angiotensin system in the feto-placental unit in preeclampsia. The Journal of Clinical Endocrinology & Metabolism. 2002;**87**(4):1871-1878.

[44] Anton L, Merrill DC, Neves LA, Stovall K, Gallagher PE, Diz DI, et al. Activation of local chorionic villi angiotensin II levels but not angiotensin (1-7) in preeclampsia. Hypertension. 2008;**51**(4):1066-1072. DOI: 10.1161/HYPERTENSIONAHA.107.103861

[45] Cooper AC, Robinson G, Vinson GP, Cheung WT, Broughton Pipkin F. The localization and expression of the renin-angiotensin system in the human placenta throughout pregnancy. Placenta. 1999;**20**(5-6):467-474. DOI: 10.1053/plac.1999.0404

[46] Kalenga MK, Thomas K, de Gasparo M, De Hertogh R. Determination of renin, angiotensin converting enzyme and angiotensin II levels in human placenta, chorion and amnion from women with pregnancy induced hypertension. Clinical Endocrinology (Oxf). 1996;**44**(4):429-433. DOI: 10.1046/j.1365-2265.1996.703525.x

[47] Li X, Shams M, Zhu J, Khalig A, Wilkes M, Whittle M, et al. Cellular localization of AT1 receptor mRNA and protein in normal placenta and its reduced expression in intrauterine growth restriction. Angiotensin II stimulates the release of vasorelaxants. Journal of Clinical Investestigation. 1998;**101**(2):442-454. DOI: 10.1172/JCI119881

[48] Shah DM, Banu JM, Chirgwin JM, Tekmal RR. Reproductive tissue renin gene expression in preeclampsia. Hypertens Pregnancy. 2000;**19**(3):341-351. DOI: 10.1081/PRG-100101996

[49] Herse F, Dechend R, Harsem NK, Wallukat G, Janke J, Qadri F, et al. Dysregulation of the circulating and tissue-based renin-angiotensin system in preeclampsia. Hypertension. 2007;**49**(3):604-611.

[50] Yagami H, Kurauchi O, Murata Y, Okamoto T, Mizutani S, Tomoda Y. Expression of angiotensin-converting enzyme in human placenta and its physiologic role in the foetal circulation. Obstetrics & Gynecology. 1994;**84**(3):453-457.

[51] Neves LA, Stovall K, Joyner J, Valdes G, Gallagher PE, Ferrario CM, et al. ACE2 and ANG-(1-7) in the rat uterus during early and late gestation. American Journal of Physiological, Regulatory, Integrative and Comparitive Physiology. 2008;**294**(1):R151–R61. DOI: 10.1152/ajpregu.00514.2007

[52] Pringle KG, Tadros MA, Callister RJ, Lumbers ER. The expression and localization of the human placental prorenin/renin-angiotensin system throughout pregnancy: roles in trophoblast invasion and angiogenesis? Placenta. 2011;**32**(12):956-962. DOI: 10.1016/j.placenta.2011.09.020

[53] Wang Y, Pringle KG, Chen YX, Zakar T, Lumbers ER. Regulation of the renin-angiotensin system (RAS) in BeWo and HTR-8/SVneo trophoblast cell lines. Placenta. 2012;**33**(8):634-639. DOI: 10.1016/j.placenta.2012.05.001

[54] Herr D, Bekes I, Wulff C. Local renin-angiotensin system in the reproductive system. Beyond the conventional Renin Angiotensin System. Front Endocrinol (Lausanne). 2013;**4**:150. DOI 10.3389/fendo.2013.00150

[55] Li XF, Ahmed A. Dual role of angiotensin II in the human endometrium. Human Reproduction. 1996;**11 Suppl 2**:95-108.

[56] Lumbers ER, Wang Y, Delforce SJ, Corbisier de Meaultsart C, Logan PC, Mitchell MD, et al. Decidualisation of human endometrial stromal cells is associated with increased expression and secretion of prorenin. Reproduction of Biological Endocrinology. 2015;**13**:129. DOI: 10.1186/s12958-015-0127-8

[57] Ahmed A, Li XF, Shams M, Gregory J, Rollason T, Barnes NM, et al. Localization of the angiotensin II and its receptor subtype expression in human endometrium and identification of a novel high-affinity angiotensin II binding site. Journal of Clinical Investestigation. 1995;**96**(2):848-857. DOI: 10.1172/JCI118131

[58] Chapman AB, Zamudio S, Woodmansee W, Merouani A, Osorio F, Johnson A, et al. Systemic and renal hemodynamic changes in the luteal phase of the menstrual cycle mimic early pregnancy. American Journal of Physiology. 1997;**273**(5 Pt 2):F777–F782.

[59] Vaz-Silva J, Carneiro MM, Ferreira MC, Pinheiro SV, Silva DA, Silva-Filho AL, et al. The vasoactive peptide angiotensin-(1-7), its receptor Mas and the angiotensin-converting enzyme type 2 are expressed in the human endometrium. Reproduction Science. 2009;**16**(3):247-256. DOI: 10.1177/1933719108327593

[60] August P, Sealey JB. Renin–Angiotensin System in Normal and Hypertensive Pregnancy and in Ovarian Function. Laragh JH, Brenner BM, editor. New York: The Raven Press; 1990.

[61] Oats JN, Broughton Pipkin F, Symonds EM. Angiotensin-converting enzyme and the renin-angiotensin system in normotensive primigravid pregnancy. Clinical and Experimental Hypertension B. 1982;**1**(1):73-91. DOI: 10.3109/10641958209037182

[62] Brown MA, Gallery ED, Ross MR, Esber RP. Sodium excretion in normal and hypertensive pregnancy: a prospective study. American Journal of Obstetrics Gynecology. 1988;**159**(2):297-307. DOI: 10.1016/S0002-9378(88)80071-1

[63] Nasjletti A, Masson GM. Studies on angiotensinogen formation in a liver perfusion system. Circulation Research. 1972;**31**(9):Suppl 2:187-20.

[64] Irani RA, Xia Y. Renin angiotensin signalling in normal pregnancy and preeclampsia. Seminars of Nephrology. 2011;**31**(1):47-58. DOI: 10.1016/j.semnephrol.2010.10.005

[65] Hill CC, Pickinpaugh J. Physiologic changes in pregnancy. Surgery Clinics of North America. 2008;**88**(2):391-401. DOI: 10.1016/j.suc.2007.12.005

[66] Gant NF, Daley GL, Chand S, Whalley PJ, MacDonald PC. A study of angiotensin II pressor response throughout primigravid pregnancy. Journal of Clinical Investestigation. 1973;**52**(11):2682-2689. DOI: 10.1172/JCI107462

[67] Langer B, Grima M, Coquard C, Bader AM, Schlaeder G, Imbs JL. Plasma active renin, angiotensin I, and angiotensin II during pregnancy and in preeclampsia. Obstetrics Gynecology. 1998;**91**(2):196-202.

[68] Iyer SN, Ferrario CM, Chappell MC. Angiotensin-(1-7) contributes to the antihypertensive effects of blockade of the renin-angiotensin system. Hypertension. 1998;**31**(1 Pt 2): 356-361. DOI: 10.1161/01.HYP.31.1.356

[69] Brosnihan KB, Neves LA, Anton L, Joyner J, Valdes G, Merrill DC. Enhanced expression of Ang-(1-7) during pregnancy. Brazilian Journal of Medical and Biological Research. 2004;**37**(8):1255-1262. DOI: S0100-879X2004000800017

[70] Merrill DC, Karoly M, Chen K, Ferrario CM, Brosnihan KB. Angiotensin-(1-7) in normal and preeclamptic pregnancy. Endocrine. 2002;**18**(3):239-245. DOI: 10.1385/ENDO: 18:3:239

[71] Neves LA, Williams AF, Averill DB, Ferrario CM, Walkup MP, Brosnihan KB. Pregnancy enhances the angiotensin (Ang)-(1-7) vasodilator response in mesenteric arteries and increases the renal concentration and urinary excretion of Ang-(1-7). Endocrinology. 2003;**144**(8):3338-3343. DOI: 10.1210/en.2003-0009

[72] Hilchey SD, Bell-Quilley CP. Association between the natriuretic action of angiotensin-(1-7) and selective stimulation of renal prostaglandin I2 release. Hypertension. 1995;**25**(6):1238-1244. DOI: 10.1161/01.HYP.25.6.1238

[73] Yang J, Shang J, Zhang S, Li H, Liu H. The role of the renin-angiotensin-aldosterone system in preeclampsia: Genetic polymorphisms and microRNA. Journal of Molecular Endocrinology. 2013;**50**(2):R53–R66. DOI: 10.1530/JME-12-0216

[74] Williams PJ, Mistry HD, Innes BA, Bulmer JN, Broughton Pipkin F. Expression of AT1R, AT2R and AT4R and their roles in extravillous trophoblast invasion in the human. Placenta. 2010;**31**(5):448-455. DOI: 10.1016/j.placenta.2010.02.014

[75] Delles C, Freel EM. Aldosterone, vascular endothelial growth factor, and preeclampsia: a mystery solved? Hypertension. 2013;**61**(5):958-960. DOI: 10.1161/HYPERTENSIONAHA.111.00767

[76] Pan PP, Zhan QT, Le F, Zheng Y-M, Jin F. Angiotensin-Converting Enzymes Play a Dominant Role in Fertility. International Journal of Molecular Sciences. 2013;**14**(10):21071-21086.

[77] Wu X, Lu K, Su Y. Renin-angiotensin system: involvement in polycystic ovarian syndrome. Zhonghua Fu Chan Ke Za Zhi. 1997;**32**(7):428-431.

[78] Celik O, Yesilada E, Hascalik S, Celik N, Sahin I, Keskin L, et al. Angiotensin-converting enzyme gene polymorphism and risk of insulin resistance in PCOS. Reproductive Biomedical Online. 2010;**20**(4):492-498. DOI: 10.1016/j.rbmo.2009.12.014

[79] Bi F-F, Li D, Cao C, Li C-Y, Yang Q. Regulation of angiotensin II type 1 receptor expression in ovarian cancer: a potential role for BRCA1. Journal of Ovarian Research. 2013;**6**(1):1.

[80] Ino K, Shibata K, Kajiyama H, Yamamoto E, Nagasaka T, Nawa A, et al. Angiotensin II type 1 receptor expression in ovarian cancer and its correlation with tumour angiogenesis and patient survival. British Journal of Cancer. 2006;**94**(4):552-560. DOI: 10.1038/sj.bjc.6602961

[81] Suganuma T, Ino K, Shibata K, Kajiyama H, Nagasaka T, Mizutani S, et al. Functional expression of the angiotensin II type 1 receptor in human ovarian carcinoma cells and its blockade therapy resulting in suppression of tumor invasion, angiogenesis, and peritoneal dissemination. Clinical Cancer Research. 2005;**11**(7):2686-2694. DOI: 10.1158/1078-0432.CCR-04-1946

[82] Organization WH, editor. International Agency for Research on Cancer (2014). World Cancer Report 2014.

[83] Piastowska-Ciesielska AW, Pluciennik E, Wojcik-Krowiranda K, Bienkiewicz A, Bednarek A, Ochedalski T. Analysis of the expression of angiotensin II type 1 receptor and VEGF in endometrial adenocarcinoma with different clinicopathological characteristics. Tumour Biology. 2012;**33**(3):767-774. DOI: 10.1007/s13277-011-0292-0

[84] Pringle KG, Delforce SJ, Wang Y, Ashton KA, Proietto A, Otton G, et al. Renin–angiotensin system gene polymorphisms and endometrial cancer. Endocrine Connections. 2016;**5**(3):128-135.

[85] Ronsmans C, Graham WJ, Lancet Maternal Survival Series steering g. Maternal mortality: who, when, where, and why. Lancet. 2006;**368**(9542):1189-1200. DOI: 10.1016/S0140-6736(06)69380-X

[86] Sibai B, Dekker G, Kupferminc M. Pre-eclampsia. Lancet. 2005;**365**(9461):785-799. DOI: 10.1016/S0140-6736(05)17987-2

[87] Bellamy L, Casas JP, Hingorani AD, Williams DJ. Pre-eclampsia and risk of cardiovascular disease and cancer in later life: Systematic review and meta-analysis. BMJ. 2007;**335**(7627):974. DOI: 10.1136/bmj.39335.385301.BE

[88] Roberts JM, Redman CW. Pre-eclampsia: More than pregnancy-induced hypertension. Lancet. 1993;**341**(8858):1447-1451. DOI: 0140-6736(93)90889-O

[89] Sibai BM. Diagnosis and management of gestational hypertension and preeclampsia. Obstetrics Gynaecology. 2003;**102**(1):181-192. DOI: 10.1016/S0029-7844(03)00475-7

[90] Spinnato JA, 2nd, Freire S, Pinto ESJL, Cunha Rudge MV, Martins-Costa S, Koch MA, et al. Antioxidant therapy to prevent preeclampsia: a randomized controlled trial. Obstetrics Gynaecology. 2007;**110**(6):1311-1318. DOI: 10.1097/01.AOG.0000289576.43441.1f

[91] Hofmeyr GJ, Lawrie TA, Atallah AN, Duley L, Torloni MR. Calcium supplementation during pregnancy for preventing hypertensive disorders and related problems. Cochrane Database Systemic Review. 2014(6):CD001059 DOI: 10.1002/14651858.CD001059.pub4

[92] Podymow T, August P. Antihypertensive drugs in pregnancy. Seminar of Nephrology. 2011;**31**(1):70-85. DOI: 10.1016/j.semnephrol.2010.10.007

[93] Wallukat G, Homuth V, Fischer T, Lindschau C, Horstkamp B, Jupner A, et al. Patients with preeclampsia develop agonistic autoantibodies against the angiotensin AT1 receptor. Journal of Clinical Investestigation. 1999;**103**(7):945-952. DOI: 10.1172/JCI4106

[94] Zhou CC, Ahmad S, Mi T, Xia L, Abbasi S, Hewett PW, et al. Angiotensin II induces soluble fms-Like tyrosine kinase-1 release via calcineurin signalling pathway in pregnancy. Circulation Research. 2007;**100**(1):88-95. DOI: 10.1161/01.RES.0000254703.11154.18

[95] Mutze S, Rudnik-Schoneborn S, Zerres K, Rath W. Genes and the preeclampsia syndrome. Journal of Perinatal Medicine. 2008;**36**(1):38-58. DOI: 10.1515/JPM.2008.004

[96] Mello G, Parretti E, Gensini F, Sticchi E, Mecacci F, Scarselli G, et al. Maternal-foetal flow, negative events, and preeclampsia: role of ACE I/D polymorphism. Hypertension. 2003;**41**(4):932-937.

[97] Ward K, Hata A, Jeunemaitre X, Helin C, Nelson L, Namikawa C, et al. A molecular variant of angiotensinogen associated with preeclampsia. NatureGenetics. 1993;**4**(1):59-61. DOI: 10.1038/ng0593-59

[98] Arngrimsson R, Purandare S, Connor M, Walker JJ, Bjornsson S, Soubrier F, et al. Angiotensinogen: A candidate gene involved in preeclampsia? Nature Genetics. 1993;**4**(2):114-115. DOI: 10.1038/ng0693-114

[99] Inoue I, Rohrwasser A, Helin C, Jeunemaitre X, Crain P, Bohlender J, et al. A mutation of angiotensinogen in a patient with preeclampsia leads to altered kinetics of the renin-angiotensin system. Journal of Biological Chemistry. 1995;**270**(19):11430-11436. DOI: 10.1074/jbc.270.19.11430

[100] Medica I, Kastrin A, Maver A, Peterlin B. Role of genetic polymorphisms in ACE and TNF-alpha gene in sarcoidosis: a meta-analysis. Journal of Human Genetics. 2007;**52**(10):836-847. DOI: 10.1007/s10038-007-0185-7

[101] Joyner J, Neves LA, Granger JP, Alexander BT, Merrill DC, Chappell MC, et al. Temporal-spatial expression of ANG-(1-7) and angiotensin-converting enzyme 2 in the kidney of normal and hypertensive pregnant rats. American Journal of Physiology. Regulatory, Integrative and Comparative Physiology. 2007;**293**(1):R169–R77. DOI: 10.1152/ajpregu.00387.2006

[102] Genest DS, Falcao S, Michel C, Kajla S, Germano MF, Lacasse AA, et al. Novel role of the renin-angiotensin system in preeclampsia superimposed on chronic hypertension and the effects of exercise in a mouse model. Hypertension. 2013;**62**(6):1055-1061. DOI: 10.1161/HYPERTENSIONAHA.113.01983

[103] Seki H. The role of the renin-angiotensin system in the pathogenesis of preeclampsia—new insights into the renin-angiotensin system in preeclampsia. Medical Hypotheses. 2014;**82**(3):362-367. DOI: 10.1016/j.mehy.2013.12.024

[104] Nartita T, Ichihara A, Matsuoka K, Takai Y, Bokuda K, Morimoto S, et al. Placental (pro)renin receptor expression and plasma soluble (pro)renin receptor levels in preeclampsia. Placenta. 2016;**37**:72-78. DOI: 10.1016/j.placenta.2015.11.007

[105] Lamarca B, Wallace K, Granger J. Role of angiotensin II type I receptor agonistic autoantibodies (AT1-AA) in preeclampsia. Current Opinion on Pharmacology. 2011;**11**(2):175-179. DOI: 10.1016/j.coph.2011.01.003

[106] Lamarca B, Wallukat G, Llinas M, Herse F, Dechend R, Granger JP. Autoantibodies to the angiotensin type I receptor in response to placental ischemia and tumor necrosis factor alpha in pregnant rats. Hypertension. 2008;**52**(6):1168-1172. DOI: 10.1161/HYPERTENSIONAHA.108.120576

[107] LaMarca B, Parrish M, Ray LF, Murphy SR, Roberts L, Glover P, et al. Hypertension in response to autoantibodies to the angiotensin II type I receptor (AT1-AA) in pregnant rats: role of endothelin-1. Hypertension. 2009;**54**(4):905-909. DOI: 10.1161/HYPERTENSIONAHA.109.137935

[108] Yia Y, Wen H, Bobst S, Day MC, Kellems RE. Maternal autoantibodies from preeclamptic patients activate angiotensin receptors on human trophoblast cells. Journal of the Society for Gynecologic Investigation. 2003;**10**(2):82-93. DOI: 10.1016/S1071-55760200259-9

[109] Dechend R, Viedt C, Muller DN, Ugele B, Brandes RP, Wallukat G, et al. AT1 receptor agonistic antibodies from preeclamptic patients stimulate NADPH oxidase. Circulation. 2003;**107**(12):1632-1639. DOI: 10.1161/01.CIR.0000058200.90059.B1

[110] Bobst SM, Day MC, Gilstrap LC, 3rd, Xia Y, Kellems RE. Maternal autoantibodies from preeclamptic patients activate angiotensin receptors on human mesangial cells and induce interleukin-6 and plasminogen activator inhibitor-1 secretion. American Journal on Hypertension. 2005;**18**(3):330-336. DOI: 10.1016/j.amjhyper.2004.10.002

[111] Zhou CC, Ahmad S, Mi T, Abbasi S, Xia L, Day MC, et al. Autoantibody from women with preeclampsia induces soluble Fms-like tyrosine kinase-1 production via angiotensin

type 1 receptor and calcineurin/nuclear factor of activated T-cells signalling. Hypertension. 2008;**51**(4):1010-1019. DOI: 10.1161/HYPERTENSIONAHA.107.097790

[112] Zhou CC, Irani RA, Zhang Y, Blackwell SC, Mi T, Wen J, et al. Angiotensin receptor agonistic autoantibody-mediated tumor necrosis factor-alpha induction contributes to increased soluble endoglin production in preeclampsia. Circulation. 2010;**121**(3):436-444. DOI: ;10.1161/CIRCULATIONAHA.109.902890

[113] Makris A, Thornton C, Thompson J, Thomson S, Martin R, Ogle R, et al. Uteroplacental ischemia results in proteinuric hypertension and elevated sFLT-1. Kidney International. 2007;**71**(10):977-984. DOI: 10.1038/sj.ki.5002175

[114] Ahmad S, Ahmed A. Elevated placental soluble vascular endothelial growth factor receptor-1 inhibits angiogenesis in preeclampsia. Circulation Research. 2004;**95**(9):884-891. DOI: 10.1161/01.RES.0000147365.86159.f5

[115] Krauss T, Pauer HU, Augustin HG. Prospective analysis of placenta growth factor (PIGF) concentrations in the plasma of women with normal pregnancy and pregnancies complicated by preeclampsia. Hypertension Pregnancy. 2004;**23**(1):101-111. DOI: 10.1081/PRG-120028286

[116] Wang A, Rana S, Karumanchi SA. Preeclampsia: The role of angiogenic factors in its pathogenesis. Physiology (Bethesda). 2009;**24**:147-158. DOI: 10.1152/physiol.00043.2008

[117] Caniggia I, Mostachfi H, Winter J, Gassmann M, Lye SJ, Kuliszewski M, et al. Hypoxia-inducible factor-1 mediates the biological effects of oxygen on human trophoblast differentiation through TGFbeta(3). Journal of Clinical Investestigation. 2000;**105**(5):577-587. DOI: 10.1172/JCI8316

[118] Nevo O, Soleymanlou N, Wu Y, Xu J, Kingdom J, Many A, et al. Increased expression of sFlt-1 in in vivo and in vitro models of human placental hypoxia is mediated by HIF-1. American Journal of Physiology. Regulatory, Integrative and Comparative Physiology. 2006;**291**(4):R1085–R1093. DOI: 10.1152/ajpregu.00794.2005

[119] Minchenko A, Caro J. Regulation of endothelin-1 gene expression in human microvascular endothelial cells by hypoxia and cobalt: role of hypoxia responsive element. Molecular and Cellular Biochemistry. 2000;**208**(1-2):53-62. DOI: 10.1023/A:1007042729486

[120] Sanchez-Elsner T, Botella LM, Velasco B, Langa C, Bernabeu C. Endoglin expression is regulated by transcriptional cooperation between the hypoxia and transforming growth factor-beta pathways. Journal of Biological Chemistry. 2002;**277**(46):43799-43808. DOI: 10.1074/jbc.M207160200

[121] Venkatesha S, Toporsian M, Lam C, Hanai J, Mammoto T, Kim YM, et al. Soluble endoglin contributes to the pathogenesis of preeclampsia. Nature Medicine. 2006;**12**(6):642-649. DOI: 10.1038/nm1429

[122] Clapp JF, 3rd. Exercise during pregnancy. A clinical update. Clinical Sports Medicine. 2000;**19**(2):273-286. DOI: 10.1016/S0278-5919(05)70203-9

[123] Genest DS, Falcao S, Gutkowska J, Lavoie JL. Impact of exercise training on preeclampsia potential preventive mechanisms. Hypertension. 2012;**60**(5):1104. DOI: 10.1161/hypertensionaha.112.194050

[124] Falcao S, Bisotto S, Michel C, Lacasse AA, Vaillancourt C, Gutkowska J, et al. Exercise training can attenuate preeclampsia-like features in an animal model. Journal of Hypertension. 2010;**28**(12):2446-2453. DOI: 10.1097/HJH.0b013e32833e97d0

Section 4

Miscellaneous Issues

Chapter 7

The Role of Renin-Angiotensin System in Ocular Inflammation and Uveitis

Ozlem Sahin and Alireza Ziaei

Additional information is available at the end of the chapter

http://dx.doi.org/10.5772/intechopen.69509

Abstract

The renin-angiotensin system (RAS) plays an important role in the pathogenesis of inflammation and autoimmune dysfunction. Uveitis is a sight-threatening intraocular inflammatory disorder caused by infectious agents, autoimmune mechanisms, exposure to toxins and many other unknown factors. Most components of RAS have been identified in every organ including the eye. The tissue-specific RAS is believed to exert diverse physiological effects locally independent of circulating angiotensin II (AT II) which functions as the effector arm of RAS causing potent proinflammatory responses via Angiotensin type 1 receptor (AT1R). AT II mediated stimulation of tissue factor (TF), the principal initiator of the clotting cascade and a major regulator of haemostasis and thrombosis rapidly inducible by inflammatory agents in several cell lines including monocytes. Activation of NFκB, a key redox-sensitive transcription factor encoding for the TF gene, plays a key role in that mechanism amplified by locally synthesized angiotensin I. (AT I) The second arm of RAS establishes systemic and local protective axis against inflammation and autoimmune dysfunction via angiotensin-converting enzyme 2 (ACE2) which is a zinc-metallopeptidase able to cleave AT II to form angiotensin-(1–7) [AT-(1–7)]. AT-(1–7), a biologically active peptide, binds to a G-protein coupled receptor Mas, and activates signaling pathways that counteract the effects of AT II by negatively effecting inflammatory responses and negatively modulating leukocyte migration, cytokine expression and release, and fibrogenic pathways. The purpose of this chapter is to analyze both pro-inflammatory and protective role of RAS in ocular inflammation and uveitis both in humans and experimental models.

Keywords: uveitis, renin, angiotensin, angiotensin converting enzyme, tissue factor

1. Introduction

The renin-angiotensin system (RAS) is a hormone system playing an important role in the pathogenesis of inflammation and autoimmune dysfunction [1]. RAS pathway elements are produced intrinsically in many diverse tissues, including the retina for controlling local inflammatory responses and maintaining local homeostasis [1]. While RAS is important for controlling normal inflammatory responses, hyperactivation of this pathway is disclosed to potentiate oxidative stress and inflammatory responses by the activation of nicotinamide adenine dinucleotide phosphate (NAD(P)H) oxidases [2]. The tissue-specific RAS is believed to exert diverse physiological effects locally independent of circulating angiotensin II (AT II), which functions as the effector arm of RAS causing potent pro-inflammatory responses via angiotensin type 1 receptor (AT1R) [1]. AT II is considered to stimulate tissue factor (TF), which induces synthesis of nuclear factor kappa-light-chain-enhancer of activated B cells (NF-κB) in several cell lines including monocytes [3]. The second arm of RAS is considered to establish systemic and local protective axis against inflammation and autoimmune dysfunction via angiotensin-converting enzyme 2 (ACE2), which cleaves AT II to angiotensin-(1–7) [2]. AT (1–7) is reported to counteract the effects of AT II by negatively affecting inflammatory responses, negatively modulating leukocyte migration, cytokine expression and release, and fibrogenic pathways [2].

Uveitis is considered as an intraocular inflammatory disorder caused by infectious agents or autoimmune mechanisms [4]. The purpose of this chapter is to analyze both pro-inflammatory and protective role of RAS in ocular inflammation and uveitis both in humans and experimental models.

2. RAS as an inflammatory cascade

Renin is considered to cleave angiotensinogen to AT1 that is further processed by ACE/ACE2 to different AT cleavage products including AT II, which is regarded as a principle effector molecule of the RAS [3]. The major functions of AT II are reported to be mediated by AT1R, which is considered to activate directly the key signaling pathways for cell growth and hypertrophy [4]. AT1R has been also shown to activate NF-κB and activator protein 1 (AP-1) to initiate the transcription of multiple proinflammatory genes [4]. AT II is disclosed to activate epidermal growth factor receptors (EGFR) to induce fibronectin synthesis and transforming growth factor beta (TGF-β) activity to promote fibrosis and extracellular matrix formation [3]. The effects of circulating and tissue RAS are considered to be controlled with RAS inhibitors, which prevent not only hypertension but also protect tissues against injury by limiting the potency of deleterious inflammatory responses [3].

Recently, several studies have revealed that modulators of the RAS-including ACE inhibitors or AT1R antagonists display beneficial effects in the treatment of cardiovascular diseases, atherosclerotic, neurodegenerative, autoimmune, and inflammatory diseases [5–8].

3. Angiotensin II and autoimmunity

The modulatory effect of AT II on T-cell responses in autoimmune diseases has been disclosed by a recent study [9]. The effect of AT II in the development of Th1/Th17-mediated multiple sclerosis (MS) has been disclosed in experimental autoimmune encephalomyelitis (EAE)[10]. Elevated levels of AT II, IFN-γ, and IL-17 cytokines have been shown in the peripheral $CD4^{+}$T cells from EAE mice [10]. AT1R is also considered to involve in experimental autoimmune uveitis (EAU) and experimental autoimmune myocarditis (EAM) through its effect on T-cell function [11]. A recent study has highlighted the role of AT1R in glomerular inflammation associated with autoimmune disease in mice leading to the inflammation resembling human systemic lupus erythematosus [12]. AT1R has also been disclosed in the pathogenesis of myelin oligodendrocyte glycoprotein-induced experimental autoimmune encephalomyelitis (MOG-EAE) [13]. The expression of renin, ACE, and AT1R has been shown to be upregulated in macrophages, DCs, and T cells during the course of the MOG-EAE [13].

4. Angiotensin II promotes inflammation and tissue injury

Inflammatory process is considered to involve activation of the endothelium of blood vessels and expression of diverse endothelial cell selectins that have been shown to lead the extravasation of specific leukocyte populations to the site of injury [14].

The expression and secretion of vascular endothelial growth factor (VEGF) by RAS and AT II have been disclosed to increase local vascular permeability [14]. AT II has also been disclosed to promote endothelial dysfunction through COX-2 activation, which generates vasoactive prostaglandins and reactive oxygen species (ROS) [15]. AT II is considered to favor the recruitment of infiltrating inflammatory cells into tissues by stimulating the production of specific cytokine/chemokines. AT II has been shown to induce the production of the potent monocyte chemoattractant MCP-1 in cultured monocytes [15]. Elevated levels of AT II associated with increased expression of MCP-1 and C–C chemokine receptor, CCR2, have been disclosed in the aorta of spontaneously hypertensive rats [16]. Modulation of MCP-1/CCR2 via AT1R blockade has been revealed to reduce vessel inflammation in hypertensive rats [16]. AT II-induced macrophage infiltration in the arterial wall was shown to be virtually absent in CCR2-deficient mice [16]. In models of progressive nephropathies, interstitial accumulation of macrophages was shown to be accompanied by increased renal expression of MCP-1, and renoprotection was provided by the ACE inhibitor lisinopril, which was considered to reduce MCP-1 expression and control inflammation [17]. Dendritic cells (DCs) and highly specialized antigen-presenting cells (APCs) were considered to mediate the pro-inflammatory activity of AT II [18]. Cultured DCs have been shown to express both AT II receptors and AT II, which were considered to enhance DCs migration, maturation, and antigen presenting ability [18]. Recent study in rats with subtotal renal ablation has disclosed blockade of AT II synthesis and its biological activity that resulted in reduction of local DC accumulation and attenuation of tubulointerstitial damage [19]. In another study considering cultured mesangial and vascular smooth muscle cells, AT II via AT1R signaling was shown to stimulate TLR-4 expression that was considered to promote cellular oxidative injury, apoptosis, and inflammation [20]. T cells were considered to show the pro-inflammatory effects of AT II via AT1R and endogenous RAS, which has been disclosed to modulate T-cell proliferation, cytoskeletal rearrangements, migration, and release of specific cytokines and chemokines [20].

5. Angiotensin II: role in immunosenesence

AT II is considered to stimulate the production of molecular oxygen species that trigger mitochondrial dysfunction and cellular injury [21]. AT II via AT1R stimulation has been shown to activate NAD(P)H oxidase to produce ROS, resulting in oxidative stress damage [21]. It has been proposed that ROSs are the most prominent molecular species involved in the aging process [22]. ROSs have been revealed to contribute significantly to various age-associated organ failures, including hypertension, cardiovascular diseases, and renal damage [22]. Hence, AT II is considered to be involved in organ senescence related to its ability to mediate the release of oxidant species [23]. Recent studies have disclosed that AT II-induced ROS production leads to functional and structural changes of blood vessels that result in vascular senescence and age-related vascular diseases [23]. Previous studies related to the long-term effects of AT II inhibition by either ACEi or ARBs disclosed protective effects on the cardiovascular system of rats and revealed the prolongation of the life span of rats [24, 25]. Another study disclosed that old mice lacking AT1R did not develop age-related cerebral circulation damage caused by the accumulation of oxygen radicals [26]. The inhibition of RAS has been disclosed to reverse age-related advanced myocardiac hypertrophy and fibrosis in old hypertensive rats, and the protective effect presumably was considered to involve the suppression of AT II-mediated oxidative stress, as disclosed by reduced expression of NAD(P)H oxidative components in the hearts of aged rats [26].

6. Further mechanisms of angiotensin II-induced inflammation: human T and natural killer cells

Co-stimulatory effects of angiotensinogen, AT I, and AT II on the proliferation of T and NK cells have been revealed [27]. T and NK cells were considered to have RAS elements, and they have been synthesizing AT II at the sites of inflammation creating a potential inflammatory amplification system [27, 28]. Th1 immune response has been disclosed to be crucial in the pathogenesis of inflammatory vascular diseases [28].

However, the interaction of AT II with Th1/Th2 cytokines during the development of inflammation is considered debatable. Recent studies have demonstrated the presence of RAS elements in human T and NK cells that they were capable to synthesize their own AT II [29]. Renin-induced inflammation has been related to the binding of AT II to the renin receptor in T cells, NK cells, and DC [29]. AT 2R which was previously considered to antagonize the actions of the AT1R and having beneficial effects in hypertension, cell growth, vascular remodeling, proliferation, and inflammation, currently, it has been thought to orchestrate the collective recruitment of leukocyte subsets to the sites of inflammation through mediating the effect of AT II [29, 30].

7. Clinical implications

New medical applications of RAS antagonists as anti-inflammatory and immunomodulatory agents without significant side-effects are being considered in the treatment of autoimmune diseases [31, 32].

7.1. Captopril suppresses inflammation in endotoxin-induced uveitis in rats

It has been suggested that ACEi captopril has a strong anti-ocular inflammatory effect in endotoxin-induced uveitis (EIU) [33]. Captopril has been shown to suppress the NF-κB activation in the iris and ciliary body cells by inhibiting the production of AT II [34]. The inhibitory effect of captopril on leucocyte infiltration, protein leakage, and other inflammatory markers in the aqueous humor including TNF-α, PGE-2, MCP-1, NO have also been revealed [35].

TNF-α is an inflammatory cytokine, which plays an important role in the recruitment of inflammatory cells, synthesis of other inflammatory cytokines, eicosanoids, and NO [35]. Anti TNF-α therapy has been used for the treatment of Behcet's disease [36]. The transcription of TNF-α was shown to be under the control of NF-κB [35, 36]. It has previously been disclosed that ACE inhibitors suppress TNF-α synthesis *in vivo* and *in vitro* and captopril was shown to successfully down regulate TNF-α in the aqueous humor by interfering the positive loop between TNF-α and NF-κB [36]. PGE2 and NO in the aqueous humor were considered to have profound effects on local inflammatory processes mainly by increasing vascular permeability and breaking down the blood-aqueous barrier in uveitis [37]. Their concentrations in the aqueous humor were disclosed to be down-regulated by captopril treatment [37]. Inhibition of both TNF-α and PGE2/NO pathways by captopril has been shown to improve EIU in rabbits [38]. Another inflammatory marker MCP-1, which is under NF-κB control, is considered as an important mediator of monocyte infiltration. MCP-1 has been shown to be over expressed in human eyes during acute anterior uveitis as well as in the rat EIU model [38]. The results of the recent studies have disclosed that captopril successfully down-regulated MCP-1 levels in anterior chamber, and it showed its anti-inflammatory properties by affecting monocyte recruitment in EIU in rats [34, 37, 38].

The beneficial effect of AT II blockers on tissue inflammation was also considered to be related to the blockage of Ang II-mediated activation of Toll-like receptors (TLRs) [39]. Drugs that limit AT II synthesis and its biological activity, ACEi lisinopril, or ARB Candesartan were disclosed to result in the suppression of Th1 and Th17 cytokine release and the induction of powerful antigen-specific regulatory T cells (Treg) through the modulation of the NF-κB pathway [40]. Administration of ARB was disclosed to suppress EAU and reduce the severity of myocardial lesions in EAM by inhibiting antigen-specific T-cell activation and contributing to the shift of Th1–Th2 immune response [41]. Chronic treatment with ACEi or ARB has been shown to reduce kidney damage associated with age, and the beneficial effect of RAS inhibition was considered to be related to the preservation of renal mitochondria [40]. Enalapril and losartan treatments have been shown to prevent the age-associated decline in the renal mitochondrial capacity for energy production and to attenuate the age-associated increase in mitochondrial oxidant production [40]. RAS inhibition was disclosed to exert a similar protective effect in the liver from aged rats through the maintenance of an adequate mitochondrial function by enhancing expression of genes responsible for mitochondrial respiration and biogenesis [41]. Aging is considered to be the result of chronic inflammation, and the use of RAS inhibitors or genetic deletion of AT1R was considered to extend the life span [41].

7.2. Oral delivery of ACE2/Ang-(1–7) bioencapsulated in plant cells protects against experimental uveitis and autoimmune uveoretinitis

Improving the systemic and local activity of the protective axis of the RAS by oral delivery of ACE2 and Ang-(1–7) bioencapsulated in plant cells has been considered as a therapeutic option for the ocular inflammation. Increased levels of ACE2 and Ang-(1–7) were observed in the retinal circulation after oral administration of ACE2 and Ang-(1–7) expressing plant cells [42]. Oral feeding of mice with bioencapsulated ACE2/Ang-(1–7) was shown significantly to reduce the incidence of EIU [42]. Treatment with bioencapsulated ACE2/Ang-(1–7) in mice disclosed dramatical decrease of cellular infiltration and retinal vasculitis in EAU [42]. It has been concluded that enhancing the protective axis of RAS by oral delivery of ACE2/Ang-(1–7) bioencapsulated in plant cells provide an innovative, highly efficient, and cost-effective therapeutic strategy for ocular inflammatory diseases [42].

8. Conclusions

Hyperactivity of the RAS resulting elevated AT II might contribute to all stages of inflammatory responses including ocular inflammation. ACE2 is more likely to establish a protective axis of RAS involving ACE2/Ang-(1–7)/Mas, which counteract the proinflammatory and hypertrophic effects of the ACE/AngII/AT1R axis. AT II might have also co-stimulatory effects on T cells, NK cells, and DC, which have specific elements of the RAS. RAS antagonists might be used in conjunction with other anti-inflammatory agents as therapy for common diseases in which inflammation plays a major pathogenic role.

Author details

Ozlem Sahin[1]* and Alireza Ziaei[2]

*Address all correspondence to: ozlem1158@yahoo.com

1 Department of Microbiology and Immunology, New York Medical College, Valhalla, New York, USA

2 Harvard Medical School, Brigham and Women's Hospital, Boston, USA

References

[1] Karnik SS, Unal H, Kemp JR, Tirupula KC, Eguchi S, et al. International Union of Basic and Clinical Pharmacology. XCIX. Angiotensin receptors: Interpreters of pathophysiological angiotensinergic stimuli. Pharmacological Reviews. 2015;**67**:754-819

[2] Marchesi C, Paradis P, Ernesto LS. Role of the renin-angiotensin system in vascular inflammation. Trends in Pharmacological Sciences. 2008;**29**:367-374

[3] Alique M, Sánchez-López E, Rayego-Mateos S, et al. Angiotensin II, via angiotensin receptor type 1/nuclear factor-κB activation, causes a synergistic effect on interleukin-1-β-induced inflammatory responses in cultured mesangial cells. J Renin Angiotensin Aldosterone Syst. 2015;**16**:23-32.

[4] Shil PK, Kwon KC, Zhu P, Verma A, Daniell H, Li Q. Oral delivery of ACE2/Ang-(1-7) bioencapsulated in plant cells protects against experimental uveitis and autoimmune uveoretinitis. Mol Ther. 2014;**22**:2069-2082.

[5] Capettini L, Monteccuco F, Mach F, Da Silva RF. Role of renin-angiotensin system in inflammation, immunity and aging. Current Pharmaceutical Design. 2012;**18**:963-970

[6] Monteccuco F, Pende A, Mach F. The renin-angiotensin system modulated inflammator processes in atheroscerosis: Evidence from basic research and clinical studies. Mediators Inflamm. 2009; **2009**: 752406.

[7] Weir MR. Effects of renin-angiotensin system inhibition end-organ protection: Can we do better? Clinical Therapeutics. 2007;**29**:1803-1824.

[8] Prisant LM. Management of hypertension in patients with cardiac disease: Use of renin-angiotensin blocking agents. The American Journal of Medicine. 2008;**121**:S8-S15.

[9] Crowley SD, Rudemiller NP. Immunologic Effects of the Renin-Angiotensin System. J Am Soc Nephrol. 2017;**28**:1350-1361.

[10] Friedrich EB, Teo KK, Böhm M. ACE inhibition in secondary prevention: Are the results controversial? Clinical Research in Cardiology. 2006;**95**:61-67.

[11] Yusuf S, Teo KK, Anderson C, et al. Effects of the angiotensin-receptor blocker telmisartan on cardiovascular events in high-risk patients intolerant to angiotensin-converting enzyme inhibitors: A randomised controlled trial. The Lancet. 2008;**372**:1174-1183.

[12] Pacurari M, Kafoury R, Tchounwou PB, et al. The renin-angiotensin-aldosterone syste in vascular inflammation ad remodelling. International Journal of Inflammation. 2014;**2014**:Article ID 689360:13

[13] Stegbauera J, Leeb DH, Seubertb S, et al. Role of the renin-angiotensin system in autoimmune inflammation of the central nervous system. Proceedings of the National Academy of Sciences. 2009;**106**:14942-14947

[14] Souza PP Fukada SY, Cunha FQ, et al. Regulation of angiotensin II receptors levels during rat induced pulpitis. Regul Pept. 2007;**140**:27-31.

[15] Luger D, et al. Either a Th17 or a Th1 effector response can drive autoimmunity: Conditions of disease induction affect dominant effector category. Journal of Experimental Medicine. 2008;**205**, 799-810.

[16] Sprovieri SR, Sens YA. Polymorphisms of the renin-angiotensin system genes in Brazilian patients with lupus nephropathy. Lupus. 2005;**14**:356-362.

[17] Valero-Esquitina V, Lucht K, Namsolleck P, et al. Direct angiotensin type 2 receptor stimulation attenuates T-cell and microglia activation and prevents demyelinization in experimental autoimmune enephalomyelitis in mice. Clincal Science. 2015;**128**:95-109.

[18] Dandona P, Dhindsa S, Ghanim H, et al. Angiotensin II and inflammation: The effect of angiotensin-converting enzyme inhibition and angiotensin II receptor blockade. Journal of Human Hypertension. 2007;**21**:20-27.

[19] Pueyo ME, Gonzalez W, Nicoletti A, et al. Angiotensin II stimulates endothelial vascular cell adhesion molecule-1 via nuclear factor-kappaB activation induced by intracellular oxidative stress. Arteriosclerosis, Thrombosis, and Vascular Biology. 2000;**20**:645-651

[20] Igase M, Strawn WB, Gallagher PE, et al. Angiotensin II AT_1 receptors regulate ACE2 and angiotensin-(1-7) expression in the aorta of spontaneously hypertensive rats. Heart and Circulatory Physiology. 2005;**289**:H1013-H1019.

[21] Remuzzi A, Fassi A, Bertani T, et al. ACE inhibition induces regression of proteinuria and halts progression of renal damage in a genetic model of progressive nephropathy. American Journal of Kidney Diseases. 1999;**34**:626-632.

[22] Nahmod KA,Vermeulen ME, Radien S, et al. Control of dendritic cell differentiation by angiotensin II. FASEB J. 2003;**17**:491-493. DOI: 10.1096:fj02-0755fje.

[23] Muller DN, Shagdarsuren E, Park JK, et al. Immunosuppressive treatment protects against angiotensin II-induced renal damage. The American Journal of Pathology. 2002;**161**:1679-1693.

[24] Griendling KK, Minieri CA, Ollerenshaw JD, et al. Angiotensin II stimulates NADH and NADPH oxidase activity in cultured vascular smooth muscle cells. Circulation Research. 1994;**74**:1141-1148.

[25] Kimura S, Zhang GX, Nishiyama A, et al. Role of NAD(P)H oxidase- and mitochondria-derived reactive oxygen species in cardioprotection of ischemic reperfusion injury by angiotensin II. Hypertension. 2005;**45**:860-866.

[26] Back P, Braeckman BP, Matthijssens F. ROS in aging Caenorhabditis elegans: Damage or signaling? Oxid Med Cell Longev. 2012;**2012**:608478.

[27] Wang JC, Bennett M. Aging and atherosclerosis mechanisms, functional consequences, and potential therapeutics for cellular senescence. Circulation Research. 2012;**111**:245-259.

[28] Tan LB, Williams SG, Goldspink DF. From CONSENSUS to CHARM – How do ACEI and ARB produce clinical benefits in chronic heart failure? International Journal of Cardiology. 2004;**94**:137-141

[29] Bai JW, Boulet G, Halpern EM, et al. Cardiovascular disease guideline adherence and self-reported statin use in longstanding type 1 diabetes: Results from the Canadian study of longevity in diabetes cohort. Cardioascular Diabetology. 2016;**15**:14.

[30] Benigni A, Cona D, Zoja C, et al. Disruption of the Ang II type 1 receptor promotes longevity in mice. Journal of Clinical Investigation. 2009;**119**:524-530.

[31] Geara AS, Azzi J, Jurewicz M, et al. The renin-angiotensin system: An old, newly discovered player in immunoregulation. Transplantation Reviews (Orlando, FL). 2009;**23**:151-158.

[32] Kossmann S, Schwenk M, Hausding M, et al. Angiotensin II-induced vascular dysfunction depends on interferon-γ-driven immune cell recruitment and mutual activation of monocytes and NK-cells. Arteriosclerosis, Thrombosis, and Vascular Biology. 2013;**33**:1313-1319.

[33] Ilieva I, Ohgami K, Jin XH, et al. Captopril suppresses inflammation in endotoxin-induced uveitis in rats. Experimental Eye Research. 2006;**83**:651-657.

[34] Di Paolo S, Schena A, Stallone G, et al. Captopril enhances transforming growth factor (TGF)-beta1 expression in peripheral blood mononuclear cells: A mechanism independent from angiotensin converting enzyme inhibition? A study in cyclosporine-treated kidney-transplanted patients. Transplantation. 2002;**74**:1710-1715.

[35] Folkersen L, Brynedal B, Diaz-Gallo LM, et al. Integration of known DNA, RNA and protein biomarkers provides prediction of anti-TNF response in rheumatoid arthritis: Results from the COMBINE study. Mol Med. 2016;**15**:22. DOI: 10.2119/molmed.2016.00078

[36] Desbois AC, Addimanda O, Bertrand A, et al. Efficacy of anti-TNF-α in severe and refractory neuro-behcet disease: An observational study. Medicine (Baltimore). 2016;**95**:e3550.

[37] Shi S, Liang D, Chen Y, et al. Gx-50 reduces β-amyloid-induced TNF-α, IL-1β, NO, and PGE2 expression and inhibits NF-κB signaling in a mouse model of Alzheimer's disease. European Journal of Immunology. 2016;**46**:665-676.

[38] Lennikov A, Kitaichi N, Noda K, et al. Amelioration of endotoxin-induced uveitis treated with an I-κB kinase β inhibitor in rats. Molecular Vision. 2012;**18**:2586-2597.

[39] Biancardi VC, Stranahan AM, Krause EG, et al. Cross talk between AT1 receptors and Toll-like receptor 4 in microglia contributes to angiotensin II-derived ROS production in the hypothalamic paraventricular nucleus. American Journal of Physiology: Heart and Circulatory Physiology. 2016;**310**:404-415.

[40] Amuchastegui SC, Azzollini N, Mister M, et al. Chronic allograft nephropathy in the rat is improved by angiotensin II receptor blockade but not by calcium channel antagonism. Journal of the American Society of Nephrology. 1998;**9**:1948-1955.

[41] El Desoky ES. Drug therapy of heart failure: An immunologic view. American Journal of Therapeutics. 2011;**18**:416-425.

[42] Shil PK, Kwon KC, Zhu P, et al. Oral delivery of ACE2/Ang-(1-7) bioencapsulated in plant cells protects against experimental uveitis and autoimmune uveoretinitis. Molecular Therapy. 2014;**22**:2069-2082.

Chapter 8

Regulation of the Renin-Angiotensin-Aldosterone System by Reactive Oxygen Species

Manuela Morato, Marta Reina-Couto, Dora Pinho, António Albino-Teixeira and Teresa Sousa

Additional information is available at the end of the chapter

http://dx.doi.org/10.5772/67016

Abstract

Angiotensin II (Ang II), the major effector of the renin-angiotensin-aldosterone system (RAAS), stimulates the production of reactive oxygen species (ROS) which are critically involved in Ang II-induced effects. Noteworthy, accumulating evidence indicates that ROS also regulate the activation of RAAS, contributing to the fine-tuning of this system under physiological conditions or to the amplification of the deleterious signaling in several pathologies. This chapter aims at giving an overview of the role of ROS in the regulation of expression, secretion and/or activity of several RAAS components.

Keywords: reactive oxygen species, superoxide, hydrogen peroxide, angiotensinogen, renin, pro(renin) receptor, angiotensin converting enzyme, angiotensin converting enzyme-2, angiotensin II, angiotensin 1–7, aldosterone, angiotensin II type 1 (AT_1) receptor, angiotensin II type 2 (AT_2) receptor, MAS receptor, regulation of expression, secretion or activity

1. Introduction

In the last two decades, reactive oxygen species (ROS) have emerged as downstream mediators of angiotensin II (Ang II) effects. The Ang II-induced activation of nicotinamide adenine dinucleotide phosphate (NADPH) oxidases within the cardiovascular system, the kidney and the brain result in increased generation of ROS, such as superoxide radical ($O_2^{\bullet-}$) and hydrogen peroxide (H_2O_2), which are involved in diverse signaling functions. Interestingly, increasing evidence suggests that ROS also act as upstream regulators of the renin-angiotensin-aldosterone system (RAAS) in various cells and tissues. In several pathological conditions, ROS have been shown to increase RAAS activation, thus creating a vicious cycle that amplifies the deleterious signaling pathways orchestrated by this endocrine system. This chapter aims at giving an overview of the interactions between ROS and RAAS, focusing on the effects of ROS on the expression, secretion and/or activity of RAAS components that may contribute to the development and progression of cardiometabolic and renal diseases.

2. ROS as regulators of the RAAS

2.1. ROS and angiotensinogen (AGT)

AGT is a 60-kDa α_2-globulin glycoprotein with 452 amino acids in humans (453 in rodents) that is mainly secreted by hepatocytes and constitutes the precursor of the RAAS [1]. AGT is a specific human substrate for renin which catalyzes the conversion of intact AGT into angiotensin I (Ang I), by releasing this decapeptide from the 63-residue NH_2-terminus.

The exact dynamics of AGT cleavage by renin has been a question of debate. In 2010, Zhou et al. suggested that the renin-cleavage site is normally in a buried position and that access and binding of renin to intact AGT would imply a conformational change that results from a disulfide bridge between two cysteines residues (Cys 18-138 in humans, Cys 18-137 in mouse) [2]—the only two conserved in all species [3, 4]. This disulfide bridge seems to be quite labile and both reduced and oxidized forms of AGT circulate in human plasma with a consistent reduced-to-oxidized ratio of 40:60 [2]. Furthermore, the study of Zhou et al. showed (although with no statistical analysis) that the affinity for renin is higher for the oxidized form of AGT when compared with the reduced form and that the affinity was even further increased in the presence of the (pro)renin receptor (PRR) [2]. These results suggest that prooxidant conditions might favor the oxidized conformation of AGT and, subsequently, activation of the RAAS. However, a very recent study of Wu et al. [5] challenged these data. They used AGT floxed mice which are almost depleted of liver-derived plasma AGT and, through the use of viral vectors specifically targeting hepatocytes, injected either wild-type AGT or AGT containing Cys18Ser and Cys137Ser mutants that were unable to form the disulfide bridge. The study showed that in mice most of the AGT exists in the oxidized bridged form and intriguingly, it was not possible to distinguish its effects on plasma renin and Ang II concentrations, in renal Ang II concentration or Ang II-dependent effects (increase in systolic blood pressure and pro-atherosclerotic effect in low-density lipoprotein (LDL) receptor$^{-/-}$ mice) [5]. So, it seems that at least in mice, the disulfide bridge is not relevant for the cleavage of AGT by renin in both the plasma and the kidney. However, species differences certainly exist and might be worth studying in the near future. In this context, it has recently been published a suggested protocol in order to modify commercially available enzyme-linked immunosorbent assay (ELISA) kits so that accurate measurements of intact AGT, in both oxidized and reduced forms, can be performed [6]. This will enable researchers to expand their studies and push forward the state-of-the-art on this field.

The evidence that ROS regulate the expression of AGT is mostly characterized in the kidney. The original study was performed in 2002, by Hsieh et al., who suggested that the mechanism through which high glucose induces AGT expression in immortalized renal proximal tubule cells (IRPTCs) was ROS generation [7]. They found that cultured IRPTCs stimulated with high-glucose medium increased the accumulation of AGT mRNA and its secretion into the culture medium. This effect was blocked by taurine (an antioxidant), tiron (an $O_2^{\bullet-}$ scavenger), MnTBAP (a manganese-dependent superoxide dismutase (SOD) mimetic) and catalase (a H_2O_2 neutralizing enzyme), thus suggesting the involvement of ROS, namely $O_2^{\bullet-}$ and H_2O_2. Indeed, the increase in AGT mRNA accumulation and secretion was also observed when IRPTCs were directly stimulated with H_2O_2 in high-glucose but not in normal-glucose conditions. The stimulatory effect of high glucose on AGT expression via ROS has been further confirmed to occur in IRPTCs by the same group [8] and suggested to occur through mitogen-activated protein kinase (MAPK) activation [7] and also protein kinase C (PKC) and hexosamine biosynthesis pathway signaling [8]. ROS also mediate the effect of TGFβ1 on AGT expression. Again in IRPTCs, it was observed that TGFβ1 induced the expression of AGT mRNA and that this effect was blocked by tiron and diphenylene iodonium (DPI, an NADPH oxidase inhibitor) pointing to a ROS-mediated effect [9]. Once more, MAPK signaling seemed to be involved since the effect was blocked by SB203580, an inhibitor of p38 MAPK [9].

The role for ROS in mediating AGT expression has also been studied through a different approach that is the use of transgenic mice overexpressing catalase, therefore reducing the levels of endogenous H_2O_2. Using this approach, it was observed that overexpression of catalase specifically in the renal proximal tubule cells (RPTCs) decreased the renal expression of AGT (evaluated by immunohistochemistry, Western Blot (WB) and polymerase chain reaction (PCR)) compared to that found in wild-type (WT) control mice. Although this was not confirmed in another study using the same approach [10], it suggests that the regulatory effect of H_2O_2 over AGT expression might be physiological, at least in the RPTCs of the mice kidney. Brezniceanu et al. expanded this view and reported that *ex vivo* exposure of RPTCs from WT mice to high glucose or to Ang II increased the generation of ROS or AGT (mRNA or protein) but this increase was not observed in cells from transgenic mice overexpressing catalase in their RPTCs [11], suggesting that ROS-mediated AGT expression might also occur in high-glucose conditions. In line with this, induction of diabetes in mice with streptozotocin (STZ, an experimental model of type I diabetes) increased the expression of AGT (mRNA and protein), plasminogen activator inhibitor-1 (a marker of ROS-inducible gene), p53 and Bax mRNA (proapoptotic markers) in RPTCs but these effects were absent when STZ-diabetes was induced in transgenic mice overexpressing catalase in their RPTCs [11]. Also, the negative impact of catalase on AGT expression was also observed when overexpression of catalase was induced in RPTCs of Akita mice (a spontaneous genetic model of type 1 diabetes), which per se showed increased AGT expression compared with WT controls [12]. This was further confirmed in another study in which overexpression of catalase markedly attenuated the increase in the urinary excretion of AGT and Ang II [10]. Even though, catalase overexpression attenuated but did not prevent the alterations seen in the diabetic kidney [11, 12]. It was suggested that endogenous H_2O_2 stimulates nuclear, but not cytoplasmatic, Nrf2 (Nuclear factor erythroid 2-related factor 2, a master regulator of redox balance in cellular cytoprotective responses) levels that, in turn, stimulate intrarenal AGT expression and RAAS activation, possibly contributing to hypertension and development of nephropathy in the Akita model of diabetes [10]. This was suggested to be a tissue-specific regulatory mechanism since *in vivo* treatment with oltipraz, an Nrf2 activator, stimulates the expression of Nrf2 and AGT in

RPTCs but not the expression of AGT mRNA in the liver [10]. Taken together, these results highlight H_2O_2 as a key element in the regulatory effect of ROS over AGT expression.

Regulation of AGT expression by ROS has also been studied in kidney structures other than the RPTCs. The Zucker diabetic fatty (ZDF) rat is an experimental model of type II diabetes that develops diabetes by 17 weeks of age with renal injury starting between 18 and 20 weeks of age and being associated with oxidative stress [13]. Ohashi et al. observed that in 18-week-old ZDF rats, the immunoreactivity against AGT was increased in the glomeruli compared with that of the lean rat and that the majority of glomerular AGT staining was found in mesangial cells, although it was also found in podocytes [13]. Moreover, in primary cultures of rat mesangial cells from ZDF rats, H_2O_2 increased the expression of AGT mRNA and protein via phosphorylation of extracellular signal-regulated kinase (ERK), Jun kinase (JNK) but not p38 MAPK and these effects were suppressed by catalase treatment [13]. Also, culturing the rat glomerular mesangial cell line HBZY-1 in high-glucose conditions increased AGT mRNA levels and increased Ang II concentration in the culture media through activation of NADPH oxidase, since the inhibitor DPI abolished these effects in high-glucose but not under normal-glucose conditions [14]. The ROS-associated stimulation of AGT expression seems to be crucial for the pathophysiology of renal damage, at least in the ZDF rat, since increased urinary excretion of 8-isoprostanes (a marker of oxidative stress) and increased kidney AGT levels precede the development of renal damage [15, 16]. More generally in the kidney, we have also previously reported that in Ang II-induced hypertension there is an associated increase in the renal medullary (not cortical) production of H_2O_2 which induces the translocation of nuclear factor kappa B (NF-κB) p50/p50 homodimer and, subsequently, increases the renal production of AGT [17]. This was shown by direct measurements of H_2O_2 production and by the urinary excretion of AGT on Ang II-hypertensive animals and corroborated by the results from PEG-catalase-treated Ang II-hypertensive rats. Interestingly, this study from our group [17] raised the possibility for H_2O_2 to be a key element in the fine-tuning processes of AGT regulation. Indeed, we have also observed that both in normotensive Wistar and spontaneously hypertensive rats (SHR), STZ-induced diabetes was associated with an increase in the medullary production and urinary excretion of H_2O_2 and an increased AGT urinary excretion but a decreased plasma AGT concentration [18]. Of note, Ang II-hypertensive rats had also decreased plasma AGT concentration on day 14 of Ang II infusion, while PEG-catalase-treated Ang II-infused rats exhibited a marked increase in plasma AGT concentration [17].

The highly reactive $O_2^{\bullet-}$ has also been implicated in the regulation of AGT expression by ROS in the kidney. Feeding Dahl salt-sensitive rats with a high-salt diet increased blood pressure, urinary excretion of thiobarbituric reactive substances (TBARS) and kidney AGT protein levels while decreased plasma AGT levels [19]. *In vivo* treatment of these rats with tempol (a SOD mimetic) totally prevented the increase in the urinary excretion of TBARS, attenuated the hypertension and although it did not affect the plasma levels of AGT, it prevented the increase in kidney AGT levels and, subsequently decreased kidney Ang II levels [19]. On the other hand, *in vivo* treatment with hydralazine was associated with similar reduction of blood pressure and no change in plasma levels of AGT, but only partially attenuated the urinary excretion of TBARS, did not prevent the increase in kidney AGT levels and actually increased kidney Ang II levels [19]. So, attenuation of ROS, namely of $O_2^{\bullet-}$, more than controlling hemodynamic-mediated renal injury, it attenuates the tissue-specific increase in renal RAAS activity seen in Dahl salt-sensitive rats on a high-salt diet [19]. In endothelial nitric oxide synthase (eNOS)$^{-/-}$ mice, a high-salt diet also elevates blood pressure and causes progressive renal injury associated with increased glomerular $O_2^{\bullet-}$ production and urinary AGT excretion and renal AGT expression (mRNA and protein) [20]. This was observed mostly in the glomeruli (endothelial and mesangial cells) although also in the renal tubules [20]. Interestingly, the increase in $O_2^{\bullet-}$ production was seen immediately since the beginning of the high-salt diet, while the increase in AGT production started only 3 days after the beginning of the high-salt diet [20]. Once more, tempol prevented these effects [20]. Besides, tempol prevented the increased expression of AGT, renin and angiotensin-converting enzyme (ACE) mRNA and increased the levels of systemic and renal ROS observed in SHR rats on a high-fat diet [21].

Although, as previously said, evidence for ROS-mediated regulation of AGT expression comes mostly from studies concerning the kidney, other tissues have recently started to be analyzed. For instance, in primary cultures of cardiac fibroblasts, H_2O_2 induced a fivefold increase in AGT mRNA expression [22] and this effect might be relevant for the development of cardiac fibrosis since it was associated with increased collagen expression [22]. Also, human placenta explants subjected to experimental hypoxia-reperfusion for 24 h or treatment with H_2O_2 under normoxia increased AGT protein expression without affecting the expression of the other RAAS components [23]. Surprisingly, in the adipose tissue, ROS seem to downregulate the expression of AGT. Indeed, during adipocyte hypertrophy, ROS production increased along with inflammatory markers such as monocyte chemoattractant protein 1 (MCP-1) and interleukin 6 but AGT mRNA and secretion into the culture medium was decreased [24]. This was observed in differentiated 3T3-L1 adipocytes and in primary adipocytes. Inversely, treatment with the antioxidant N-acetylcysteine (NAC) suppressed the ROS production, inhibited the increase of the MCP-1 expression of hypertrophied adipocytes and increased AGT mRNA level [24]. Similar results were obtained in the obese db/db mice. In fact, compared with their lean littermates, the obese db/db mice showed decreased AGT mRNA in epididymal adipose tissue, but increased systemic and local tumor necrosis factor α (TNF-α) and oxidative stress [24]. Again, treatment with NAC reduced oxidative stress, interleukin 6 and TNF-α, but increased the AGT mRNA level in the epididymal adipose tissue, while liver AGT mRNA levels were not altered [24]. In this study, Okada et al. raised the hypothesis that tissue-specific decrease of AGT in obese adipose tissue may serve as a defense against further exacerbation of adiposity [24]. In line with this, we just recently observed (Morato et al., unpublished observations) that in obese prepubertal children, the duration of obesity seems to trigger a systemic H_2O_2/AGT pathway (eventually originated from the adipose tissue) that might help to control plasma AGT levels and, subsequently, Ang II-mediated increase in renal AGT expression and, thus, renal RAAS activation. Moreover, this interplay seems to be implicated in renal tissue remodeling since urinary excretion of AGT was associated with the urinary excretion of profibrotic cytokines endothelin 1 (ET-1) and transforming growth factor β (TGF-β) [25]. So, further studies are needed to expand the knowledge concerning the regulation of AGT expression by ROS in different tissues and experimental models of disease so that the big picture can be taken.

Figure 1 summarizes the role of ROS in the regulation of AGT.

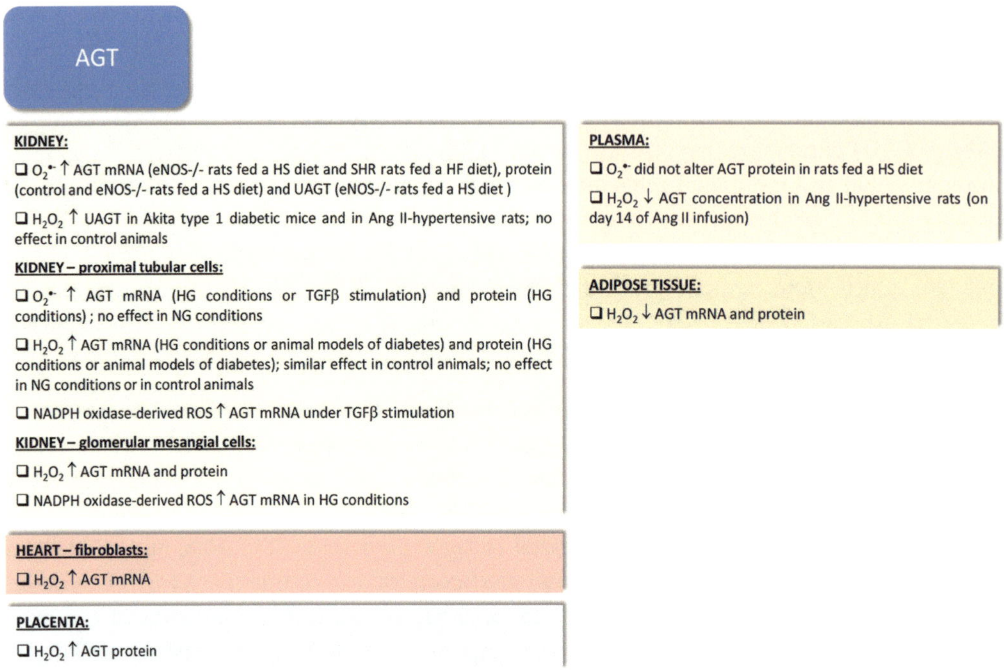

Figure 1. Regulation of AGT by ROS. AGT, angiotensinogen; Ang II, angiotensin II; eNOS, endothelial nitric oxide synthase; HF, high-fat; HS, high-salt; NG, normal glucose; TGFβ, transforming growth factor beta; ROS, reactive oxygen species; SHR, spontaneously hypertensive rats; UAGT, urinary AGT.

2.2. ROS, renin and the prorenin receptor

Renin is the enzyme responsible for the initiation of the RAAS pathway. It is an aspartyl protease with high specificity toward AGT which is its only known substrate [26, 27]. Renin catalyzes the rate-limiting step of Ang II formation, cleaving 10 amino acids from the NH_2-terminus of AGT with resulting production of Ang I which is subsequently transformed into Ang II by ACE [28, 29]. Circulating active renin is predominantly derived from the juxtaglomerular (JG) cells in the renal afferent arterioles [26, 27, 30]. In the kidney, renin can also be synthesized, although to a lesser extent, in the renal proximal and connecting tubules and in the collecting duct [26, 31]. There are also extrarenal sources of renin where renin is generated as part of the tissue-specific RAAS, but in much lower levels than in the kidney [26].

Renin is initially produced as a preprorenin protein that is further cleaved originating prorenin. This renin precursor is either directed to dense-core secretory granules for controlled exocytosis or constitutively secreted [26, 32]. Directly released prorenin accounts for 80–90% of the total renin in human circulation [26, 30, 32]. Therefore, questions have arisen regarding the physiological role of prorenin, namely if circulating prorenin can be activated into renin, or if it acts independently of the formation of active renin, for example by binding to a specific receptor [26, 33]. This receptor has been identified and named PRR and can bind both prorenin and renin [26, 33, 34]. The catalytic activity of renin is fourfold increased when renin is bound to PRR [26]. The binding of prorenin to PRR also confers enzymatic activity to prorenin which then becomes able to convert AGT into Ang I, without proteolytic removal of the prosegment

http://dx.doi.org/10.5772/67016

[26, 33, 34]. Binding of prorenin and renin to PRR also triggers a range of intracellular events in the receptor-expressing cells, contributing to the upregulation of profibrotic genes [26, 33, 34]. Activation of renin occurs by proteolytic cleavage of prorenin within the secretory granules [26, 32]. It is currently not known if prorenin can be activated in the extracellular space, but it has been reported that it can be taken up by some tissues and contribute to the local production of angiotensin peptides [32, 35].

The initial evidence of the involvement of ROS in the regulation of renin came from the studies of Galle et al. [36–38]. The existence of ROS-producing cells in the close vicinity to JG cells led these authors to question if ROS modulate renin release [37]. In these studies, performed in primary cultured mouse JG cells, renin activity was measured by radioimmunoassay both in cells and supernatants and the renin release rates were expressed as the percentage of extracellular renin activity compared to the total renin activity [36–38]. The viability of cells after the incubation periods was tested and shown to be preserved [36–38]. It was found that the prolonged exposure (20 h) of JG cells to the $O_2^{\bullet-}$-generating xanthine/xanthine oxidase (XOD) reaction had a stimulatory effect on renin release. This increase was only modestly inhibited by the $O_2^{\bullet-}$-removing enzyme, SOD, but was eliminated by catalase, an H_2O_2-neutralizing enzymatic defense [37]. Furthermore, H_2O_2 applied exogenously for 20 h dose-dependently stimulated renin release and this effect was also prevented by catalase. Therefore, it was concluded that H_2O_2 or a subsequently formed reaction product, such as the hydroxyl radical ($^{\bullet}OH$), promotes renin release [37]. In subsequent studies, these authors investigated the effects of the treatment for 20 h with native and oxidized LDL and lipoprotein A (LpA) on renin release in JG cells, as well as the contribution of ROS to the putative lipoprotein-stimulated renin release [36, 38]. They observed that although renin release was not affected by native LDL or LpA, it was markedly stimulated by oxidized LDL and LpA, with oxidized LpA being about 30-fold more potent than oxidized LDL [36, 38]. SOD further enhanced the oxidized LpA-stimulated renin release but partly inhibited the renin release induced by oxidized LDL [38]. Catalase abolished the stimulatory effect of oxidized LpA on renin release, both in the absence and presence of SOD. The oxidized LDL-induced renin release was strongly inhibited by catalase and completely prevented in the presence of both catalase and SOD [38]. These findings indicate that oxidized LDL and LpA are stimulants of renin release by a mechanism that involves the formation of ROS [36, 38]. This conclusion was further reinforced by the observation that high-density lipoprotein (HDL) prevents the stimulatory effect of oxidized lipoproteins on renin release and $O_2^{\bullet-}$ in JG cells [36], which is in accordance to the now well-established antioxidant activity of HDL [39].

Recent evidence also indicates that ROS promote renin release. In primary cultures of mouse JG cells, the exposure for 60 min to an $O_2^{\bullet-}$-generating reaction mixture with hypoxanthine and XOD significantly increased renin release [40]. Tempol prevented this stimulatory effect but did not change basal renin release [40]. Furthermore, the incubation with exogenous H_2O_2 for 60 min enhanced the renin release rate and treatment of JG cells with catalase reduced the basal renin release rate by 45%. These results indicate that ROS such as $O_2^{\bullet-}$ and H_2O_2 can acutely stimulate renin release [40]. Further work by the same group showed that this effect of H_2O_2 on renin release is most likely mediated by cyclic adenosine monophosphate (cAMP) [41]. Moreover, since the NADPH oxidase isoform (Nox) 4 was shown to be expressed in JG cells and silencing of this isoform resulted in a significant reduction of renin release, it was suggested that endogenously Nox4-derived H_2O_2 in JG cells promotes renin release [42]. *In vivo* experiments were also performed in mice to test the hypothesis that the augmentation of H_2O_2 in the renal cortex stimulates renin release and increases blood pressure. A subcapsular renal catheter connected to an osmotic mini pump to achieve a concentration of 1 μM H_2O_2 was implanted in mice. Two days after the infusion, the systolic blood pressure, measured by radiotelemetry, was shown to be increased by 22 ± 2 mmHg and there was a twofold increase in plasma renin concentration [42]. Overall, these results indicate that renal cortical ROS might contribute to arterial hypertension by increasing renin release [40, 42]. In addition, increased ROS generation appears to reverse the inhibitory influence of other hormones on renin release [43]. Leptin, an adipocyte-derived hormone, exhibits natriuretic effects on normotensive, nonobese animals [43, 44]. However, the natriuretic response to the infusion of leptin appears to be attenuated in animal models of arterial hypertension or obesity [43–45], which are known to be associated with oxidative stress [17, 46–49]. Since the infusion of leptin tends to elevate blood pressure and increased renin levels might contribute to this effect [43, 50], experiments were performed to evaluate the effects of leptin on renin release, under normal conditions or during high oxidative stress [43]. It was observed that leptin treatment for 1 hour reduced renin release in JG cells. However, in cells pretreated with H_2O_2, leptin significantly promoted renin release [43]. These results suggest that increased ROS levels change the impact of leptin on renin release [43] and are in accordance with previous observations that plasma renin activity is positively correlated with systemic leptin concentration in hypertension [51, 52].

In physiological conditions, renin expression and release are under a negative feedback in response to Ang II, macula densa sodium chloride concentration and renal perfusion pressure [26, 53]. The cytokine TNF-α was shown to mediate the drinking and pressor responses to Ang II and to markedly inhibit renin expression [54–56]. Since TNF-α can increase ROS generation and contribute to oxidative stress [57, 58], Itani et al. using an *in vitro* model of JG cells (As4.1 cells) tested the hypothesis that TNF-α increases the production of ROS which in turn inhibit renin mRNA expression [54]. They observed that treatment with TNF-α increased the production of both $O_2^{\bullet-}$ and H_2O_2 in these cells and that NAC reduced the H_2O_2 generation induced by TNF-α [54]. NAC itself had no effect on renin mRNA expression but prevented its attenuation in cells treated with TNF-α [54]. Moreover, H_2O_2 was found to negatively regulate renin mRNA expression and the renin-promoter activity through a mechanism independent of NF-κB activation [54].

The *in vivo* effects of antioxidants or inhibitors of ROS production on renin expression and activity have also been studied in animal models of hypertension. In order to test the hypothesis that in hypertension the increased ROS generation modifies type 1 nitric oxide synthase (NOS1) and cyclooxygenase-2 (COX-2) expression in the JG apparatus, thereby altering renin synthesis and secretion, the NADPH oxidase inhibitor apocynin was given for 3–7-week old Wistar-Kyoto (WKY) and SHR rats [59]. Untreated SHR rats exhibited higher oxidative stress and NOS1 immunoreactivity and lower COX-2 immunoreactivity, renin mRNA expression, renin immunoreactivity and plasma renin activity than the untreated WKY rats [59]. Apocynin treatment reduced oxidative stress and the immunoreactivity of NOS1 and renin in JG apparatus but did not alter COX-2 immunoreactivity, renin mRNA expression, or plasma renin activity in SHR rats and was devoid of effects on all these parameters in WKY rats [59]. These results suggest that the increased ROS generation in SHR is responsible for the induction of NOS1 expression and augmented nitric oxide (NO) synthesis, thereby increasing local renin expression. Indeed, NO appears to be involved not only in the stimulation of renin secretion but also in the recruitment of renin-expressing cells [60, 61]. Another study in SHR rats evaluated if the antihypertensive response to tempol is related to a decrease in plasma renin activity and in the urinary excretion of isoprostanes, NO metabolites, ET-1, or catecholamines [62]. Tempol administered for 12 days reduced the urinary excretion of isoprostanes, doubled the plasma renin activity and did not alter the urinary excretion of ET-1, NO metabolites, or catecholamines [62]. Although these authors suggested that the increase in plasma renin activity with tempol was due to the decrease in blood pressure [62], the putative contribution of H_2O_2 to this effect in plasma renin activity should be also considered. As a SOD mimetic, tempol converts $O_2^{\bullet-}$ into H_2O_2 and previous studies have shown that increased H_2O_2 production counteracts the putative protective effects of tempol in hypertension [48, 49, 63].

The effects of a lower dose of tempol on renin activity and expression were also investigated in SHR rats fed a high-fat diet. Tempol was given to 8-week old SHR rats fed a high-fat diet for 12 weeks [21]. The administration of high-fat diet was associated with increased systolic blood pressure, unaltered plasma renin activity, increased oxidative stress and reduced urinary excretion of NO metabolites in SHR [21]. Furthermore, these rats also exhibited increases in the JG renin immunoreactivity and in the renal cortical mRNA and protein expression of renin [21]. Treatment with tempol reduced oxidative stress, improved the urinary excretion of NO metabolites, did not alter plasma renin activity, but significantly reduced the impact of the high-fat diet on the other renin parameters evaluated in that study [21]. Thus, increased $O_2^{\bullet-}$ production appears to enhance intrarenal renin expression in SHR rats fed a high-fat diet. In contrast, no changes were observed in renin expression or immunoreactivity in SHR fed a normal-fat diet or in WKY rats fed a normal or a high-fat diet [21].

In addition to the studies demonstrating a role for ROS in the regulation of renin expression and release, there is also evidence that PRR is upregulated in conditions of enhanced ROS generation. In STZ-induced diabetic Sprague-Dawley rats, the renal mRNA and protein expression of PRR, as well as the PRR immunostaining in glomeruli and tubules, were significantly increased compared to control rats [64]. Treatment of STZ-diabetic rats with DPI or with the Ang II type 1 (AT_1) receptor blocker valsartan for 1 week prevented the increases in renal PRR mRNA, protein and immunoreactivity [64]. These results indicate that in diabetes the upregulation of renal PRR results from the activation of both AT_1 receptor and the ROS-generating NADPH oxidase [64].

The modulation of PRR expression by ROS was also studied in a model of enhanced ROS generation induced by the deletion of DJ-1, a multifunctional antioxidant protein that scavenges ROS and also regulates the expression of several genes by directly interacting with histone deacetylase [65–69]. DJ-1-knockout mice (DJ-$1^{-/-}$) had increased renal mRNA, protein and immunoreactivity of PRR, increased ERK1/2 activation in response to prorenin and increased fibrotic gene expression compared to the WT animals (DJ-$1^{+/+}$) [66]. A decreased histone deacetylase 1 recruitment at the PRR promoter and a reduction of its histone acetylation were also observed in DJ-$1^{-/-}$ mice [66]. Furthermore, mesangial cells derived from DJ-$1^{-/-}$ mice animals exhibited increased H_2O_2 generation compared with those from DJ-1$^{+/+}$ mice [66]. The effects on PRR expression and epigenetic regulation were induced by the treatment with H_2O_2 and reversed by the addition of the antioxidant NAC in DJ-1$^{+/+}$ mesangial cells. Furthermore, silencing of PRR by transfecting mesangial cells with siRNA-PRR markedly reduced the expression of fibrotic genes [66]. Therefore, it was concluded that the reduction of DJ-1 protein might hasten renal damage via H_2O_2-mediated epigenetic regulation of PRR expression [66].

Evidence for the regulation of renin and the (pro)renin receptor by ROS is presented in **Figure 2**.

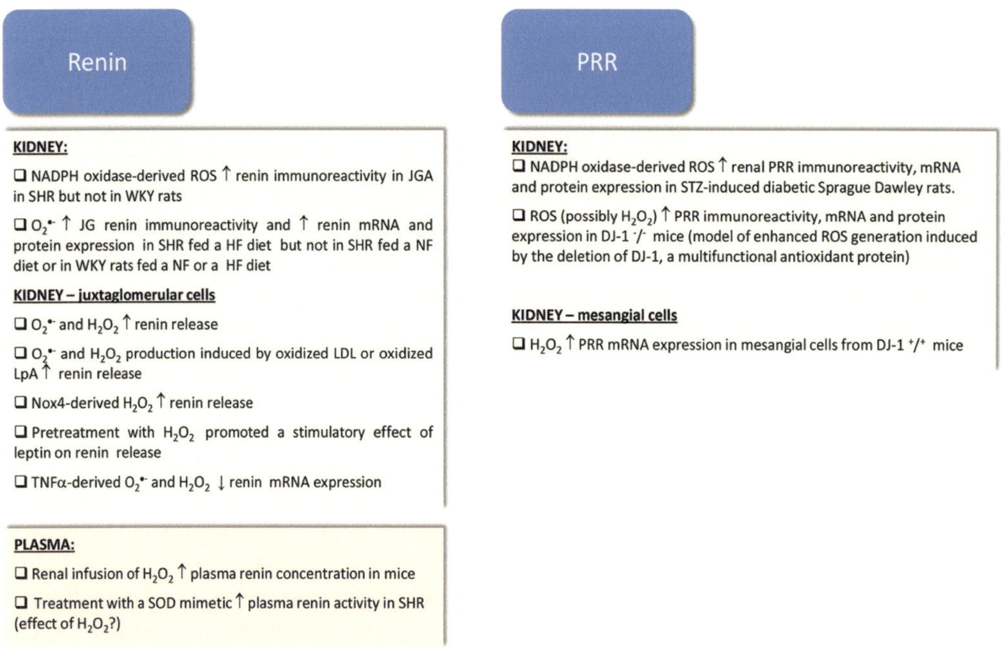

Figure 2. Regulation of renin and pro(renin) receptor by ROS. JG, juxtaglomerular; JGA, juxtaglomerular apparatus; LDL, low-density lipoprotein; LpA, lipoprotein A; PRR, pro (renin) receptor; ROS, reactive oxygen species; SOD, superoxide dismutase; SHR, spontaneously hypertensive rats; STZ, streptozotocin; TNFα, tumoral necrosis factor alpha; WKY, Wistar Kyoto.

2.3. ROS, ACE and ACE2

ACE is a 1306-amino acid 140 kDa zinc-containing metalloprotease that acts as a dipeptidyl carboxypeptidase, hydrolyzing the physiologically inactive decapeptide Ang I to the physiologically active octapeptide Ang II [70], thus being crucial for the formation of the major effector of the RAAS. ACE also inactivates the vasodilator bradykinin [70]. ACE has two catalytic domains: NH_2- and COOH-terminus that are highly homologous although the preferential catalytic conditions and the rate of hydrolysis might differ for the same substrate [71]. In 2000, two independent research groups came out with a homologous form of ACE (40–42% homology)—the angiotensin-converting enzyme 2 (ACE2)—which is also a zinc metalloprotease with carboxypeptidase activity [72, 73]. However, ACE2 is a mono-carboxypeptidase and so, it catalyzes the conversion of Ang I or Ang II to the nonapeptide angiotensin (1–9) [Ang (1–9)] or the heptapeptide angiotensin (1–7) [Ang (1–7)], respectively [72]. As the affinity of ACE2 for Ang II is 400-fold higher than that for Ang I, the formation of Ang (1–7) predominates [74, 75]. The ACE2/Ang (1–7)/MAS axis has been highlighted as the counterregulatory arm of the RAAS [76]. The balance between the activities of ACE and ACE2 will determine, respectively, the relative levels of Ang II and Ang (1–7) at the surface of the correspondent receptors and, thus, the net effect of the RAAS.

The first evidence concerning a putative role of ROS on ACE activity comes from a study of Tominaga et al., in 1988, who observed that the thiol-oxidizing agent diamide markedly increased the activity of ACE in crude extracts of rat renal cortex, heart and brain while causing a moderate increase in ACE activity in the lung and aorta and no alteration in plasma ACE activity [77]. By that time, no particular ROS was identified as being responsible for the reported effect. However, in 1993 Chen and Catravas [78] reported that *in vitro* H_2O_2 or the ROS-generating system XOD decreased the activity of ACE in cultured bovine pulmonary endothelial cells, contrary to what was expected from the results of the pioneering study. Moreover, Chen and Catravas observed that H_2O_2 was also responsible for the decrease in ACE activity when neutrophils were activated with phorbol 12-myristate 13-acetate (PMA) [78]. Indeed, they characterized the effect as being the result of the production of H_2O_2 and its intracellular conversion into $^{\bullet}OH$ through the iron-catalyzed Haber-Weiss reaction since the inhibitory effect of activated neutrophils on ACE activity was prevented by catalase and by a cell-permeable scavenger of $^{\bullet}OH$, an iron-chelator and a thiol reducing agent [78]. These results were confirmed in another study using purified ACE from bovine lungs, which showed that H_2O_2 decreased ACE activity at least in part through the generation of $^{\bullet}OH$ from H_2O_2 since an iron chelator attenuated the effect [79]. When tested directly, $^{\bullet}OH$ decreased ACE activity at high concentrations and this effect was prevented by scavengers of $^{\bullet}OH$ and by thiol-reducing agents, thus suggesting oxidation of the thiol groups of ACE [79]. Interestingly, this study revealed that the inhibitory effect was more marked on the COOH-domain than on the NH_2-domain of ACE [79]. Another *in vitro* study showed that neither $O_2^{\bullet-}$ nor H_2O_2 or $^{\bullet}OH$ altered the activity of purified ACE [80]. In contrast to these studies but in line with the study of Tominaga et al. [77], recently it has been reported that in human umbilical vein endothelial cells, H_2O_2 increased the expression of ACE via the cAMP/protein kinase A (PKA)/cAMP response-element binding pathway, although there was also decreased cell viability due to increased apoptosis [81]. These apparent contradictory results have not raised discussion in the literature. Eventually, they might represent an example of species-dependent effect since the only two studies that reported decreased ROS-mediated ACE activity used bovine or rabbit cells while all the others, concerning mostly rats and mice, reported ROS-mediated increases in ACE expression and activity, as already referred above and will be further presented below. Indeed, NADPH oxidase, SOD, or H_2O_2 have been associated with increased ACE expression and/or activity. Alternatively but less probably, it might be that the $^{\bullet}OH$ would have the opposite effect on ACE than the other ROS, putatively reflecting a fine-tuning regulatory network. The fact that some studies evaluated ACE activity while others quantified ACE expression might also contribute to the apparent controversial data. Unfortunately, not so many studies have addressed this question and so, further studies are needed in order to fully characterize the role of ROS in regulating ACE expression and/or activity.

A role for NADPH oxidase was evident from a study using rats subjected to unilateral nephrectomy (UNX) subjected to an albumin overload, which show overt proteinuria [82]. These rats have serum ACE activity similar to that found in controls but they show increased expression of ACE (mRNA and protein) in the renal cortex, especially in RPTCs; treatment with apocynin had no effect on serum ACE activity but attenuated the increase in renal ACE expression [82]. In another model of renal damage, it was characterized that kidney cells (the NRK52E line) exposed to albumin activated by advanced oxidation protein products (AOPPs) (usually generated by the reaction of proteins with hypochlorous acid) show increased expression (mRNA and protein) and activity of ACE via activation of cluster of differentiation 36 (CD36) and the receptor for advanced glycation end products and the PKCα-NADPH oxidase pathway [83]. Consistently, in Sprague-Dawley rats with UNX and daily intravenous injections of albumin activated by AOPPs for 3 weeks, renal ACE expression (mRNA and protein) and activity increased, mainly in PTCs, although plasma levels and activity of ACE did not change [83]. Treatment with apocynin attenuated the increase in renal ACE expression and activity [83]. Also, DPI prevented the increase in ACE mRNA levels induced by high glucose in the glomerular mesangial cell line HBZY-1 [14].

The above referred study of Chen and Catravas [78] excluded a role of $O_2^{\bullet -}$, hypochlorous acid, peroxynitrite, or proteases in the decrease of ACE activity found in PMA-activated neutrophils from New Zealand rabbits since the effect was not altered by SOD, an MPO inhibitor, hypochlorous acid scavengers, an inhibitor of NO synthesis and proteinases inhibitors. However, tempol abolished the increase in renal ACE mRNA levels observed in SHR rats fed with a high-fat diet in comparison with those in a normal-fat diet [21]. Interestingly, normotensive WKY rats fed a high-fat diet showed the same renal ACE mRNA levels as those normotensive rats on a normal-fat diet [21]. Similarly, obese Zucker rats show higher expression of ACE (mRNA and protein) than lean controls and tempol treatment normalized the differences found in obese Zucker rats [84]. Furthermore, $O_2^{\bullet -}$ has also been implicated in the increased expression of ACE protein in the hypothalamic paraventricular nucleus (PVN) of the Sprague-Dawley rat intravenous infused with Ang II since the effect was attenuated by bilateral microinjections of tempol [85].

The increased expression of ACE protein was also found in the PVN of Sprague-Dawley rats fed a high-salt diet compared with the normal-salt fed rats [86]. Interestingly, bilateral microinjections of PEG-catalase into the PVN attenuated this increase while microinjections of aminotriazole (a catalase inhibitor) augmented it, thus suggesting a role for endogenous H_2O_2 in the regulation of ACE expression [86]. H_2O_2-mediated increase in ACE expression was also reported to occur in the diabetic Akita mice, in which the higher renal ACE expression (mRNA and protein) was normalized by overexpression of catalase in the RPTCs [12].

If a regulatory effect of ROS on ACE expression and/or activity has been the aim of some studies, evidence for an impact of ROS on ACE2 expression and/or activity is still quite scarce. The above referred study on the diabetic Akita mice showed a decrease in the renal ACE2 expression (mRNA and protein) that was normalized by overexpression of catalase specifically in the RPTCs [12]. Curiously, the obese Zucker rats show lower expression of ACE2 (mRNA and protein) besides higher expression of ACE than the lean controls and these differences were normalized by tempol treatment [84]. Interestingly, overexpression of catalase in the RPTCs [12] or tempol treatment in Zucker lean rats [84] did not alter the expression of either ACE or ACE2. Taken together, these results suggest that endogenous SOD and H_2O_2 might be crucial for the regulation of ACE and ACE2 expression in the context of diabetes although not in the physiological context. Another very recent study focused on the vascular activity of ACE2 through the characterization of the relaxant effect mediated by Ang II on rat carotid rings [87]. In this setup, Ang II caused a biphasic response over a precontraction induced by phenylephrine: a contraction (for nM range Ang II) followed by a relaxation that came to the previous phenylephrine-induced tone and even further to a tension that was below that of the phenylephrine-induced contraction (for μM range Ang II). This second part of the Ang II-mediated relaxation reflects ACE2 activity since it was the only part of the response to Ang II that was blocked by a MAS receptor antagonist and considering that ACE2 is the only enzyme responsible for the conversion of Ang II in Ang (1–7) (the endogenous agonist of the MAS receptor). The authors observed that in control rats, this Ang II-mediated vasorelaxation (reflecting ACE2 activity) was not altered by apocynin, tiron, or PEG-catalase. However, in STZ-diabetic rats, the ACE2/Ang (1–7)/MAS-mediated vasorelaxant effect was usually absent but it was restored by apocynin, tiron and PEG-catalase, suggesting that NADPH oxidase-$O_2^{\bullet -}$-H_2O_2 play a significant role in this effect, namely through ROS-mediated inhibition of ACE2 activity [87].

Figures 3 and **4** summarize the role of ROS in the regulation of ACE and ACE2, respectively.

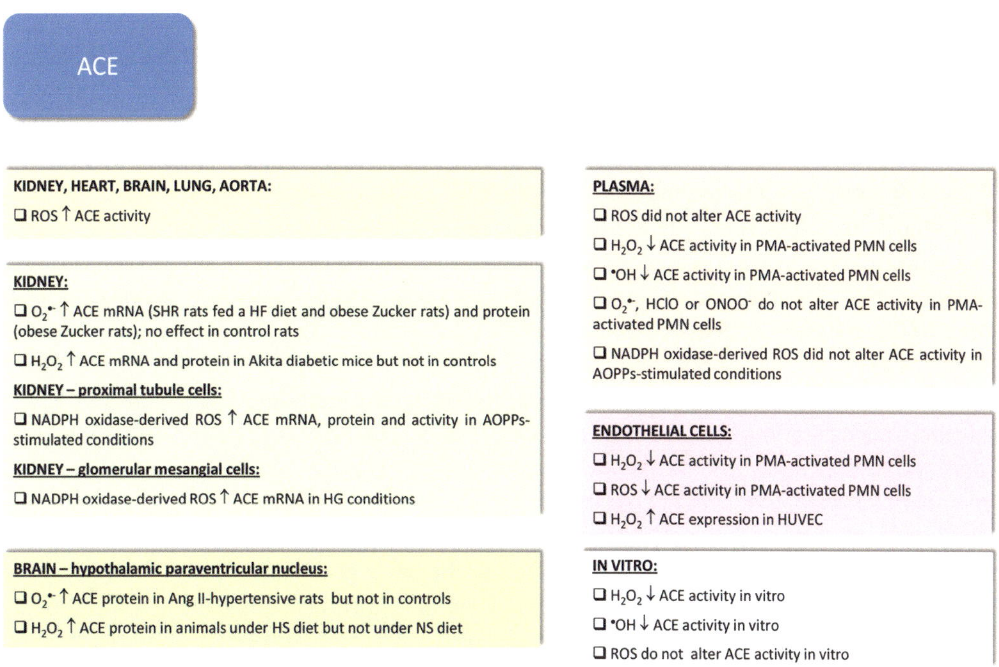

Figure 3. Regulation of ACE by ROS. ACE, angiotensin converting enzyme; AngII, angiotensin II; AOPPs, advanced oxidation protein products; HF, high fat; HG, high glucose; HS, high salt; HUVEC, human umbilical vein endothelial cells; NS, normal salt; PMA, phorbol myristate acetate; PMN, polymorphonuclear neutrophils; ROS, reactive oxygen species; SHR, Spontaneously Hypertensive Rats.

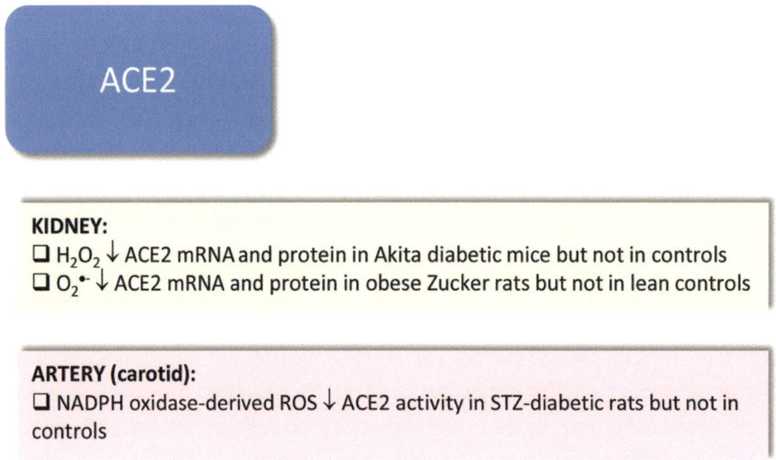

Figure 4. Regulation of ACE2 by ROS. ACE2, angiotensin converting enzyme 2; ROS, reactive oxygen species; STZ, streptozotocin.

2.4. ROS, Ang II, Ang (1–7) and aldosterone

Ang II, the most important peptide of the RAAS, is mainly formed from the precursor AGT by the sequential action of renin and ACE. Other angiotensin-derived peptides also exhibit biological activity, including angiotensin 2–8 (Ang III), angiotensin 3–8 (Ang IV) and Ang (1–7). Ang III and Ang IV are products from the catabolism of Ang II at the NH_2-terminus by aminopeptidases A and N. In human tissues there are several alternative ACE-independent pathways for Ang II formation, including proteinases such as chymase, kallikrein, cathepsin G and elastase-2 whose clinical significance is not yet explored [88, 89]. Ang II binds to two receptor subtypes, the AT_1 and Ang II type 2 (AT_2) receptors, that belong to the G-protein-coupled receptor (GPCR) family but differ in terms of tissue distribution and cell signaling pathways. Most of the known vasoactive, mitogenic, proinflammatory and profibrotic effects of Ang II are mediated by the activation of AT_1 receptor, but it can also bind to the AT_2 receptor thereby triggering opposite effects to those elicited by the AT_1 receptor [90–92]. Importantly, Ang II-AT_1 receptor interaction stimulates the activation of NADPH oxidase, a major source of ROS in the heart, vasculature, kidneys and central nervous system [93]. Under pathological conditions, characterized by RAAS activation, such as arterial hypertension, diabetes, atherosclerosis and heart failure, there is an Ang II-induced increase in the expression and/or activity of several Nox, leading to higher ROS generation and oxidative stress [93–100]. Ang (1–7), an active peptide of this system that typically opposes the effects of Ang II in the cardiovascular system, is formed primarily from Ang II through the action of ACE2 at the COOH-terminus but may also be formed by the cleavage of Ang I by neutral endopeptidases [28, 101, 102]. Many of Ang (1–7) counteracting actions on AT_1 receptor-mediated effects occur via the MAS receptor. However, this peptide may also interact with AT_2 and AT_1 receptors. Ang (1–7) seems to play a protective role in cardiometabolic and renal diseases due to its antihypertensive, antiproliferative, antifibrotic, antiarrhytmic, antithrombotic, antidiabetic, natriuretic and diuretic effects [28, 101–105]. Moreover, it also has antioxidant and anti-inflammatory actions [106–108].

Interestingly, both Ang II and Ang (1–7) content appear to be modulated by ROS. In cardiac fibroblasts from young adult male Sprague Dawley rats, treatment with H_2O_2 for 3 hours caused a threefold increase in secreted Ang II levels [22]. Oxidative stress induced by *in vitro* or *in vivo* treatment with high concentrations of albumin or with AOPP-modified albumin also resulted in increased Ang II levels in cultured RPTCs or in the renal cortex of UNX rats [82, 83]. Noteworthy, treatment with apocynin reduced the Ang II content in the renal cortex of UNX rats subjected to high concentrations of albumin or AOPP-modified albumin [82, 83]. In SHR fed a high-fat diet for 12 weeks there was also an increase in renal immunoreactivity and concentration of Ang II which was counteracted by tempol treatment but no changes were observed in SHR fed a normal-fat diet or in WKY fed a normal- or a high-fat diet [21]. Obese Zucker rats exhibited a similar concentration of Ang II and reduced Ang (1–7) content in the renal cortex, as compared to lean Zucker rats. Obese rats had also increased diuretic and natriuretic responses to AT_1 receptor blockade and decreased natriuretic response to Ang (1–7). In obese Zucker rats, but not in lean controls, treatment with tempol significantly decreased renal cortical Ang II content, augmented Ang (1–7) concentration and reverted the increase in AT_1 receptor-mediated effect and the decrease in the natriuretic response to Ang (1–7) [84]. Moreover, the enhanced Ang II immunostaining observed in proximal convoluted tubules and cortical collecting ducts of Sprague Dawley rats subjected to acute sodium overload was also normalized by tempol treatment. The concomitant decrease of hypoxia-inducible factor 1α and increase of eNOS expression induced by tempol administration to these rats suggest oxidative stress inhibition [109]. Type 1 diabetic Akita mice had unchanged serum Ang II concentration, higher urinary Ang II levels and lower urinary content of Ang (1–7) compared to nonAkita WT mice. Renal mRNA and protein expression of ACE and ACE2 in Akita mice followed a similar pattern to that observed for urinary Ang II and urinary Ang (1–7), respectively. The overexpression of catalase in RPTCs of Akita mice did not alter serum Ang II levels but reduced the renal ACE expression and urinary Ang II content and normalized renal expression of ACE2 and urinary Ang (1–7) levels [12]. Additionally, in cultured rat mesangial cells, treatment with high glucose induced an increase in ROS generation, as well as an elevation in the mRNA expression of AGT, ACE and AT_1 receptor and in Ang II concentration in the media. Incubation with DPI reduced ROS generation and the mRNA expression of RAAS components in these cells [14]. The exposure of cultured vascular smooth muscle cells (VSMCs) to high-glucose media significantly decreased Ang (1–7) concentration in cell lysates compared to that observed under normal-glucose conditions. High glucose also induced an upregulation of Nox1 mRNA and protein expression, while decreasing the expression of Nox4. Treatment with DPI, apocynin, or catalase reverted the lowering effect of high-glucose on Ang (1–7) content but caused a significant reduction of Ang (1–7) in cells exposed to normal-glucose media. These results suggest that high glucose stimulates the production of Nox1-derived ROS that causes a reduction in Ang 1–7 content. In contrast, under normal glucose conditions, Nox1- or Nox4-derived ROS appear to contribute to maintain the physiological concentrations of Ang (1–7) [110]. The changes in Ang II or Ang (1–7) content observed in these studies probably result from the ROS modulation of renin, AGT, ACE, or ACE2, although for Ang II we cannot exclude an effect of ROS on other alternative pathways responsible for its production.

Aldosterone is a steroid hormone primarily produced and secreted by zona glomerulosa in the adrenal cortex in response to Ang II stimulation through the AT_1 receptor [111]. Its synthesis from cholesterol involves a series of hydroxylation and oxidation reactions by members of the cytochrome P450 super family such as aldosterone synthase (CYP11B2), the key enzyme that catalyzes the final step of aldosterone synthesis and is excessively produced in the type 1 form of familial primary aldosteronism (PA) [112]. Patients with PA exhibit an increased susceptibility to cardiovascular complications, including left ventricular hypertrophy, stroke, nonfatal myocardial infarction, atrial fibrillation, as well as higher levels of oxidative stress markers than essential hypertensive patients, which decrease after specific treatment of PA [113, 114]. Noteworthy, ROS seem to be upstream regulators of aldosterone synthesis. In a study performed in human and rat adrenal cortical cells, Ang II increased CYP11B2 activity, mRNA and protein with simultaneous elevation of oxidative stress by-products, NADPH oxidase activity and H_2O_2 levels. These Ang II-induced effects were abolished or attenuated by pretreatment of cells with either the AT_1 receptor antagonist losartan, the antioxidants PEG-catalase and NAC, the Nox inhibitor VAS-2870, siRNA silencing of Nox1, 2 and 4, or inhibitors of phospholipase C (PLC) and PKC. Importantly, treatment with H_2O_2 mimicked the facilitatory effects of Ang II on CYP11B2 activity, mRNA and protein expression and these changes were absent or attenuated in PEG-catalase pretreated cells, suggesting that H_2O_2 is a key regulator of aldosterone production [115].

Plasma aldosterone levels were also shown to be modulated by the induction of heme oxygenase-1 (HO-1), an important antioxidant pathway [116–118]. In a rat model of renovascular hypertension treatment with cobalt protoporphyrin markedly increased the expression and activity of HO-1 and these effects were accompanied by a marked attenuation of the development of hypertension, decreased oxidative stress and reduced plasma aldosterone concentration [116]. Although the mechanisms contributing to a lower aldosterone synthesis by HO-1 induction remain to be clarified, the authors speculated that HO-1 might inhibit the CYP450 enzymes required for aldosterone formation, by limiting the availability of heme or by increasing the production of carbon monoxide [116]. Of note, heme is a prooxidant molecule that has been shown to contribute to increased generation of ROS and lipid peroxidation, while the HO-1 product carbon monoxide appears to possess antioxidant properties [116, 118].

Secretory products derived from visceral adipocytes have also been shown to upregulate aldosterone synthase expression and stimulate adrenal aldosterone synthesis thus suggesting a direct link between obesity and hypertension [119–122]. In fact, several clinical studies have already observed elevated plasma aldosterone levels in obese patients [121, 122]. In an experimental model of obesity, it was also shown that the enhanced blood pressure response to Ang II was associated with an increase in circulating aldosterone. Ang II infusion induced a more prominent increase in plasma aldosterone levels and blood pressure in obese Zucker rats that in lean controls. These results corroborate the hypothesis that aldosterone contributes to obesity-related hypertension [123]. Furthermore, even though the basal circulating aldosterone concentration was similar in lean and obese Zucker rats [84, 123], treatment with tempol significantly reduced serum aldosterone levels, in addition to its antioxidant and blood pressure lowering effects, in obese but not in lean Zucker rats [84]. Of note, although the link between obesity and increased systemic aldosterone concentration has not been consistently evidenced, it has been reported that in obesity-induced hypertension an intrarenal RAAS might operate independently of the systemic RAAS, contributing to increased aldosterone action [21, 124]. Chung et al. demonstrated that SHR fed a high-fat diet for 12 weeks exhibited increased renal cortical expression of several RAAS components and augmented 24-h urinary excretion of aldosterone, despite the absence of changes in plasma renin activity or plasma aldosterone concentration. These SHR rats had also higher blood pressure and renal oxidative stress, as well as lower fractional excretion of sodium, than those maintained on a normal-fat diet. Importantly, tempol significantly attenuated the high-fat diet-induced increases in the renal expression of RAAS components and in urinary aldosterone excretion and blunted or attenuated the changes in oxidative stress, blood pressure and sodium reabsorption [21]. These findings emphasize the importance of ROS as regulators of renal RAAS components, including aldosterone and suggest that the use of a SOD mimetic might be an effective therapy to prevent the progression of hypertension in obese subjects. Indeed, in the remnant kidney rat model, an experimental model of progressive nephropathy, treatment with NAC had a protective effect also attributable to a decrease in oxidative stress and plasma aldosterone levels [125]. The beneficial effect that NAC had on glomerular filtration rate was more impressive than the modest reduction in proteinuria and was independent of blood pressure reduction [125]. Additionally, the combination of NAC and spironolactone was found to confer additive protection in the same model, improving blood pressure control and renal function more than did NAC or spironolactone alone, thus suggesting that antioxidant/antihypertensive combinations could be important therapeutic strategies to attenuate the aggravation of chronic renal disease [125].

The classical genomic pathway whereby aldosterone exerts its effects involves the binding to the cytosolic mineralocorticoid receptor (MR) within the renal cortical collecting duct cells and subsequent translocation of this aldosterone-MR complex to the nucleus, thereby promoting the transcription of genes that regulate electrolyte and fluid balance resulting in sodium reabsorption, water retention and potassium and magnesium loss, with consequent volume expansion and blood pressure rise [102]. It is well known now that inappropriate regulation of the aldosterone/MR system contributes to sodium retention and hypertension and to the development of renal injury [126]. These adverse actions of aldosterone in the kidney appear to involve the production of ROS that activate the MAPK pathway in renal cortical tissues, which in turn causes renal injury [127, 128]. Interestingly, MR activation and subsequent renal injury may be triggered by other ligands and/or pathological conditions besides aldosterone [129]. In Dahl salt-sensitive rats, glomerular MR was activated by high-salt-feeding-induced oxidative stress and this effect was suppressed by tempol. *In vitro* luciferase assays also confirmed that oxidative stress can accelerate MR transcriptional activity in the glomeruli cells [129]. Moreover, MR activation was sustained by high ROS production even after reducing salt intake. Therefore, oxidative stress appears to limit the therapeutic effects of salt restriction, an important therapeutic strategy for salt-sensitive hypertensive patients [129]. Since previous studies also demonstrated that ROS stimulate aldosterone production [21, 115, 125], the use of antioxidants might be an effective strategy to protect the kidney from the overactivation of the aldosterone/MR system.

The main effects of ROS on AngII, Ang (1–7) and aldosterone are depicted in **Figures 5** and **6**, respectively.

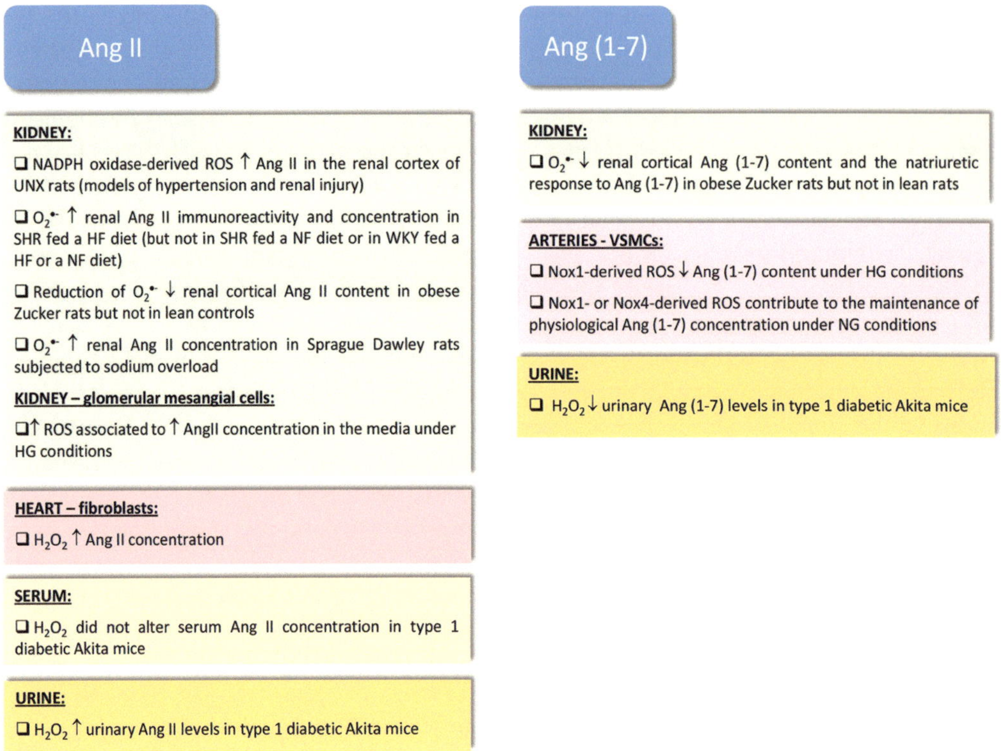

Figure 5. Regulation of AngII and Ang (1–7) by ROS. Ang (1–7), angiotensin 1–7; Ang II, angiotensin II; HF, high-fat; HG, high-glucose; NF, normal-fat; ROS, reactive oxygen species; SHR, Spontaneously Hypertensive Rats; UNX, uninephrectomized; WKY, Wistar Kyoto.

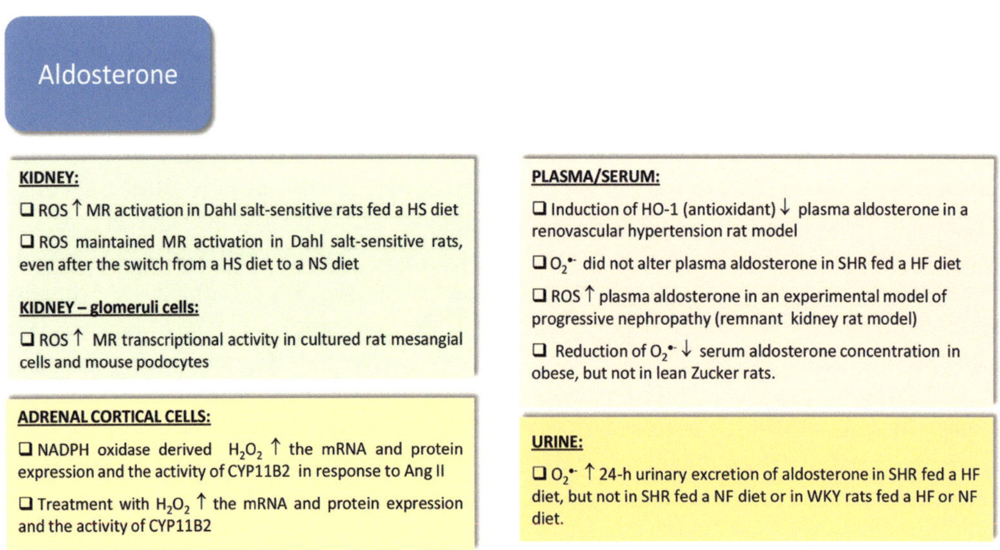

Figure 6. Regulation of aldosterone by ROS. Ang II, angiotensin II; HF, high-fat; HO-1, heme oxygenase-1; HS, high-salt; MR, mineralocorticoid receptor; NF, normal-fat; NS, normal-salt; ROS, reactive oxygen species; SHR, Spontaneously Hypertensive Rats; WKY, Wistar Kyoto.

2.5. ROS and Ang receptors

Ang II, the major effector of the RAAS, elicits its actions by binding to the AT_1 or to the AT_2 receptor, which belong to the GPCR superfamily [91]. The AT_1 receptor actually comprises two isoforms, the AT_{1A} receptor and AT_{1B} receptor subtypes that share 95% amino acid sequence homology. Although they have been considered pharmacologically identical, there appears to be differences in their tissue distribution and transcriptional regulation [91]. Furthermore, several studies have suggested that in vascular tissues, AT_1 receptors are AT_{1B} prejunctionally and AT_{1A} postjunctionally [130–133]. AT_1 receptor activation initiates several signaling pathways, including those associated with heterotrimeric G-proteins, G-protein independent β-arrestin, nonreceptor and receptor tyrosine kinases, ROS and small guanosine triphosphate (GTP) binding proteins, which contribute for the wide range of responses to Ang II [91]. One important feature of the AT_1 receptor is the rapid phosphorylation and internalization that occur following stimulation by Ang II [91, 134]. This physiological mechanism limits the functional availability of AT_1 receptors on the cell surface, thus avoiding exaggerated responsiveness to Ang II [134]. Several physiological and pathological factors, including Ang II, ROS, cytokines, growth factors and hormones, regulate AT_1 receptors in all organs [91, 134, 135].

The AT_2 receptor shares only 34% amino acid sequence homology with the AT_1 receptor and exhibits obvious differences in its tissue-specific expression, signaling pathways, pharmacological features and regulation of receptor function [91]. Signal transduction mechanisms initiated by AT_2 receptor activation are unusual for a GPCR and markedly different from those driven by AT_1 receptor. Of note, the AT_2 receptor does not undergo desensitization and internalization on stimulation by Ang II [91]. The AT_2 receptor signaling involves G_i/G_o activation, protein phosphatases, scaffold proteins, NO/cyclic guanosine monophosphate (cGMP), ion channel protein and constitutive activity (ligand-independent actions). The AT_2 receptor is expressed in low levels in normal nongrowing cells [91].

There is evidence that AT_1 and AT_2 receptors mediate opposite actions in response to Ang II. AT_1 receptor activation induces several effects such as vasoconstriction, enhancement of sympathetic outflow, aldosterone release, sodium reabsorption, ROS generation, inflammation, cell proliferation and extracellular matrix formation that contribute to cardiovascular and renal dysfunction under conditions of enhanced AT_1 receptor stimulation [90, 91]. In contrast, AT_2 receptor appears to play a beneficial role in cardiovascular disease due to its vasodilatory, natriuretic, apoptotic, anti-proliferative, antifibrotic and anti-inflammatory effects [90, 91, 136]. Of note, some of these AT_2 receptor actions appear to be best detected under partial AT_1 receptor blockade [91, 102]. Given the protective effects of AT_2 receptor activation, research is being conducted in order to develop specific agonists of AT_2 receptors [102]. The compound 21 is one of these drugs, but unexpectedly it had no effect or even increased blood pressure, an effect that may be related to the fact that in SHR the AT_2 receptors may present an AT_1 receptor-like profile [102, 137]. Nevertheless, AT_2 receptor agonists may be useful to protect against tissue injury [102, 136].

ACE2 transforms Ang II into Ang (1–7), which has been shown to exert vasodilatory, antiproliferative, natriuretic, antithrombotic and antiarrhytmic actions. The MAS receptor, an orphan GPCR, appears to mediate many of these effects and has therefore been proposed as a candidate receptor for this RAAS peptide [91]. Indeed, MAS-knockout mice exhibit changes in heart rate and blood pressure variability, impaired cardiac and renal function accompanied by profibrotic changes, increased expression of proinflammatory molecules and several metabolic changes such as augmented abdominal fat mass, dyslipidemia, increased insulin and leptin concentration and altered response of adipocytes to insulin [91]. Nevertheless, deletion of the MAS gene may confer protection against salt-induced hypertension and cardiac or renal ischemia-reperfusion injury [91]. Activation of MAS receptor by Ang (1–7) is thought to involve the production of arachidonic acid and nitric oxide synthase (NOS) activation. The potential protective effects of MAS activation by Ang (1–7) make this receptor an attractive drug target [91].

The majority of studies evaluating the regulation of AT_1 receptors by ROS has been performed in the kidney and has demonstrated a stimulating effect of these species on AT_1 receptors [14, 17, 21, 82–84, 138–141]. In adult male Sprague Dawley rats treated for 2 or 3 weeks with L-buthionine sulfoximine (BSO), a prooxidant agent that inhibits the synthesis of glutathione (GSH) [142], the increase in oxidative stress and blood pressure was accompanied by the upregulation of the mRNA, protein and ligand binding of the AT_1 receptor in renal proximal tubules when compared to normotensive controls [138, 139]. Furthermore, incubation with Ang II had a markedly higher impact on AT_1 receptor signaling and on the activation of the sodium transporters Na^+/K^+-ATPase and Na^+/H^+ exchanger 3 in renal proximal tubules from BSO-treated rats than in those from control rats [138, 139]. Treatment for 2 or 3 weeks with tempol decreased oxidative stress and normalized AT_1 receptor mRNA, protein and ligand binding [138, 139]. Furthermore, tempol also reduced AT_1 receptor signaling and activation of sodium transporters in response to Ang II [138, 139]. Overall, the restoration of AT_1 expression and signaling with the antioxidant tempol might have contributed to the normalization of blood pressure in BSO-treated rats [138, 139]. The protective effects of tempol on AT_1 receptor regulation were also evidenced in obese Zucker rats and in SHR fed a high-fat diet [21, 84]. Obese Zucker rats showed higher basal blood pressure values than age-matched lean Zucker rats, as well as an age-dependent increase in blood pressure that was not observed in lean rats [84]. Obese rats also exhibited increased systemic and renal cortical oxidative stress, augmented AT_1-receptor-mediated effects on sodium and water excretion and increased renal cortical mRNA and protein expression of the AT_1 receptor [84]. Tempol treatment for 4 weeks prevented the age-dependent increase in blood pressure in obese Zucker rats, although their blood pressure values remained higher than in lean Zucker rats [84]. Tempol also ameliorated oxidative stress, reversed the AT_1-receptor-mediated actions on sodium and water excretion and decreased the renal cortical mRNA and protein expression of AT_1 receptor in obese Zucker rats but did not alter these parameters in lean Zucker rats [84]. Data from *in vitro* assays were also in agreement with the *in vivo* findings. RPTCs from 14-week-old obese Zucker rats, compared to those from lean Zucker rats, showed a higher protein expression of the AT_1 receptor which was normalized by the *in vitro* treatment with tempol for 24 hours [84]. A significantly higher renal cortical protein expression of AT_1 receptor was also observed in SHR fed a high-fat diet for 12 weeks, starting at the age of 8 weeks. This effect was not verified in SHR fed a normal-fat diet or in WKY rats fed a normal- or a high-fat diet for the same period of time [21]. Furthermore, in SHR fed a high-fat diet and simultaneously treated with tempol, there was a significant reduction in renal cortical AT_1 receptor protein expression [21]. Beneficial effects of tempol have also been demonstrated in a rat aging model [140]. Aged (21 months old) Fischer 344 Brown Norway F1 (FBN) rats exhibited increased oxidative stress, evidenced by the augmented plasma isoprostanes concentration, decreased urinary antioxidant capacity and increased expression of NADPH oxidase-gp91phox in renal proximal tubular homogenate, when compared to adult (3 months old) FBN rats [140]. These effects were accompanied by exaggerated AT_1 receptor-mediated actions on urine flow and urinary sodium excretion [140]. Tempol treatment for 3 or 4 weeks reduced oxidative stress and normalized the AT_1 receptor-mediated effects on diuresis and urinary sodium excretion in aged but not in adult FBN rats [140].

The impact of ROS on AT_1 receptor regulation has also been studied in *in vivo* or *in vitro* models of diabetes [14, 141]. In STZ-induced diabetic male Sprague Dawley rats, treatment with recombinant human extracellular SOD for 4 weeks, beginning 2 weeks after STZ, prevented the decrease in renal SOD activity and the increase in protein expression of the renal AT_1 receptor induced by STZ intraperitoneal injection [141]. In the rat glomerular mesangial cell line HBZY-1 exposed to a high-glucose medium, ROS generation and the AT_1 receptor mRNA levels were significantly augmented when compared to the effects observed in cells cultured in the normal-glucose medium [14]. These effects were abolished by DPI or by application of NaHS, a donor of the gas transmitter hydrogen sulfide which is also known to exhibit antioxidative properties [14, 143]. Intriguingly, in the same study these authors observed a downregulation, instead of an upregulation, of the AT_1 receptor mRNA expression in the kidney of diabetic male Sprague Dawley rats, 3 weeks after STZ injection [14]. Treatment with NaHS during the 3rd week abolished the decrease in mRNA levels of the AT_1 receptor in STZ-induced diabetic rats, but did not alter the AT_1 receptor expression in nondiabetic rats [14].

A study of our group in a model of arterial hypertension induced by the infusion of Ang II in male Sprague Dawley rats showed that Ang II increased H_2O_2 production and the protein expression of Nox4 and AT_1 receptor in the renal medulla, but not in the renal cortex [17]. Noteworthy, treatment of Ang II-infused rats with PEG-catalase from day 7 to day 14 significantly reduced H_2O_2 production and the expression of Nox4 and AT_1 receptors in the renal medulla, thus suggesting that Ang II-derived H_2O_2 in the renal medulla stimulates the expression of Nox4 and AT_1 receptors[17].

The upregulation of intrarenal AT_1 receptor has also been evidenced in models of renal disease. Female WKY rats subjected to UNX and treated with bovine serum albumin for 4 weeks had increased $O_2^{\bullet-}$ generation and upregulation of AT_1 receptor mRNA and protein in the renal cortex [82]. Treatment of protein-overload UNX rats with apocynin for 3 weeks reduced renal cortical $O_2^{\bullet-}$ production and AT_1 receptor mRNA and protein levels [82]. Similar effects were also observed in male Sprague Dawley rats subjected to UNX and treated with AOPP-modified albumin [83]. These UNX rats treated with AOPP-modified albumin also showed increased renal cortical $O_2^{\bullet-}$ generation, as well as an augmented expression of the mRNA and protein of AT_1 receptor [83]. As previously observed in protein-overload UNX rats, treatment with apocynin also reduced the production of $O_2^{\bullet-}$ and the mRNA and protein levels of the AT_1 receptor in the renal cortex of AOPP-albumin-challenged rats [83]. The effects observed for the *in vivo* treatment with high levels of albumin or with AOPP-modified albumin on ROS production and AT_1 receptor expression were also reproduced in *in vitro* assays using cultured RPTCs (NRK52E) [82, 83].

In the heart, the mechanisms linking oxidative stress to altered AT_1 expression were investigated in fibroblasts prepared from young adult (2–3 months old) male Sprague Dawley rats

[22]. Treatment of cardiac fibroblasts with H_2O_2 caused a sixfold increase in AT_1 receptor mRNA levels in 3 hours, which were reduced to twofold at the end of 12 hours. AT_1 receptor protein expression was also significantly increased with maximum values reached at 6 and 12 hours of H_2O_2 treatment [22]. The preincubation of cardiac fibroblasts with the NADPH inhibitors DPI or VAS2870 abolished the H_2O_2-induced increase in AT_1 receptor mRNA and protein levels. Treatment with DPI also inhibited the H_2O_2-induced increase in intracellular ROS in cardiac fibroblasts [22]. Further experiments also showed that H_2O_2 induced the activation of NF-κB and activator protein 1 (AP-1) in cardiac fibroblasts and that preincubation of these cells for 60 min with the NF-κB inhibitor BAY-11-7085 or with the AP-1 inhibitor SR11302 prior to H_2O_2 treatment attenuated the AT_1 mRNA and protein expression. These data demonstrate that the H_2O_2-induced increase of AT_1 receptor mRNA and protein expression in cardiac fibroblasts involves the activation of NF-κB and AP-1 [22]. In subsequent experiments, H_2O_2 was also shown to increase by threefold the local secretion of Ang II. In addition, treatment with Ang II augmented the AT_1 receptor mRNA and protein expression in cardiac fibroblasts and these effects were significantly reduced by pretreatment with VAS2870. Therefore, it was concluded that Ang II increases the AT_1 receptor mRNA and protein expression in cardiac fibroblasts via NADPH oxidase-dependent ROS [22]. Moreover, H_2O_2 treatment significantly increased collagen mRNA and protein expression in these cells and the AT_1 receptor antagonist candesartan decreased these effects [22]. Overall, these findings suggest the existence of a positive feedback loop involving the reciprocal regulation of ROS, Ang II and the AT_1 receptor, which sustains the Ang II pathological signaling in the heart [22].

There have been contradictory reports regarding the effects of ROS on the AT_1 receptor regulation in the vasculature [135, 144]. In a study aimed at characterizing the second messengers used by Ang II in the regulation of AT_1 receptor gene expression, Nickenig et al. showed that treatment with Ang II caused a significant release of ROS in VSMCs and a downregulation in AT_1 receptor mRNA and density in cultured VSMCs isolated from the thoracic aorta of 6–10-week old female WKY rats. Coincubation with DPI significantly inhibited the Ang II-induced ROS release and the downregulation in AT_1 receptor mRNA [135]. VSMCs were also incubated with a mixture of H_2O_2 and ferric nitrilotriacetate or with xanthine oxidase plus purine in order to evaluate if ROS have direct effects on AT_1 receptor expression. Both H_2O_2 and xanthine oxidase induced a dose-dependent downregulation in AT_1 receptor mRNA. H_2O_2 also decreased the AT_1 receptor protein expression [135]. Further experiments demonstrated that although H_2O_2 did not alter the AT_1 receptor mRNA transcription rate it caused a marked decrease in the AT_1 receptor mRNA half-life, thus suggesting that ROS destabilize the AT_1 receptor mRNA [135]. These findings identify ROS as possible mediators of Ang II-induced downregulation of the AT_1 receptor and suggest that ROS-mediated negative feedback regulation of AT_1 receptor is a cellular self-protecting mechanism that limits the potential pathological effects of the exposure of VSMCs to high concentrations of ROS generated in response to prolonged AT_1 receptor activation [135]. In contrast to these results, Bhatt et al. demonstrated that augmented vascular oxidative stress caused an upregulation of the AT_1 receptor in human aortic smooth muscle cells and in arteries from 11 to 12 weeks old SHR [144]. Treatment of these cells for 24 hours with BSO or with H_2O_2 for 3 hours failed to induce a significant increase in AT_1 receptor mRNA. However, the combination of these oxidants elicited a twofold increase in the AT_1 receptor mRNA, as well as an increase in oxidative stress. These effects were prevented by the simultaneous treatment with catalase. Moreover, in the presence of p65 siRNA, the oxidant treatment did not increase the AT_1 receptor mRNA [144]. In SHR, but not in WKY rats, vascular oxidative stress was also increased, as evidenced by augmented H_2O_2 levels and was associated with increased vascular protein expression of NF-κB and AT_1 receptor and enhanced vasoconstriction in response to Ang II. Treatment with the antioxidant and NF-κB inhibitor pyrrolidine dithiocarbamate (PDTC) for 6–7 weeks reduced blood pressure, vascular H_2O_2 levels, p65 overexpression, AT_1 receptor expression and Ang II-induced vasoconstriction [144]. Together, these results indicate that under conditions of enhanced oxidative stress there is an upregulation of vascular AT_1 receptor that possibly involves ROS-induced NF-κB activation. Furthermore, the blood pressure lowering the effect of PDTC might have resulted from the normalization of vascular AT_1 receptor expression and prevention of exaggerated vasoconstriction to Ang II [144]. In addition to the stimulation of vascular AT_1 receptor expression, ROS may also enhance the vascular response to Ang II by increasing the functional availability of AT_1 receptors [134]. Under physiological conditions, AT_1 receptors are rapidly desensitized and internalized on stimulation by Ang II, thus avoiding an excessive responsiveness to Ang II [91, 134]. However, in pathological conditions such as arterial hypertension this mechanism might be compromised thus resulting in sustained activation of AT_1 receptors [134]. Bagi et al. tested the hypothesis that the acute exposure of resistance arteries to high intraluminal pressure increases the constriction to Ang II via a ROS-mediated improvement in the functional availability of AT_1 receptors [134]. In this study, performed in gracilis arterioles isolated from male Wistar rats, they observed that the transient exposure of the vessels to high intraluminal pressure (160 mmHg) significantly increased the constrictions to the second application of Ang II. This response was reduced by the AT_1 receptor antagonist telmisartan but not by the selective AT_2 receptor blocker PD123,319. In addition, preincubation of the arterioles with tiron or with PEG-catalase prevented the high intraluminal pressure-induced increase of arteriolar constrictions to the second application of Ang II [134]. Furthermore, the transient exposure to H_2O_2 resulted in augmented vessel constriction in response to the second application of Ang II. Overall, these findings indicate that ROS, especially H_2O_2, contribute to the high pressure-induced increase of the vasoconstriction to Ang II. This pathological feedforward mechanism may therefore lead to increased vascular resistance and amplify the hypertensive state [134].

The effects of oxidative stress on AT_1 receptor expression were also studied in macrophages, since Ang II is a proatherogenic molecule and both oxidative stress and AT_1 receptor expression are increased in hypercholesterolaemia [145–147]. In mouse peritoneal macrophages (MPMs) harvested from the E^0 mice, an animal model of severe hypercholesterolemia and atherosclerosis caused by apolipoprotein E deficiency, there was an age-dependent increase in lipid peroxide content accompanied by an age-dependent increase in the AT_1 receptor mRNA and protein expression [146]. MPMs obtained from 3.5 months old E^0 mice treated for 6 weeks with the potent antioxidant vitamin E had lower lipid peroxides concentration and reduced AT_1 receptor mRNA expression, compared to MPMs harvested from untreated E^0 mice [146]. To further demonstrate the role of oxidative stress in the regulation of macrophage AT_1 receptor, the GSH content was manipulated by the supplementation for 5 weeks with BSO or with L-2-oxothiazolidine-4-carboxylic acid (OTC), a precursor of GSH synthesis. It was observed that the reduction in macrophage GSH content was associated with increased AT_1

receptor mRNA expression, whereas the elevation of macrophage GSH levels caused a lower expression of AT_1 receptor mRNA. Similar effects of BSO and OTC on the AT_1 receptor mRNA expression were shown in MPMs obtained from control BALB/c mice [146]. Moreover, oxidized LDL, but not native LDL, caused a significant dose-dependent increase in AT_1 receptor mRNA and protein levels in MPMs from BALB/c mice [146]. These results suggest that oxidative stress enhances the proatherogenic effects of Ang II by inducing the overexpression of AT_1 receptors in arterial macrophages [146].

The regulation of AT_1 receptor by oxidative stress was also investigated in the central nervous system of male New Zealand white rabbits with chronic heart failure (CHF) [148]. It is well known that activation of the RAAS and of the sympathetic nervous system in CHF critically contributes to the development and progression of this pathological syndrome [148–151]. Previous studies have shown that CHF animals exhibit an upregulation of central AT_1 receptor and that the stimulation of sympathetic outflow by central Ang II treatment is mediated by oxidative stress via stimulation of NADPH oxidase-derived ROS production [148, 152–154]. Furthermore, NADPH oxidase-derived ROS in the rostral ventrolateral medulla (RVLM) are involved in the Ang II-induced pressor responses [155]. Therefore, Liu et al. evaluated the relationship between oxidative stress, antioxidant treatment and AT_1 receptor regulation in a neuronal cell line and in the RVLM of CHF rabbits. They observed that treatment of CATH.a cells with Ang II markedly increased the AT_1 receptor mRNA expression, NADPH oxidase activity and $O_2^{\bullet -}$ generation [148]. These effects on the AT_1 receptor expression and oxidative stress were inhibited by the AT_1 receptor antagonist losartan, apocynin and tempol, thus suggesting that there is a positive feedback mechanism whereby Ang II upregulates the AT_1 receptor expression via increased ROS production [148]. In the RVLM of CHF rabbits that received an intracerebroventricular infusion of tempol for 7 days AT_1 receptor mRNA and protein expression was significantly reduced when compared to vehicle-infused CHF rabbits. Furthermore, they also verified that the RVLM AP-1 binding activity that was previously shown to be increased in CHF rabbits, compared to sham rabbits, was decreased by the intracerebroventricular administration of tempol to CHF rabbits [148]. Collectively, these findings indicate that ROS play a major role in the central upregulation of AT_1 receptor expression in CHF.

Currently, there is a lack of studies regarding the regulation of AT_2 and MAS receptors by ROS. To our knowledge, only one study explored the impact of oxidative stress on AT_2 and MAS receptor expression. The evaluation of mRNA and protein expression of RAAS components in the renal cortex of 10-week-old male obese Zucker rats revealed that there was an increase in the AT_1 receptor accompanied by augmented AT_2 receptor expression and lower expression of MAS receptor, compared to lean Zucker rats [84]. In addition, obese rats also exhibited a greater diuretic and natriuretic response to the AT_2 receptor agonist CGP-42112A and a lower Ang (1–7)-mediated natriuresis than lean rats [84]. Treatment with tempol for 4 weeks further increased AT_2 receptor expression, as well as the AT_2 receptor-mediated diuretic and natriuretic responses in obese, but not lean rats. It also decreased AT_1 receptor expression and increased MAS receptor expression and the diuretic effect of Ang (1–7) in obese rats but not in lean Zucker rats [84]. In agreement with the *in vivo* data, cultured RPTCs obtained from 14-week-old obese Zucker rats showed higher protein expressions of AT_1 and AT_2 receptors, but decreased protein expression of MAS receptor when compared with cells from lean Zucker rats [84]. *In vitro* treatment with tempol for 24 hours reduced AT_1 receptor expression, increased the expression of MAS receptor and further increased the expression of AT_2 receptor expression [84]. These results suggest that in obesity the supplementation with antioxidants may correct the balance between natriuretic and antinatriuretic components of the renal RAAS [84].

Figures 7 and **8** summarize the effects of ROS on Ang receptors.

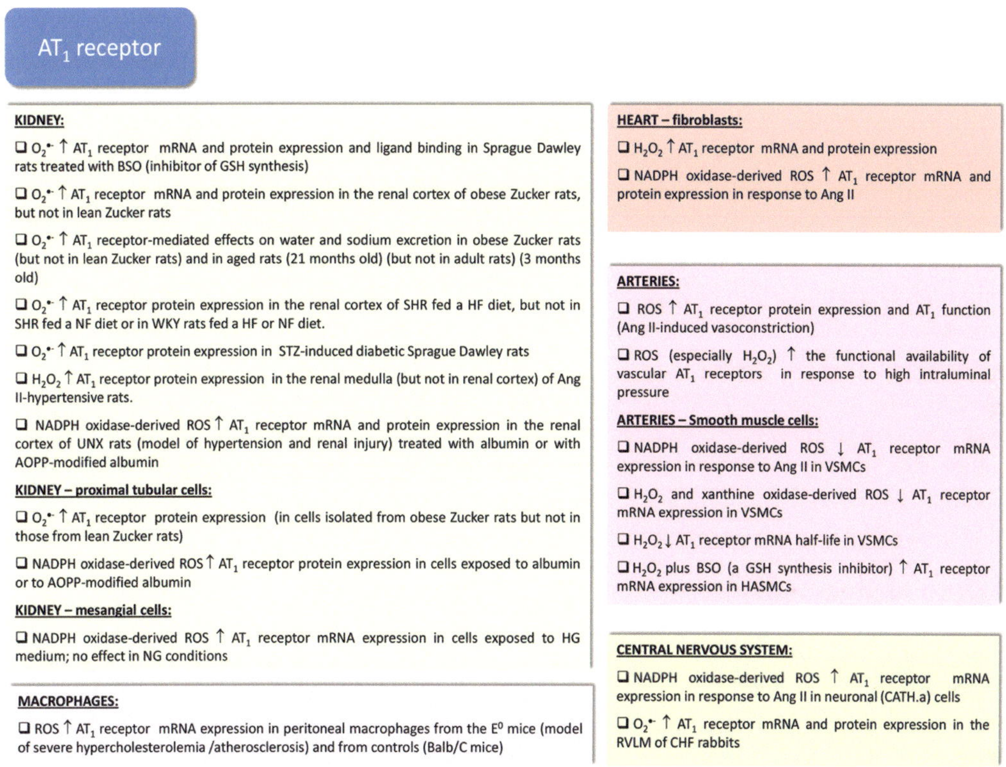

Figure 7. Regulation of AT_1 receptor by ROS. Ang II, angiotensin II; AOPP, advanced oxidation protein products; BSO, L-buthionine sulfoximine; CHF, chronic heart failure; GSH, glutathione (reduced form) HASMCs, human aortic smooth muscle cells; HF, high-fat; HG, high-glucose; NF, normal-fat; NG, normal-glucose; ROS, reactive oxygen species; RVLM, rostral ventrolateral medulla; SHR, Spontaneously Hypertensive Rat; STZ, streptozotocin; UNX, uninephrectomized; VSMCs, vascular smooth muscle cells; WKY, Wistar Kyoto.

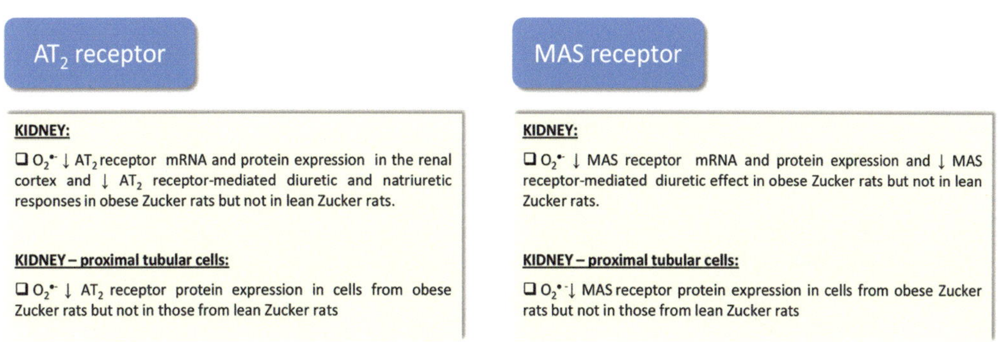

Figure 8. Regulation of AT_2 receptor and MAS receptor by ROS.

3. Conclusions

A plethora of experimental evidence indicates that ROS are important upstream regulators of the expression, secretion and/or activity of RAAS components. The majority of the referred studies suggests that under conditions of increased ROS availability there is an enhanced RAAS activation that is attenuated or abolished by treatment with antioxidants or inhibitors of ROS production. Nevertheless, there are also some reports of negative regulation of RAAS constituents by oxidant species that might serve as physiological protective mechanisms limiting the overactivation of this system and consequent deleterious effects on cell and organ functions. Importantly, in experimental pathological conditions associated with increased oxidative stress, such as arterial hypertension, obesity, diabetes, heart failure and renal disease, ROS have been shown to promote RAAS upregulation, thereby inducing a positive feedback loop that aggravates the cardiometabolic and/or renal injury. Currently, there is a lack of clinical studies evaluating the impact of the manipulation of ROS levels by antioxidants or inhibitors of ROS production on the expression, secretion and activity of RAAS components. The elucidation of the role of ROS in the regulation of RAAS in human physiological and pathological conditions, as well as the development of dual antioxidant-cardiovascular acting drugs and comparison of their clinical efficacy over currently used agents, would be important to improve the therapeutic strategies for many pathologies for which the blockade of RAAS appears to be insufficient to prevent disease-associated morbidity and mortality due to the existence of escape mechanisms.

Acknowledgements

Teresa Sousa was supported by the Portuguese Foundation for Science and Technology (FCT) (SFRH/BPD/112005/2015).

Abbreviations

AP-1	activator protein 1
AOPPs	advanced oxidation protein products
CYP11B2	aldosterone synthase
AT_1	Ang II type 1
AT_2	Ang II type 2
Ang (1–7)	angiotensin (1–7)
Ang (1–9)	angiotensin (1–9)
Ang III	angiotensin 2–8
Ang IV	angiotensin 3–8
ACE	angiotensin-converting enzyme
Ang I	angiotensin I
Ang II	angiotensin II
ACE2	angiotensin-converting enzyme 2
AGT	angiotensinogen
CHF	chronic heart failure
CD36	cluster of differentiation 36

http://dx.doi.org/10.5772/67016

cAMP	cyclic adenosine monophosphate
cGMP	cyclic guanosine monophosphate
COX-2	cyclooxygenase-2
DPI	diphenylene iodonium
$DJ\text{-}1^{-/-}$	DJ-1-knockout mice
eNOS	endothelial nitric oxide synthase
ET-1	endothelin 1
ELISA	enzyme-linked immunosorbent assay
ERK	extracellular signal-regulated kinase
FBN	Fischer 344 Brown Norway F1
GSH	glutathione
GPCR	G-protein-coupled receptor
GTP	guanosine triphosphate
HO-1	heme oxygenase-1
HDL	high-density lipoprotein
H_2O_2	hydrogen peroxide
$^{\bullet}OH$	hydroxyl radical
PVN	hypothalamic paraventricular nucleus
IRPTCs	immortalized renal proximal tubule cells
JNK	Jun Kinase
JG	juxtaglomerular
OTC	L-2-oxothiazolidine-4-carboxylic acid
BSO	L-buthionine sulfoximine
LpA	lipoprotein A
LDL	low-density lipoprotein
MR	mineralorticoid receptor
MAPK	mitogen activated protein kinase
MCP-1	monocyte chemoattractant protein 1
MPMs	mouse peritoneal macrophages
NAC	N-acetylcysteine
Nox	NADPH oxidase isoform
NADPH	nicotinamide adenine dinucleotide phosphate
NO	nitric oxide
NOS	nitric oxide synthase
Nrf2	Nuclear factor erythroid 2-related factor 2
NF-κB	nuclear factor kappa B
PMA	phorbol 12-myristate 13-acetate
PLC	phospholipase C
PCR	polymerase chain reaction
PA	primary aldosteronism
PRR	(pro)renin receptor (PRR)
PKA	protein kinase A
PKC	protein kinase C
PDTC	pyrrolidine dithiocarbamate
ROS	reactive oxygen species

RPTCs	renal proximal tubule cells
RAAS	renin-angiotensin-aldosterone system
RVLM	rostral ventrolateral medulla
SHR	spontaneously hypertensive rats
STZ	streptozotocin
SOD	superoxide dismutase
$O_2^{\bullet -}$	superoxide radical
TBARS	thiobarbituric reactive substances
TGFβ	transforming growth factor β
TNFα	tumor necrosis factor α
NOS1	type 1 nitric oxide synthase
UNX	unilateral nephrectomy
VSMCs	vascular smooth muscle cells
WB	Western Blot
WT	wild-type
WKY	Wistar-Kyoto
XOD	xanthine/xanthine oxidase
ZDF	Zucker Diabetic Fatty

Author details

Manuela Morato[1,2,3], Marta Reina-Couto[2,3,4], Dora Pinho[2,3], António Albino-Teixeira[2,3]* and Teresa Sousa[2,3]*

*Address all correspondence to: tsousa@med.up.pt and albinote@med.up.pt

1 Laboratory of Pharmacology, Department of Drug Sciences, Faculty of Pharmacy of Porto, University of Porto, Portugal

2 Department of Biomedicine—Unit of Pharmacology and Therapeutics, Faculty of Medicine, University of Porto, Porto, Portugal

3 MedInUP—Center for Drug Discovery and Innovative Medicines, University of Porto, Porto, Portugal

4 Intermediate Care Unit of Intensive Care Department, Centro Hospitalar de São João, EPE, Porto, Portugal

References

[1] Celerier J, Schmid G, Le Caer JP, et al. Characterization of a human angiotensinogen cleaved in its reactive center loop by a proteolytic activity from Chinese hamster ovary cells. J Biol Chem 2000;275(14):10648–54.

[2] Zhou A, Carrell RW, Murphy MP, et al. A redox switch in angiotensinogen modulates angiotensin release. Nature 2010;468(7320):108–11.

[3] Gimenez-Roqueplo AP, Celerier J, Schmid G, Corvol P, Jeunemaitre X. Role of cysteine residues in human angiotensinogen. Cys232 is required for angiotensinogen-pro major basic protein complex formation. J Biol Chem 1998;273(51):34480–7.

[4] Streatfeild-James RM, Williamson D, Pike RN, Tewksbury D, Carrell RW, Coughlin PB. Angiotensinogen cleavage by renin: importance of a structurally constrained N-terminus. FEBS Lett 1998;436(2):267–70.

[5] Wu C, Xu Y, Lu H, et al. Cys18-Cys137 disulfide bond in mouse angiotensinogen does not affect AngII-dependent functions in vivo. Hypertension 2015;65(4):800–5.

[6] Satou R, Kobori H, Katsurada A, Miyata K, Navar LG. Quantification of intact plasma AGT consisting of oxidized and reduced conformations using a modified ELISA. Am J Physiol Renal Physiol 2016. [Epub ahead from print]

[7] Hsieh TJ, Zhang SL, Filep JG, Tang SS, Ingelfinger JR, Chan JS. High glucose stimulates angiotensinogen gene expression via reactive oxygen species generation in rat kidney proximal tubular cells. Endocrinology 2002;143(8):2975–85.

[8] Hsieh TJ, Fustier P, Wei CC, et al. Reactive oxygen species blockade and action of insulin on expression of angiotensinogen gene in proximal tubular cells. J Endocrinol 2004;183(3):535–50.

[9] Brezniceanu ML, Wei CC, Zhang SL, et al. Transforming growth factor-beta 1 stimulates angiotensinogen gene expression in kidney proximal tubular cells. Kidney Int 2006;69 (11):1977–85.

[10] Abdo S, Shi Y, Otoukesh A, et al. Catalase overexpression prevents nuclear factor erythroid 2-related factor 2 stimulation of renal angiotensinogen gene expression, hypertension and kidney injury in diabetic mice. Diabetes 2014;63(10):3483–96.

[11] Brezniceanu ML, Liu F, Wei CC, et al. Catalase overexpression attenuates angiotensinogen expression and apoptosis in diabetic mice. Kidney Int 2007;71(9):912–23.

[12] Shi Y, Lo CS, Chenier I, et al. Overexpression of catalase prevents hypertension and tubulointerstitial fibrosis and normalization of renal angiotensin-converting enzyme-2 expression in Akita mice. Am J Physiol Renal Physiol 2013;304(11):F1335–46.

[13] Ohashi N, Urushihara M, Satou R, Kobori H. Glomerular angiotensinogen is induced in mesangial cells in diabetic rats via reactive oxygen species—ERK/JNK pathways. Hypertens Res 2010;33(11):1174–81.

[14] Xue H, Yuan P, Ni J, et al. H(2)S inhibits hyperglycemia-induced intrarenal renin-angiotensin system activation via attenuation of reactive oxygen species generation. PLoS One 2013;8(9):e74366.

[15] Miyata K, Ohashi N, Suzaki Y, Katsurada A, Kobori H. Sequential activation of the reactive oxygen species/angiotensinogen/renin-angiotensin system axis in renal injury of type 2 diabetic rats. Clin Exp Pharmacol Physiol 2008;35(8):922–7.

[16] Suzaki Y, Ozawa Y, Kobori H. Intrarenal oxidative stress and augmented angiotensinogen are precedent to renal injury in Zucker diabetic fatty rats. Int J Biol Sci. 2006;3(1):40–6. [Research Support, N.I.H., Extramural Research Support, Non-U.S. Gov't].

[17] Sousa T, Oliveira S, Afonso J, et al. Role of H(2)O(2) in hypertension, renin-angiotensin system activation and renal medullary disfunction caused by angiotensin II. Br J Pharmacol 2012;166(8):2386–401.

[18] Patinha D, Afonso J, Sousa T, Morato M, Albino-Teixeira A. Diabetes-induced increase of renal medullary hydrogen peroxide and urinary angiotensinogen is similar in normotensive and hypertensive rats. Life Sci 2014;108(2):71–9.

[19] Kobori H, Nishiyama A. Effects of tempol on renal angiotensinogen production in Dahl salt-sensitive rats. Biochem Biophys Res Commun 2004;315(3):746–50.

[20] Nakamura T, Kataoka K, Tokutomi Y, et al. Novel mechanism of salt-induced glomerular injury: critical role of eNOS and angiotensin II. J Hypertens 2011;29(8):1528–35.

[21] Chung S, Park CW, Shin SJ, et al. Tempol or candesartan prevents high-fat diet-induced hypertension and renal damage in spontaneously hypertensive rats. Nephrol Dial Transplant 2010;25(2):389–99.

[22] Anupama V, George M, Dhanesh SB, Chandran A, James J, Shivakumar K. Molecular mechanisms in H_2O_2-induced increase in AT1 receptor gene expression in cardiac fibroblasts: a role for endogenously generated Angiotensin II. J Mol Cell Cardiol 2016;97:295–305.

[23] Kurlak LO, Mistry HD, Cindrova-Davies T, Burton GJ, Broughton Pipkin F. Human placental renin-angiotensin system in normotensive and pre-eclamptic pregnancies at high altitude and after acute hypoxia-reoxygenation insult. J Physiol 2016;594(5):1327–40.

[24] Okada S, Kozuka C, Masuzaki H, et al. Adipose tissue-specific dysregulation of angiotensinogen by oxidative stress in obesity. Metabolism 2010;59(9):1241–51.

[25] Correia-Costa L, Morato M, Sousa T, et al. Urinary fibrogenic cytokines ET-1 and TGF-beta1 are associated with urinary angiotensinogen levels in obese children. Pediatr Nephrol 2016;31(3):455–64.

[26] Castrop H, Hocherl K, Kurtz A, Schweda F, Todorov V, Wagner C. Physiology of kidney renin. Physiol Rev 2010;90(2):607–73.

[27] Hackenthal E, Paul M, Ganten D, Taugner R. Morphology, physiology and molecular biology of renin secretion. Physiol Rev 1990;70(4):1067–116.

[28] Putnam K, Shoemaker R, Yiannikouris F, Cassis LA. The renin-angiotensin system: a target of and contributor to dyslipidemias, altered glucose homeostasis and hypertension of the metabolic syndrome. Am J Physiol Heart Circ Physiol 2012;302(6):H1219–30.

[29] Verdecchia P, Angeli F, Mazzotta G, Gentile G, Reboldi G. The renin angiotensin system in the development of cardiovascular disease: role of aliskiren in risk reduction. Vasc Health Risk Manag 2008;4(5):971–81.

[30] Friis UG, Madsen K, Stubbe J, et al. Regulation of renin secretion by renal juxtaglomerular cells. Pflugers Arch 2013;465(1):25–37.

[31] Kobori H, Nangaku M, Navar LG, Nishiyama A. The intrarenal renin-angiotensin system: from physiology to the pathobiology of hypertension and kidney disease. Pharmacol Rev 2007;59(3):251–87.

[32] Kurtz A. Control of renin synthesis and secretion. Am J Hypertens 2012;25(8):839–47.

[33] Jan Danser AH, Batenburg WW, van Esch JH. Prorenin and the (pro)renin receptor–an update. Nephrol Dial Transplant 2007;22(5):1288–92.

[34] Nguyen G. Renin, (pro)renin and receptor: an update. Clin Sci (Lond) 2011;120(5):169–78.

[35] Peters J, Farrenkopf R, Clausmeyer S, et al. Functional significance of prorenin internalization in the rat heart. Circ Res 2002;90(10):1135–41.

[36] Galle J, Heinloth A, Schwedler S, Wanner C. Effect of HDL and atherogenic lipoproteins on formation of O2- and renin release in juxtaglomerular cells. Kidney Int 1997;51(1): 253–60.

[37] Galle J, Herzog C, Schollmeyer P, Wanner C. Oxygen-derived radicals stimulate renin release of isolated juxtaglomerular cells. FEBS Lett 1994;351(3):314–6.

[38] Galle J, Stunz P, Schollmeyer P, Wanner C. Oxidized LDL and lipoprotein(a) stimulate renin release of juxtaglomerular cells. Kidney Int 1995;47(1):45–52.

[39] Soran H, Schofield JD, Durrington PN. Antioxidant properties of HDL. Front Pharmacol 2015;6:222.

[40] Mendez M. Superoxide and hydrogen peroxide acutely stimulates renin release from mouse juxtaglomerular (JG) cells. Hypertension 2011;58(5):e98.

[41] Mendez M. Abstract 489: hydrogen peroxide stimulates renin release from mouse juxtaglomerular cells by enhancing cAMP. Hypertension 2013;62(Suppl 1):A489–A.

[42] Mendez M. Renal cortical hydrogen peroxide (H_2O_2) stimulates renin release from juxtaglomerular (JG) cells and increases blood pressure: role of JG cell NOX4. The FASEB 2016;30(1):1218.7.

[43] Mendez M. Abstract P084: oxidative stress preconditioning is required for leptin to stimulate renin release from mouse juxtaglomerular cells. Hypertension 2015;66(Suppl 1):AP084–AP.

[44] Bravo PE, Morse S, Borne DM, Aguilar EA, Reisin E. Leptin and hypertension in obesity. Vasc Health Risk Manag 2006;2(2):163–9.

[45] Villarreal D, Reams G, Freeman RH, Taraben A. Renal effects of leptin in normotensive, hypertensive and obese rats. Am J Physiol 1998;275(6 Pt 2):R2056–60.

[46] Correia-Costa L, Sousa T, Morato M, et al. Oxidative stress and nitric oxide are increased in obese children and correlate with cardiometabolic risk and renal function. Br J Nutr 2016;116(5):805–15.

[47] Le Lay S, Simard G, Martinez MC, Andriantsitohaina R. Oxidative stress and metabolic pathologies: from an adipocentric point of view. Oxid Med Cell Longev 2014;2014:908539.

[48] Sousa T, Afonso J, Carvalho F, Albino-Teixeira A. Lipid peroxidation and antioxidants in arterial hypertension. In: Catala A, editor. Lipid peroxidation. Rijeka, Croatia: InTech; 2012: 345–92.

[49] Sousa T, Pinho D, Morato M, et al. Role of superoxide and hydrogen peroxide in hypertension induced by an antagonist of adenosine receptors. Eur J Pharmacol 2008;588(2–3):267–76.

[50] Kuo JJ, Jones OB, Hall JE. Chronic cardiovascular and renal actions of leptin during hyperinsulinemia. Am J Physiol Regul Integr Comp Physiol 2003;284(4):R1037–42.

[51] Adamczak M, Kokot F, Wiecek A. Relationship between plasma renin profile and leptinaemia in patients with essential hypertension. J Hum Hypertens 2000;14(8):503–9.

[52] Uckaya G, Ozata M, Sonmez A, et al. Plasma leptin levels strongly correlate with plasma renin activity in patients with essential hypertension. Horm Metab Res 1999;31(7):435–8.

[53] Muller MW, Todorov V, Kramer BK, Kurtz A. Angiotensin II inhibits renin gene transcription via the protein kinase C pathway. Pflugers Arch 2002;444(4):499–505.

[54] Itani H, Liu X, Sarsour EH, et al. Regulation of renin gene expression by oxidative stress. Hypertension 2009;53(6):1070–6.

[55] Sriramula S, Haque M, Majid DS, Francis J. Involvement of tumor necrosis factor-alpha in angiotensin II-mediated effects on salt appetite, hypertension and cardiac hypertrophy. Hypertension 2008;51(5):1345–51.

[56] Todorov V, Muller M, Schweda F, Kurtz A. Tumor necrosis factor-alpha inhibits renin gene expression. Am J Physiol Regul Integr Comp Physiol 2002;283(5):R1046–51.

[57] De Keulenaer GW, Alexander RW, Ushio-Fukai M, Ishizaka N, Griendling KK. Tumour necrosis factor alpha activates a p22phox-based NADH oxidase in vascular smooth muscle. Biochem J 1998;329 (Pt 3):653–7.

[58] Morgan MJ, Liu ZG. Reactive oxygen species in TNFalpha-induced signaling and cell death. Mol Cells 2010;30(1):1–12.

[59] Paliege A, Pasumarthy A, Mizel D, Yang T, Schnermann J, Bachmann S. Effect of apocynin treatment on renal expression of COX-2, NOS1 and renin in Wistar-Kyoto and spontaneously hypertensive rats. Am J Physiol Regul Integr Comp Physiol 2006;290(3): R694–700.

[60] Neubauer B, Machura K, Kettl R, Lopez ML, Friebe A, Kurtz A. Endothelium-derived nitric oxide supports renin cell recruitment through the nitric oxide-sensitive guanylate cyclase pathway. Hypertension 2013;61(2):400–7.

[61] Sayago CM, Beierwaltes WH. Nitric oxide synthase and cGMP-mediated stimulation of renin secretion. Am J Physiol Regul Integr Comp Physiol 2001;281(4):R1146–51.

[62] Welch WJ, Mendonca M, Blau J, et al. Antihypertensive response to prolonged tempol in the spontaneously hypertensive rat. Kidney Int 2005;68(1):179–87.

[63] Chen YF, Cowley AW, Jr., Zou AP. Increased H(2)O(2) counteracts the vasodilator and natriuretic effects of superoxide dismutation by tempol in renal medulla. Am J Physiol Regul Integr Comp Physiol 2003;285(4):R827–33.

[64] Siragy HM, Huang J. Renal (pro)renin receptor upregulation in diabetic rats through enhanced angiotensin AT1 receptor and NADPH oxidase activity. Exp Physiol 2008;93 (5):709–14.

[65] Cuevas S, Zhang Y, Yang Y, et al. Role of renal DJ-1 in the pathogenesis of hypertension associated with increased reactive oxygen species production. Hypertension 2012;59 (2):446–52.

[66] Lee DY, Kim HS, Won KJ, et al. DJ-1 regulates the expression of renal (pro)renin receptor via reactive oxygen species-mediated epigenetic modification. Biochim Biophys Acta 2015;1850(2):426–34.

[67] Niki T, Takahashi-Niki K, Taira T, Iguchi-Ariga SMM, Ariga H. DJBP: A novel DJ-1-binding protein, negatively regulates the androgen receptor by recruiting histone deacetylase complex and DJ-1 antagonizes this inhibition by abrogation of this complex. Mol Cancer Res 2003;1(4):247–61.

[68] Opsahl JA, Hjornevik LV, Bull VH, et al. Increased interaction between DJ-1 and the Mi-2/ nucleosome remodelling and deacetylase complex during cellular stress. Proteomics 2010;10(7):1494–504.

[69] Wilson MA. The role of cysteine oxidation in DJ-1 function and dysfunction. Antioxid Redox Signal 2011;15(1):111–22.

[70] Lanzillo JJ, Stevens J, Dasarathy Y, Yotsumoto H, Fanburg BL. Angiotensin-converting enzyme from human tissues. Physicochemical, catalytic and immunological properties. J Biol Chem 1985;260(28):14938–44.

[71] Jaspard E, Wei L, Alhenc-Gelas F. Differences in the properties and enzymatic specificities of the two active sites of angiotensin I-converting enzyme (kininase II). Studies with bradykinin and other natural peptides. J Biol Chem 1993;268(13):9496–503.

[72] Donoghue M, Hsieh F, Baronas E, et al. A novel angiotensin-converting enzyme-related carboxypeptidase (ACE2) converts angiotensin I to angiotensin 1–9. Circ Res 2000;87(5): E1–9.

[73] Tipnis SR, Hooper NM, Hyde R, Karran E, Christie G, Turner AJ. A human homolog of angiotensin-converting enzyme. Cloning and functional expression as a captopril-insensitive carboxypeptidase. J Biol Chem 2000;275(43):33238–43.

[74] Rice GI, Thomas DA, Grant PJ, Turner AJ, Hooper NM. Evaluation of angiotensin-converting enzyme (ACE), its homologue ACE2 and neprilysin in angiotensin peptide metabolism. Biochem J 2004;383(Pt 1):45–51.

[75] Vickers C, Hales P, Kaushik V, et al. Hydrolysis of biological peptides by human angiotensin-converting enzyme-related carboxypeptidase. J Biol Chem 2002;277(17): 14838–43.

[76] Bader M. ACE2, angiotensin-(1–7) and Mas: the other side of the coin. Pflugers Arch 2013;465(1):79-85.

[77] Tominaga M, Song GB, Ikemoto F, Yamamoto K. Effect of oxidation on the activity of angiotensin converting enzyme in the rat kidney, heart and brain. Clin Exp Hypertens A 1988;10(6):1271–8.

[78] Chen X, Catravas JD. Neutrophil-mediated endothelial angiotensin-converting enzyme dysfunction: role of oxygen-derived free radicals. Am J Physiol 1993;265(3 Pt 1):L243–9.

[79] Michel B, Grima M, Nirina LB, et al. Inhibitory effect of reactive oxygen species on angiotensin I-converting enzyme (kininase II). Clin Exp Pharmacol Physiol 2001;28 (3):212–8.

[80] Kumar KV, Das UN. Effect of cis-unsaturated fatty acids, prostaglandins and free radicals on angiotensin-converting enzyme activity in vitro. Proc Soc Exp Biol Med 1997;214 (4):374–9.

[81] Mu X, He K, Sun H, et al. Hydrogen peroxide induces overexpression of angiotensin-converting enzyme in human umbilical vein endothelial cells. Free Radic Res 2013;47 (2):116–22.

[82] Cao W, Zhou QG, Nie J, et al. Albumin overload activates intrarenal renin-angiotensin system through protein kinase C and NADPH oxidase-dependent pathway. J Hypertens 2011;29(7):1411–21.

[83] Cao W, Xu J, Zhou ZM, Wang GB, Hou FF, Nie J. Advanced oxidation protein products activate intrarenal renin-angiotensin system via a CD36-mediated, redox-dependent pathway. Antioxid Redox Signal 2013;18(1):19–35.

[84] Luo H, Wang X, Chen C, et al. Oxidative stress causes imbalance of renal renin angiotensin system (RAS) components and hypertension in obese Zucker rats. J Am Heart Assoc 2015;4(2): pii: e001559.

[85] Su Q, Qin DN, Wang FX, et al. Inhibition of reactive oxygen species in hypothalamic paraventricular nucleus attenuates the renin-angiotensin system and proinflammatory cytokines in hypertension. Toxicol Appl Pharmacol 2014;276(2):115–20.

[86] Zhang M, Qin DN, Suo YP, et al. Endogenous hydrogen peroxide in the hypothalamic paraventricular nucleus regulates neurohormonal excitation in high salt-induced hypertension. Toxicol Lett 2015;235(3):206–15.

[87] Pernomian L, Gomes MS, Restini CB, de Oliveira AM. MAS-mediated antioxidant effects restore the functionality of angiotensin converting enzyme 2-angiotensin-(1–7)-MAS axis in diabetic rat carotid. Biomed Res Int 2014;2014:640329.

[88] Becari C, Oliveira EB, Salgado MC. Alternative pathways for angiotensin II generation in the cardiovascular system. Braz J Med Biol Res 2011;44(9):914–9.

[89] Kramkowski K, Mogielnicki A, Buczko W. The physiological significance of the alternative pathways of angiotensin II production. J Physiol Pharmacol 2006;57(4):529–39.

[90] Balakumar P, Jagadeesh G. A century old renin-angiotensin system still grows with endless possibilities: AT1 receptor signaling cascades in cardiovascular physiopathology. Cell Signal 2014;26(10):2147–60.

[91] Karnik SS, Unal H, Kemp JR, et al. International Union of Basic and Clinical Pharmacology. XCIX. Angiotensin Receptors: interpreters of pathophysiological angiotensinergic stimuli [corrected]. Pharmacol Rev 2015;67(4):754–819.

[92] Singh KD, Karnik SS. Angiotensin Receptors: Structure, Function, Signaling and Clinical Applications. J Cell Signal 2016;1(2): pii: 111.

[93] Garrido AM, Griendling KK. NADPH oxidases and angiotensin II receptor signaling. Mol Cell Endocrinol 2009;302(2):148–58.

[94] Gorin Y, Block K. Nox4 and diabetic nephropathy: with a friend like this, who needs enemies? Free Radic Biol Med 2013;61:130–42.

[95] Grote K, Drexler H, Schieffer B. Renin-angiotensin system and atherosclerosis. Nephrol Dial Transplant 2004;19(4):770–3.

[96] Hsueh WA, Wyne K. Renin-Angiotensin-aldosterone system in diabetes and hypertension. J Clin Hypertens (Greenwich) 2011;13(4):224–37.

[97] Munzel T, Gori T, Keaney JF, Jr., Maack C, Daiber A. Pathophysiological role of oxidative stress in systolic and diastolic heart failure and its therapeutic implications. Eur Heart J 2015;36(38):2555–64.

[98] Nguyen Dinh Cat A, Touyz RM. Cell signaling of angiotensin II on vascular tone: novel mechanisms. Curr Hypertens Rep 2011;13(2):122–8.

[99] Sedeek M, Hebert RL, Kennedy CR, Burns KD, Touyz RM. Molecular mechanisms of hypertension: role of Nox family NADPH oxidases. Curr Opin Nephrol Hypertens 2009;18(2):122–7.

[100] van Thiel BS, van der Pluijm I, te Riet L, Essers J, Danser AH. The renin-angiotensin system and its involvement in vascular disease. Eur J Pharmacol 2015;763(Pt A):3–14.

[101] Santos RA. Angiotensin-(1–7). Hypertension 2014;63(6):1138–47.

[102] Te Riet L, van Esch JH, Roks AJ, van den Meiracker AH, Danser AH. Hypertension: renin-angiotensin-aldosterone system alterations. Circ Res 2015;116(6):960–75.

[103] DelliPizzi AM, Hilchey SD, Bell-Quilley CP. Natriuretic action of angiotensin(1–7). Br J Pharmacol 1994;111(1):1–3.

[104] Iusuf D, Henning RH, van Gilst WH, Roks AJ. Angiotensin-(1–7): pharmacological properties and pharmacotherapeutic perspectives. Eur J Pharmacol 2008;585(2–3):303–12.

[105] Santos SH, Giani JF, Burghi V, et al. Oral administration of angiotensin-(1–7) ameliorates type 2 diabetes in rats. J Mol Med (Berl) 2014;92(3):255–65.

[106] Liu C, Lv XH, Li HX, et al. Angiotensin-(1–7) suppresses oxidative stress and improves glucose uptake via Mas receptor in adipocytes. Acta Diabetol 2012;49(4):291–9.

[107] Simoes ESAC, Teixeira MM. ACE inhibition, ACE2 and angiotensin-(1–7) axis in kidney and cardiac inflammation and fibrosis. Pharmacol Res 2016;107:154–62.

[108] Zhang F, Liu C, Wang L, Cao X, Wang YY, Yang JK. Antioxidant effect of angiotensin (17) in the protection of pancreatic beta cell function. Mol Med Rep 2016;14(3):1963–9.

[109] Roson MI, Della Penna SL, Cao G, et al. Different protective actions of losartan and tempol on the renal inflammatory response to acute sodium overload. J Cell Physiol 2010;224(1):41–8.

[110] Lavrentyev EN, Malik KU. High glucose-induced Nox1-derived superoxides downregulate PKC-betaII, which subsequently decreases ACE2 expression and ANG(1–7) formation in rat VSMCs. Am J Physiol Heart Circ Physiol 2009;296(1):H106–18.

[111] Tomaschitz A, Pilz S, Ritz E, Obermayer-Pietsch B, Pieber TR. Aldosterone and arterial hypertension. Nat Rev Endocrinol 2010;6(2):83–93.

[112] Lisurek M, Bernhardt R. Modulation of aldosterone and cortisol synthesis on the molecular level. Mol Cell Endocrinol 2004;215(1–2):149–59.

[113] Milliez P, Girerd X, Plouin PF, Blacher J, Safar ME, Mourad JJ. Evidence for an increased rate of cardiovascular events in patients with primary aldosteronism. J Am Coll Cardiol 2005;45(8):1243–8.

[114] Stehr CB, Mellado R, Ocaranza MP, et al. Increased levels of oxidative stress, subclinical inflammation and myocardial fibrosis markers in primary aldosteronism patients. J Hypertens 2010;28(10):2120–6.

[115] Rajamohan SB, Raghuraman G, Prabhakar NR, Kumar GK. NADPH oxidase-derived H (2)O(2) contributes to angiotensin II-induced aldosterone synthesis in human and rat adrenal cortical cells. Antioxid Redox Signal 2012;17(3):445–59.

[116] Botros FT, Schwartzman ML, Stier CT, Jr., Goodman AI, Abraham NG. Increase in heme oxygenase-1 levels ameliorates renovascular hypertension. Kidney Int 2005;68(6):2745–55.

[117] Otterbein LE, Foresti R, Motterlini R. Heme oxygenase-1 and carbon monoxide in the heart: the balancing act between danger signaling and pro-survival. Circ Res 2016;118 (12):1940–59.

[118] Parfenova H, Leffler CW, Basuroy S, Liu J, Fedinec AL. Antioxidant roles of heme oxygenase, carbon monoxide and bilirubin in cerebral circulation during seizures. J Cereb Blood Flow Metab 2012;32(6):1024–34.

[119] Ehrhart-Bornstein M, Lamounier-Zepter V, Schraven A, et al. Human adipocytes secrete mineralocorticoid-releasing factors. Proc Natl Acad Sci USA 2003;100(24):14211–6.

[120] Huby AC, Antonova G, Groenendyk J, et al. Adipocyte-derived hormone leptin is a direct regulator of aldosterone secretion, which promotes endothelial dysfunction and cardiac fibrosis. Circulation 2015;132(22):2134–45.

[121] El-Gharbawy AH, Nadig VS, Kotchen JM, et al. Arterial pressure, left ventricular mass and aldosterone in essential hypertension. Hypertension 2001;37(3):845–50.

[122] Thakur V, Richards R, Reisin E. Obesity, hypertension and the heart. Am J Med Sci 2001;321(4):242–8.

[123] Muller-Fielitz H, Lau M, Johren O, Stellmacher F, Schwaninger M, Raasch W. Blood pressure response to angiotensin II is enhanced in obese Zucker rats and is attributed to an aldosterone-dependent mechanism. Br J Pharmacol 2012;166(8):2417–29.

[124] Lamounier-Zepter V, Ehrhart-Bornstein M, Bornstein SR. Mineralocorticoid-stimulating activity of adipose tissue. Best Pract Res Clin Endocrinol Metab 2005;19(4):567–75.

[125] Shimizu MH, Coimbra TM, de Araujo M, Menezes LF, Seguro AC. N-acetylcysteine attenuates the progression of chronic renal failure. Kidney Int 2005;68(5):2208–17.

[126] Nagase M. Activation of the aldosterone/mineralocorticoid receptor system in chronic kidney disease and metabolic syndrome. Clin Exp Nephrol 2010;14(4):303–14.

[127] Munoz-Durango N, Fuentes CA, Castillo AE, et al. Role of the Renin-Angiotensin-Aldosterone System beyond Blood Pressure Regulation: Molecular and Cellular Mechanisms Involved in End-Organ Damage during Arterial Hypertension. Int J Mol Sci 2016;17(7): pii: E797.

[128] Rafiq K, Hitomi H, Nakano D, Nishiyama A. Pathophysiological roles of aldosterone and mineralocorticoid receptor in the kidney. J Pharmacol Sci 2011;115(1):1–7.

[129] Kitada K, Nakano D, Liu Y, et al. Oxidative stress-induced glomerular mineralocorticoid receptor activation limits the benefit of salt reduction in Dahl salt-sensitive rats. PLoS One 2012;7(7):e41896.

[130] Guimaraes S, Carneiro C, Brandao F, Pinheiro H, Albino-Teixeira A, Moura D. A pharmacological differentiation between postjunctional (AT1A) and prejunctional (AT1B) angiotensin II receptors in the rabbit aorta. Naunyn Schmiedebergs Arch Pharmacol 2004;370(4):262–9.

[131] Guimaraes S, Pinheiro H. Functional evidence that in the cardiovascular system AT1 angiotensin II receptors are AT1B prejunctionally and AT1A postjunctionally. Cardiovasc Res 2005;67(2):208–15.

[132] Morato M, Pinho D, Sousa T, Guimaraes S, Moura D, Albino-Teixeira A. Pre- and postjunctional effects of angiotensin II in hypertension due to adenosine receptor blockade. Eur J Pharmacol 2006;531(1–3):209–16.

[133] Nap A, Balt JC, Mathy MJ, Pfaffendorf M, van Zwieten PA. Different AT1 Receptor Subtypes at Pre- and Postjunctional Sites: AT1A versus AT1B Receptors. J Cardiovasc Pharmacol 2004;43(1):14–20.

[134] Bagi Z, Erdei N, Koller A. High intraluminal pressure via H2O2 upregulates arteriolar constrictions to angiotensin II by increasing the functional availability of AT1 receptors. Am J Physiol Heart Circ Physiol 2008;295(2):H835–41.

[135] Nickenig G, Strehlow K, Baumer AT, et al. Negative feedback regulation of reactive oxygen species on AT1 receptor gene expression. Br J Pharmacol 2000;131(4):795–803.

[136] Dhande I, Ma W, Hussain T. Angiotensin AT2 receptor stimulation is anti-inflammatory in lipopolysaccharide-activated THP-1 macrophages via increased interleukin-10 production. Hypertens Res 2015;38(1):21–9.

[137] Moltzer E, Verkuil AV, van Veghel R, Danser AH, van Esch JH. Effects of angiotensin metabolites in the coronary vascular bed of the spontaneously hypertensive rat: loss of angiotensin II type 2 receptor-mediated vasodilation. Hypertension 2010;55(2):516–22.

[138] Banday AA, Lokhandwala MF. Oxidative stress-induced renal angiotensin AT1 receptor upregulation causes increased stimulation of sodium transporters and hypertension. Am J Physiol Renal Physiol 2008;295(3):F698–706.

[139] Banday AA, Lokhandwala MF. Oxidative stress causes renal angiotensin II type 1 receptor upregulation, Na+/H+ exchanger 3 overstimulation and hypertension. Hypertension 2011;57(3):452–9.

[140] Chugh G, Lokhandwala MF, Asghar M. Oxidative stress alters renal D1 and AT1 receptor functions and increases blood pressure in old rats. Am J Physiol Renal Physiol 2011;300(1):F133–8.

[141] Kuo CW, Shen CJ, Tung YT, et al. Extracellular superoxide dismutase ameliorates streptozotocin-induced rat diabetic nephropathy via inhibiting the ROS/ERK1/2 signaling. Life Sci 2015;135:77–86.

[142] Vaziri ND, Wang XQ, Oveisi F, Rad B. Induction of oxidative stress by glutathione depletion causes severe hypertension in normal rats. Hypertension 2000;36(1):142–6.

[143] Zhang Y, Tang ZH, Ren Z, et al. Hydrogen sulfide, the next potent preventive and therapeutic agent in aging and age-associated diseases. Mol Cell Biol 2013;33(6):1104–13.

[144] Bhatt SR, Lokhandwala MF, Banday AA. Vascular oxidative stress upregulates angiotensin II type I receptors via mechanisms involving nuclear factor kappa B. Clin Exp Hypertens 2014;36(6):367–73.

[145] Ferroni P, Basili S, Falco A, Davi G. Oxidant stress and platelet activation in hypercholesterolemia. Antioxid Redox Signal 2004;6(4):747–56.

[146] Keidar S, Heinrich R, Kaplan M, Aviram M. Oxidative stress increases the expression of the angiotensin-II receptor type 1 in mouse peritoneal macrophages. J Renin Angiotensin Aldosterone Syst 2002;3(1):24–30.

[147] Yang BC, Phillips MI, Mohuczy D, et al. Increased angiotensin II type 1 receptor expression in hypercholesterolemic atherosclerosis in rabbits. Arterioscler Thromb Vasc Biol 1998;18(9):1433–9.

[148] Liu D, Gao L, Roy SK, Cornish KG, Zucker IH. Role of oxidant stress on AT1 receptor expression in neurons of rabbits with heart failure and in cultured neurons. Circ Res 2008;103(2):186–93.

[149] Goldsmith SR. Angiotensin II and sympathoactivation in heart failure. J Card Fail 1999;5 (2):139–45.

[150] Goldsmith SR, Garr M, McLaurin M. Regulation of regional norepinephrine spillover in heart failure: the effect of angiotensin II and beta-adrenergic agonists in the forearm circulation. J Card Fail 1998;4(4):305–10.

[151] Zucker IH, Xiao L, Haack KK. The central renin-angiotensin system and sympathetic nerve activity in chronic heart failure. Clin Sci (Lond) 2014;126(10):695–706.

[152] Campese VM, Shaohua Y, Huiquin Z. Oxidative stress mediates angiotensin II-dependent stimulation of sympathetic nerve activity. Hypertension 2005;46(3):533–9.

[153] Gao L, Wang W, Li YL, et al. Sympathoexcitation by central ANG II: roles for AT1 receptor upregulation and NAD(P)H oxidase in RVLM. Am J Physiol Heart Circ Physiol 2005;288(5):H2271–9.

[154] Liu D, Gao L, Roy SK, Cornish KG, Zucker IH. Neuronal angiotensin II type 1 receptor upregulation in heart failure: activation of activator protein 1 and Jun N-terminal kinase. Circ Res 2006;99(9):1004–11.

[155] Chan SH, Hsu KS, Huang CC, Wang LL, Ou CC, Chan JY. NADPH oxidase-derived superoxide anion mediates angiotensin II-induced pressor effect via activation of p38 mitogen-activated protein kinase in the rostral ventrolateral medulla. Circ Res 2005;97 (8):772–80.

Chapter 9

Current Research of the Renin-Angiotensin System Effect on Stem Cell Therapy

Elham Ahmadian, Aziz Eftekhari and
Ahmad Yari Khosroushahi

Additional information is available at the end of the chapter

http://dx.doi.org/10.5772/67726

Abstract

The renin-angiotensin system (RAS) is a chief regulator of the cardiovascular system and body fluid homeostasis. Stem/progenitor cell therapy has pointed towards a novel tool for medical and therapeutic intervention. In addition to the physiological and pathological role of the RAS and its pharmacological inhibitors, the proliferation, differentiation in stem cells is mediated through various cell-signalling pathways. This book chapter reviews the new role of RAS components, distinct from other common roles by considering its regulating impact on the several signalling pathways involved in different body tissues, as well as in stem cell therapy.

Keywords: stem cell, progenitor cell, renin-angiotensin system, pancreatic stem cells, cardiac stem cells

1. Introduction

The concept that the renin-angiotensin system (RAS) is involved in the regulation of stem (progenitor) cell function is novel. This is beyond the conventional notion of the RAS acting as a potent vasoconstrictor responsible for blood pressure regulation and body fluid homeostasis. The expression of RAS components during human embryonic development has been addressed in the literature. The existence of RAS components in different organs and tissues suggests the presence of local RAS in addition to the circulating common RAS, which has paracrine effects mediating stem (progenitor) cell function. Moreover, recent evidence has shown the expression of major RAS components such as angiotensinogen, renin, angiotensin-converting enzyme (ACE), angiotensin receptors type 1 and 2 and angiotensin-(1–7) during growth, proliferation and differentiation of stem cells. Improvement of the stem cell functionality and making them ideal candidates in different kinds of disorders has been a new research field in the last decade. Meanwhile, the effect of RAS on stem cell growth, proliferation and function is an emerging attempt among researchers. Ang II receptor activation increases the proliferation of several progenitor cells, such as mouse bone marrow-derived stem cells and human cord blood cells. Accordingly, manipulation of the RAS may alter and/or have beneficial effects on the efficacy of stem cell therapy.

2. Stem cells

The term stem cell stands for the population of immature precursor cells, which are able to renew themselves and be the source of de novo replacement for many body tissues. Stem cells are classified into two main groups: embryonic stem cells (ESCs) and adult stem cells. ESCs can be obtained from the inner cell mass of the embryonal blastocyst. Although they are easily achieved, some disadvantages restrict their application. Adult stem cells such as mesenchymal and haematopoietic stem cells (HSCs) are obtained from mature tissues. Due to their plasticity, adult stem cells produce cell lineage different from their original organ. Thus, adult stem cells seem to be an appropriate candidate for organ regeneration in different kinds of diseases or lost/damaged organs. **Table 1** represents the main stem cell and their advantages and disadvantages.

Stem cell type	Origin	Advantages	Disadvantages
Embryonic stem cell	Blastocyst stage of an embryo	- High expansion - Pluripotent	- Ethical objection - Risk of rejection - Risk of teratocarcinoma
Adult stem cell	Mature tissue	- Easily obtained - No ethical objection - High compatibility	- Lack of specific identification markers

Table 1. Main stem cell and their advantages and disadvantages.

3. The RAS and ESCs

ESCs are pluripotent cells capable of differentiation into different cells such as cardiomyocytes, and endothelial cells have been considered as a source of regenerative medicine [1]. For instance, ESC-derived endothelial cells have therapeutic effects via the increment of angiogenesis and heart functionality [2]. PI3/Akt-signalling pathway has been shown to be linked with human ESC-derived cardiomyocyte proliferation in vitro [3]. RAS stimulation activates PI3/AKT pathway, while the inhibition of RAS increases Akt phosphorylation [4], which might influence the proliferation of ESCs. High survival rate after transplantation is another main, noteworthy issue about ESCs [5].

RAS is a novel regulatory candidate, which controls the development of ESCs into different cell types. It has been reported that the expression AT1 receptors were detected in an early stage of human ESCs differentiation. Since the addition of Ang II results in the phosphorylation of extracellular signal-regulated kinase (ERK) 1/2 and Jun N-terminal (JNK) 1/2, this peptide is capable of acting as signalling molecules and thus it could regulate differentiation [6]. Moreover, Ang II has been shown to increase glucose uptake in ESCs [7] and induce mitogenic effect, possibly through protein kinase C and mitogen-activated protein kinase (MAPK)-signalling pathways. Interestingly, exposure to a high glucose niche in the presence of Ang II has been shown to produce a synergistic impact on ESC proliferation [8].

4. The RAS and mesenchymal stem cells

Mesenchymal stem cells (MSCs) as multipotent cells are mainly found in bone marrow and adipose tissue and can differentiate into various cell types [9]. Simple isolation, high immune prevalence and angiogenic-inducing properties have made MSCs suitable candidates for stem cell therapy of different kinds of diseases [10]. Besides, these MSCs exert paracrine effects causing the modulation of a large number of cellular responses, such as survival, proliferation, migration and gene expression [11]. Diminishing oxidative stress and suppression of the TGF-β/Smad2-signalling pathway are some of these paracrine effects [12, 13]. In the rat pulmonary hypertension model, MSCs have shown superiority regarding the lowering of blood pressure and ventricular overload; hence, MSC transplantation in chronic lung disease with pulmonary hypertension has pointed towards a new therapeutic option [14]. Concomitant percutaneous trans-luminal renal angioplasty with MSC therapy has been reported to decrease inflammation, fibrinogenesis and vascular remodelling in atherosclerotic renal artery stenosis of swine [15]. Also, MSCs have the ability to recognize inflammation lesions, and Ang II effects the migration and homing of these cells to the site of injury [16]. Dysregulation of the RAS decreases the paracrine therapeutic potential of MSCs [17].

Expression of renin, AT1 and AT2 receptors has been implicated with the regulation of MSCs differentiation to adipocytes, while the differentiated cell produces significant amounts of endogenous RAS [18]. Indeed, endogenous blockade of AT1 receptor inhibited adipogenesis of MSCs [18]. These outcomes are in line with clinical observations that RAS blockade acts as a protective factor against the onset of obesity-induced diabetes mellitus type 2 [19]. Ang II also has been shown to stimulate the synthesis of vascular endothelial growth factor (VEGF) that is an angiogenic agent in MSCs [20]. Additionally, MSCs have been suggested as a promising regenerative medicine for treating ischaemic heart disease and diabetes [21]. Hence, it is probable that Ang II-induced production of VEGF might be a contributing underlying mechanism of the beneficial consequences obtained following MSC transplantation.

5. The RAS and endothelial progenitor cells

The identification of circulating endothelial progenitor cells (EPCs) has introduced the concept of postnatal vasculogenesis. EPCs could originate from haematopoietic stem cells (HSCs) or MSCs [22, 23]. Also, the EPCs existing in the adventitial layer of vessels have the ability to differentiate into adult endothelial cells [24]. Different factors such as ischaemia, vascular damage and even physical exercise result in the recruitment of circulating EPCs and thus neovascularization and restoration of endothelial functionality [25, 26]. In this context, the improvement of myocardial perfusion after EPC transplantation has been observed in clinical trials [27]. Several mechanisms have been suggested regarding EPCs mobilization. For instance, it was observed that ischaemic lesions release angiogenic factors like VEGF and activate MAPK or the RAS-signalling pathways [28], which increase EPCs migration.

Despite the important role of vascular endothelium in cardiovascular disease (CVD), their limited regeneration capacity remains a vital problem. EPCs improve angiogenesis and participate in endothelium recovery subsequent to vascular injuries [29]. Cardiovascular diseases (CVDs) are directly related to both the decline of EPC mobilization and the number of EPCs present in the damaged site. In this context, Ang II stimulates EPCs migration to ischaemic regions and commences vascularization through VEGF-associated endothelial nitric oxide synthase [30]. The activation of NAPH and subsequent ROS (reactive oxygen species) generation constitutes the stimulatory impact of Ang II on EPCs that is required for normal EPC function. However, the long-term activation of NADPH and oxidative stress is concomitant with cell senescence [31]. Moreover, acute high-dose exposure to Ang II has been shown to negatively modulate EPC function in the hind limb ischaemic rat model [32].

6. The vascular RAS and erythropoiesis

RAS has been shown to result in progenitor cell senescence and suppression of differentiation and adherence in bone marrow-derived EPCs in Ang II infusion models. This inhibitory impact could be attenuated by the administration of AT1 receptor antagonists [31]. Previous reports have proved the crucial role of Ang II during erythropoiesis [33]. In studies using transgenic mice expressing human renin and angiotensinogen, a drastic rise in levels of erythropoietin was observed, which is a glycoprotein hormone that controls erythropoiesis. Genetic ablation of AT1 receptor from these mice reduced erythropoietin levels and restored haematocrit levels [34]. Also, ACE blockade has been concomitant with haematocrit decrease in vivo [35]. The idea of ACE and/or Ang II being contributed to erythropoiesis was further confirmed by a recent research in which ACE marked haematopoietic stem cells from human embryonic, fetal and adult haematopoietic tissues [36]. However, the mechanism of Ang II-associated regulation of erythropoiesis is mainly unclear. Most of these effects are observed during early phases of erythropoiesis [37]. As mentioned above, some researchers imply that Ang II acts indirectly via its effect on erythropoietin levels [38], whereas others do not agree with this link [39]. The other possible mechanism is proposed to be the involvement of JAK (Janus kinase)/STAT (signal transducer and activator of transcription) pathway. JAK/STAT pathway is known to be activated by Ang II [40].

http://dx.doi.org/10.5772/67726

7. Current research on the RAS in pancreatic stem cells

The local RAS is not only involved in the physiology of pancreas, but it also influences the pancreatic stem cell (PSC) functionality. RAS has been shown to be associated with pancreatic islet cell function and proliferation and differentiation of PSCs/progenitor cells during development [41]. Different stem/progenitor cells have been reported to be differentiated into insulin-expressing cells, which make them appropriate candidates for islet cell transplantation. Regarding the potential role of RAS in stem cell differentiation, it is possible that RAS-modulated stem cell could be a new source of pancreatic β-cells. Both exocrine and endocrine pancreas are known to have local RAS components [42]. In exocrine part, AT1 receptor activation turns on signalling pathways such as ROS generation and activation of pro-inflammatory, vasoactive and growth factor receptors [43, 44]. Therefore, Ang II might result in fibrosis and inflammation of exocrine pancreas through the AT1 receptor. Hence, blockade of RAS has been considered a potential therapeutic opportunity for some pancreas disorders.

In the endocrine portion of pancreas, RAS has been shown to be a key regulator of insulin and islet physiology [43]. AT1 receptor stimulation leads to β-cells, decreased islet blood flow and insulin secretion, while AT2 receptor activation results in β-cell proliferation and islet blood flow and insulin secretion enhancement [19]. Moreover, the ACE2/Ang-(1–7)/Mas axis, which has been attracting more research attention recently, is present in several local tissues and mainly acts as a negative modulator of ACE/Ang II/AT1R signalling. Similar to AT2 receptor activation, ACE2 overexpression in the pancreas of type 2 diabetic animals restored glucose homeostasis, as evidenced by diminished blood glucose levels, elevated insulin secretion and β-cell proliferation [45].

PSCs exist in both developing and adult pancreas in three major pancreas sections, that is, ductal endothelium, islet and acinar tissues [46]. Embryo, foetus and adult pancreas as well as bone marrow-derived MSCs are probable sources for PSCs. Transplantation of mouse or human PSCs into diabetic mice has been revealed to reduce their diabetes [46].

A novel well-defined area of research is the developmental control of RAS on cell proliferation in tumours and in tissue regeneration. Both the ACE/AngII/AT1R signalling and the alternative RAS arm (ACE2/Ang-(1–7)/Mas) interact with different growth factors; hence, they might contribute to cell proliferation and angiogenesis in neoplasms, including pancreatic cancers [47–49]. It has been demonstrated that RAS inhibition seems to be a promising therapeutic approach for the mitigation of pathophysiological circumstances of the pancreas including diabetes [50], pancreatitis [43] and pancreatic cancer [51]. Transplantation of human fetal pancreatic progenitor cell has been shown to reverse hyperglycaemia and glucose intolerance in diabetic mice [52]. ROS production has a close relation with RAS activation, and ROS-signalling pathway is associated with stem/progenitor cell proliferation, differentiation and function [53]. So, it is an interesting probability that the elevation of RAS-induced differentiation of pancreatic progenitor cells towards an endocrine lineage might offer a basis for therapy in terms of islet replacement treatments for diabetes.

MSCs have been suggested as an appropriate substitute to islet transplantation for promoting regeneration of endogenous pancreatic progenitor cells to achieve permanent normal blood glucose level in patients with type 1 diabetes [54]. Local RAS in pancreatic islet could regulate PSC differentiation and thus lead to the beneficial outcomes following MSC transplantation. In a study, these kinds of pancreatic progenitor cells have shown to differentiate into insulin-secreting cells.

RAS components like angiotensinogen and renin are expressed after the beginning of pancreatic progenitor cells differentiation, but they are not present in undifferentiated cells. These results indicate that a functional RAS exists in pancreatic progenitor cells and in mature islets that could be modulating cellular differentiation. The mitogenic behaviour related to the Ang II bindings of AT1 receptors has been proposed to regulate reprogramming of pancreatic cells and the differentiation plasticity [55]. However, it is unclear whether AT2 receptor activation reveals counter-regulatory role in this context. Furthermore, it is hypothesized that the ACE2/Ang-(1–7)/Mas axis plays an essential role in pancreatic stem cell differentiation as previous studies have shown the involvement of ACE2 arm in the proliferation and differentiation of other stem cells [56].

8. Current research on the RAS in cardiac stem cells

Regarding the intracellular signalling pathway of Ang II, RAS effect on cardiovascular stem/progenitor cell transplantation has largely been investigated. Among the regenerative medicine-based therapies in the cardiovascular system, induced pluripotent stem cells (iPSCs), which are artificially derived from an adult non-differentiated somatic cell, are a field of research study. In spite of different origin, they resemble ESCs in their growth and gene expression profile [57]. Also, Ang II receptors are expressed in iPSCs, which induce the proliferation and differentiation of pluripotent stem cells to several kinds of stem cells. As mentioned before, Ang II stimulates cell-signalling cascade through ROS production which in turn instigates stem cell proliferation [58]. In a study, the administration of Tempol (ROS generation-blocking agent) in Ang II-treated pluripotent stem cells has attenuated the proliferation of stem cells and DNA synthesis suggesting the role of oxidative-signalling pathway in RAS-associated cell proliferation. The other signalling pathway linked to the differentiation of iPSCs and Ang II is JAK/STAT pathway [59].

Ang II is also able to induce ESCs differentiation. In this context, the effect of AT1 receptor activation on collagen IV protein has been investigated [18]. Collagen IV is an extracellular matrix protein having a role in cell adhesion, growth, migration and differentiation. Collagen IV has been shown to be involved in the differentiation of ESCs to smooth muscle cell.

Up-regulation of several transcription factors such as egr-1, c-fos/c-jun, Stat91, NFk-B, which has a fundamental role in stem cell differentiation, is mediated through PI3/Akt pathway. Ang II is the upstream cascade of PI3/Akt82-84. NFk-B is markedly up-regulated in Ang II-treated cells, proposing that there is NFk-B involvement in ESC differentiation into the smooth muscle cells [60].

The TGF-β/Smad pathway plays a key role in the cellular responses to Ang II. Ang II activates TGF-β secretion in various tissues, such as fibroblasts and smooth muscle cells that induce interstitial fibrosis in the heart and kidney. Besides, TGF-β/Smad pathway is highly engaged to vascular fibrosis and arteriosclerosis [61] and gives rise to the differentiation of MSCs to smooth muscle cell. Furthermore, TGF-β secretion is connected with the MAPK/ERK cascade, and Ang II in this pathway interferes with TGF-β production, thus leading to the differentiation of MSCs to smooth muscle cells [62].

Regarding owning various paracrine effects, MSC transplantation has gained great importance in cardiovascular disease [63]. The supportive effects of vascular VEGF have been recognized in the migration, invasion of extracellular matrix, proliferation, survival of MSCs, and they contribute to MSCs' paracrine effects [64, 65]. In this context, all pathways increasing VEGF would give rise to the function of MSCs. Ang II increases VEGF mRNA and protein expression in MSCs [20], which is associated with Akt-signalling pathway. Pre-treatment of MSCs with the Akt inhibitor (LY292002) has been shown to reduce Ang II-induced VEGF expression. So, local Ang II, as a cytokine, might boost VEGF generation in MSC grafts and upgrade the transplantation effectiveness.

The excess RAS expression is detected in CVDs such as myocardial infarction, hypertension, heart failure and atherosclerosis [66]. On the other hand, RAS inhibition via ACE inhibitors (ACEIs) and angiotensin receptor blockers (ARBs) has been widely examined in cardiovascular disease beyond their effects in lowering the blood pressure [67]. Despite the daily increasing use of regenerative medicine in treating different disorders, the functionality of stem cell transplantation is not sufficient in animal models and clinical trials [68].

Therefore, clarifying the mechanisms that enhance the graft efficacy seems important. Researchers have investigated the effect of RAS inhibition on stem cell therapy of cardiovascular system [69].

The insulin-like growth factor 1-1 secreted from stem cells has a close relationship with the RAS and down-regulates the local RAS through the attenuation of the p53 gene [70]. The IGF-1 has an anti-apoptotic effect on cardiomyocytes in ischaemic heart disease and also enhances differentiation and survival of stem cells after transplantation [71]. In acute MI in cardiomyocytes, ACEIs up-regulate the IGF-1 receptors; thus, the concurrent use of perindopril in bone marrow stem cell transplantation increases the paracrine effects of the IGF-1, which abolishes apoptosis through increased Bcl2 expression and improves cardiac function [72]. Also, pretreatment of MSCs with ARBs before transplantation increases their trans-differentiation efficacy and also improves the systolic function of the heart [73].

9. Limitations and future directions

Comprehensive elucidation of the complexity of the regulatory network that drives stem cell therapy will require extensive effort and time. The accretion of daily increasing research and obtained ideas will undoubtedly assist the current research field of stem/progenitor cell therapy. Regenerative progenitor cell therapy has emerged as a possible alternative for pharmacotherapy in different human diseases. A major problem in this field is insufficient efficacy during stem cell transplantation. In order to improve the efficiency of regenerative medicine, researchers examined the impact of the modulation of various cell-signalling pathways, including the RAS. Effects of Ang II in stem cell proliferation and differentiation have been documented in the literature. The presence of the RAS components in progenitor cells and many tissues may regulate growth and development and thus might contribute to the preparation of various progenitor cells for clinical transplantation.

Acknowledgements

The moral support of the Faculty of Pharmacy and Drug Applied Research Center of Tabriz University of Medical Sciences in Tabriz, Iran, is gratefully acknowledged.

Author details

Elham Ahmadian[1,2,3], Aziz Eftekhari[1,2] and Ahmad Yari Khosroushahi[2,4*]

*Address all correspondence to: yarikhosroushahia@tbzmed.ac.ir

1 Department of Pharmacology and Toxicology, Tabriz University of Medical Science, Tabriz, Iran

2 Drug Applied Research Center, Tabriz University of Medical Sciences, Tabriz, Iran

3 Student Research Committee, Tabriz University of Medical Science, Tabriz, Iran

4 Department of Pharmacognosy, Tabriz University of Medical Sciences, Tabriz, Iran

References

[1] Mummery, C.L., et al., Differentiation of human embryonic stem cells and induced pluripotent stem cells to cardiomyocytes a methods overview. Circulation Research, 2012. **111**(3): pp. 344-358.

[2] Lundy, S.D., et al., Structural and functional maturation of cardiomyocytes derived from human pluripotent stem cells. Stem Cells and Development, 2013. **22**(14): pp. 1991-2002.

[3] McDevitt, T.C., Laflamme, M.A., and Murry, C.E., Proliferation of cardiomyocytes derived from human embryonic stem cells is mediated via the IGF/PI 3-kinase/Akt signaling pathway. Journal of Molecular and Cellular Cardiology, 2005. **39**(6): pp. 865-873.

[4] Cheng, W.H., et al., Renin activates PI3K-Akt-eNOS signalling through the angiotensin AT1 and Mas receptors to modulate central blood pressure control in the nucleus tractus solitarii. British Journal of Pharmacology, 2012. **166**(7): pp. 2024-2035.

[5] van Laake, L.W., et al., Human embryonic stem cell-derived cardiomyocytes survive and mature in the mouse heart and transiently improve function after myocardial infarction. Stem Cell Research, 2007. **1**(1): pp. 9-24.

[6] Huang, Z., et al., Angiotensin II type 1 and bradykinin B2 receptors expressed in early stage epithelial cells derived from human embryonic stem cells. Journal of Cellular Physiology, 2007. **211**(3): pp. 816-825.

[7] Han, H.J., et al., ANG II-stimulated DNA synthesis is mediated by ANG II receptor-dependent Ca2+/PKC as well as EGF receptor-dependent PI3K/Akt/mTOR/p70S6K1 signal pathways in mouse embryonic stem cells. Journal of Cellular Physiology, 2007. **211**(3): pp. 618-629.

[8] Kim, Y.H. and Han, H.J., Synergistic effect of high glucose and ANG II on proliferation of mouse embryonic stem cells: involvement of PKC and MAPKs as well as AT1 receptor. Journal of Cellular Physiology, 2008. **215**(2): pp. 374-382.

[9] Trivedi, P., et al., Mesenchymal stem cell therapy for treatment of cardiovascular disease: helping people sooner or later. Stem Cells and Development, 2010. **19**(7): pp. 1109-1120.

[10] Jiang, S., et al., Transcriptional profiling of young and old mesenchymal stem cells in response to oxygen deprivation and reparability of the infarcted myocardium. Journal of Molecular and Cellular Cardiology, 2008. **44**(3): pp. 582-596.

[11] Choi, Y.-H., Kurtz, A., and Stamm, C., Mesenchymal stem cells for cardiac cell therapy. Human Gene Therapy, 2010. **22**(1): pp. 3-17.

[12] Eirin, A., et al., Adipose tissue-derived mesenchymal stem cells improve revascularization outcomes to restore renal function in swine atherosclerotic renal artery stenosis. Stem Cells, 2012. **30**(5): pp. 1030-1041.

[13] Ahmadian, E., Jafari, S., and Khosroushahi, A.Y., Role of angiotensin II in stem cell therapy of cardiac disease. Journal of Renin-Angiotensin-Aldosterone System, 2015. **16**(4); pp. 702-711.

[14] Hansmann, G., et al., Mesenchymal stem cell-mediated reversal of bronchopulmonary dysplasia and associated pulmonary hypertension. Pulmonary Circulation, 2012. **2**(2): pp. 170-181.

[15] Ebrahimi, B., et al., Mesenchymal stem cells improve medullary inflammation and fibrosis after revascularization of swine atherosclerotic renal artery stenosis. PLoS One, 2013. **8**(7): p. e67474.

[16] de Resende, M.M., Stodola, T.J., and Greene, A.S., Role of the renin angiotensin system on bone marrow-derived stem cell function and its impact on skeletal muscle angiogenesis. Physiological Genomics, 2010. **42**(3): pp. 437-444.

[17] Resende, M.M., Stodola, T.J., and Greene, A.S., Role of the renin angiotensin system on bone marrow-derived stem cell function and its impact on skeletal muscle angiogenesis after electrical stimulation. The FASEB Journal, 2009. **23**(1_MeetingAbstracts): p. 1030.10.

[18] Matsushita, K., et al., Local renin angiotensin expression regulates human mesenchymal stem cell differentiation to adipocytes. Hypertension, 2006. **48**(6): pp. 1095-1102.

[19] Wang, L. and Leung, P.S., The role of renin-angiotensin system in cellular differentiation: implications in pancreatic islet cell development and islet transplantation. Molecular and Cellular Endocrinology, 2013. **381**(1): pp. 261-271.

[20] Shi, R.-Z., et al., Angiotensin II induces vascular endothelial growth factor synthesis in mesenchymal stem cells. Experimental Cell Research, 2009. **315**(1): pp. 10-15.

[21] Xu, Y.-X., et al., Mesenchymal stem cell therapy for diabetes through paracrine mechanisms. Medical Hypotheses, 2008. **71**(3): pp. 390-393.

[22] Asahara, T., Kawamoto, A., and Masuda, H., Concise review: circulating endothelial progenitor cells for vascular medicine. Stem Cells, 2011. **29**(11): pp. 1650-1655.

[23] Sata, M., et al., Hematopoietic stem cells differentiate into vascular cells that participate in the pathogenesis of atherosclerosis. Nature Medicine, 2002. **8**(4): pp. 403-409.

[24] Richardson, M.R. and Yoder, M.C., Endothelial progenitor cells: quo vadis? Journal of Molecular and Cellular Cardiology, 2011. **50**(2): pp. 266-272.

[25] Corselli, M., et al., The tunica adventitia of human arteries and veins as a source of mesenchymal stem cells. Stem Cells and Development, 2011. **21**(8): pp. 1299-1308.

[26] Lam, C.-F., et al., Transplantation of endothelial progenitor cells improves pulmonary endothelial function and gas exchange in rabbits with endotoxin-induced acute lung injury. Anesthesia & Analgesia, 2011. **112**(3): pp. 620-627.

[27] Traverse, J.H., et al., Effect of intracoronary delivery of autologous bone marrow mononuclear cells 2 to 3 weeks following acute myocardial infarction on left ventricular function: the LateTIME randomized trial. JAMA, 2011. **306**(19): pp. 2110-2119.

[28] Jiang, H., et al., Palmitic acid promotes endothelial progenitor cells apoptosis via p38 and JNK mitogen-activated protein kinase pathways. Atherosclerosis, 2010. **210**(1): pp. 71-77.

[29] Lee, P. and Poh, K.K., Endothelial progenitor cells in cardiovascular diseases. World Journal of Stem Cells, 2014. **6**(3): pp. 355-366.

[30] Hiasa, K., et al., Gene transfer of stromal cell–derived factor-1a enhances ischemic vasculogenesis and angiogenesis via vascular endothelial growth factor/endothelial nitric oxide synthase–related pathway next-generation chemokine therapy for therapeutic neovascularization. Circulation, 2004. **109**(20): pp. 2454-2461.

[31] Kobayashi, K., Imanishi, T., and Akasaka, T., Endothelial progenitor cell differentiation and senescence in an angiotensin II-infusion rat model. Hypertension Research, 2006. **29**(6): pp. 449-455.

[32] You, D., et al., Combination of the angiotensin-converting enzyme inhibitor perindopril and the diuretic indapamide activate postnatal vasculogenesis in spontaneously hyper-

tensive rats. Journal of Pharmacology and Experimental Therapeutics, 2008. **325**(3): pp. 766-773.

[33] Hubert, C., et al., The hematopoietic system: a new niche for the renin–angiotensin system. Nature Clinical Practice Cardiovascular Medicine, 2006. **3**(2): pp. 80-85.

[34] Kato, H., et al., Enhanced erythropoiesis mediated by activation of the renin-angiotensin system via angiotensin II type 1a receptor. The FASEB Journal, 2005. **19**(14): pp. 2023-2025.

[35] Savary, K., et al., Role of the renin-angiotensin system in primitive erythropoiesis in the chick embryo. Blood, 2005. **105**(1): pp. 103-110.

[36] Jokubaitis, V.J., et al., Angiotensin-converting enzyme (CD143) marks hematopoietic stem cells in human embryonic, fetal, and adult hematopoietic tissues. Blood, 2008. **111**(8): pp. 4055-4063.

[37] Naito, M., et al., Effects of an angiotensin II receptor antagonist and angiotensin-converting enzyme inhibitors on burst forming units-erythroid in chronic hemodialysis patients. American Journal of Nephrology, 2003. **23**(5): pp. 287-293.

[38] Freudenthaler, S., et al., Angiotensin II increases erythropoietin production in healthy human volunteers. European Journal of Clinical Investigation, 1999. **29**(10): pp. 816-823.

[39] Chew, C., Weise, M., and Disney, A., The effect of angiotensin II receptor antagonist on the exogenous erythropoietin requirement of haemodialysis patients. Nephrology Dialysis Transplantation, 1999. **14**(8): pp. 2047-2049.

[40] Durik, M., Pessôa, B.S., and Roks, A.J., The renin–angiotensin system, bone marrow and progenitor cells. Clinical Science, 2012. **123**(4): pp. 205-223.

[41] Leung PS . Current research progress in the pancreas. In: Advances in experimental medicine and biology book series. The renin-angiotensin system. Dordrech: Springer; 2010. p. 1-207.

[42] Leung, P.S. and Carlsson, P.-O., Pancreatic islet renin angiotensin system: its novel roles in islet function and in diabetes mellitus. Pancreas, 2005. **30**(4): pp. 293-298.

[43] Chan, Y.C. and Leung, P.S., The renin–angiotensin system and reactive oxygen species: implications in pancreatitis. Antioxidants & Redox Signaling, 2011. **15**(10): pp. 2743-2755.

[44] Iwai, M. and Horiuchi, M., Devil and angel in the renin–angiotensin system: ACE–angiotensin II–AT1 receptor axis vs. ACE2–angiotensin-(1-7)–Mas receptor axis. Hypertension Research, 2009. **32**(7): pp. 533-536.

[45] Bindom, S.M., et al., Angiotensin I–converting enzyme type 2 (ACE2) gene therapy improves glycemic control in diabetic mice. Diabetes, 2010. **59**(10): pp. 2540-2548.

[46] Jiang, F.-X. and Morahan, G., Pancreatic stem cells: from possible to probable. Stem Cell Reviews and Reports, 2012. **8**(3): pp. 647-657.

[47] Ager, E.I., Neo, J., and Christophi, C., The renin–angiotensin system and malignancy. Carcinogenesis, 2008. **29**(9): pp. 1675-1684.

[48] Ni, L., et al., Angiotensin-(1-7) inhibits the migration and invasion of A549 human lung adenocarcinoma cells through inactivation of the PI3K/Akt and MAPK signaling pathways. Oncology Reports, 2012. **27**(3): pp. 783-790.

[49] Zhou, L., et al., Angiotensin-converting enzyme 2 acts as a potential molecular target for pancreatic cancer therapy. Cancer Letters, 2011. **307**(1): pp. 18-25.

[50] Cheng, Q., et al., Combination of the dipeptidyl peptidase IV inhibitor LAF237 [(S)-1-[(3-hydroxy-1-adamantyl) ammo] acetyl-2-cyanopyrrolidine] with the angiotensin II type 1 receptor antagonist valsartan [N-(1-oxopentyl)-N-[[2'-(1H-tetrazol-5-yl)-[1, 1'-biphenyl]-4-yl] methyl]-L-valine] enhances pancreatic islet morphology and function in a mouse model of type 2 diabetes. Journal of Pharmacology and Experimental Therapeutics, 2008. **327**(3): pp. 683-691.

[51] Lau, S.T., and Leung, P.S., Role of the RAS in pancreatic cancer. Current Cancer Drug Targets, 2011. **11**(4): pp. 412-420.

[52] Suen, P., et al., PDZ-domain containing-2 (PDZD2) is a novel factor that affects the growth and differentiation of human fetal pancreatic progenitor cells. The International Journal of Biochemistry & Cell Biology, 2008. **40**(4): pp. 789-803.

[53] Diehn, M., et al., Association of reactive oxygen species levels and radioresistance in cancer stem cells. Nature, 2009. **458**(7239): pp. 780-783.

[54] Milanesi, A., et al., β-Cell regeneration mediated by human bone marrow mesenchymal stem cells. PloS One, 2012. **7**(8): p. e42177.

[55] Saleem, S., et al., β1 integrin/FAK/ERK signalling pathway is essential for human fetal islet cell differentiation and survival. The Journal of Pathology, 2009. **219**(2): pp. 182-192.

[56] Burns, W.C., et al., Angiotensin II mediates epithelial-to-mesenchymal transformation in tubular cells by ANG 1-7/MAS-1-dependent pathways. American Journal of Physiology-Renal Physiology, 2010. **299**(3): pp. F585-F593.

[57] Yu, J. and Thomson, J.A., Pluripotent stem cell lines. Genes & Development, 2008. **22**(15): pp. 1987-1997.

[58] Chan, E.C., et al., Regulation of cell proliferation by NADPH oxidase-mediated signaling: potential roles in tissue repair, regenerative medicine and tissue engineering. Pharmacology & Therapeutics, 2009. **122**(2): pp. 97-108.

[59] Kristensen, D.M., Kalisz, M., and Nielsen, J.H., Cytokine signalling in embryonic stem cells. Apmis, 2005. **113**(11-12): pp. 756-772.

[60] Huang, D., et al., Angiotensin II promotes poly (ADP-ribosyl) ation of c-Jun/c-Fos in cardiac fibroblasts. Journal of Molecular and Cellular Cardiology, 2009. **46**(1): pp. 25-32.

[61] Wang, W., et al., Essential role of Smad3 in angiotensin II–induced vascular fibrosis. Circulation Research, 2006. **98**(8): pp. 1032-1039.

[62] Jeon, E.S., et al., Sphingosylphosphorylcholine induces differentiation of human mesenchymal stem cells into smooth-muscle-like cells through a TGF-β-dependent mechanism. Journal of Cell Science, 2006. **119**(23): pp. 4994-5005.

[63] Williams, A.R., et al., Intramyocardial stem cell injection in patients with ischemic cardiomyopathy functional recovery and reverse remodeling. Circulation Research, 2011. **108**(7): pp. 792-796.

[64] Xu, M., et al., In vitro and in vivo effects of bone marrow stem cells on cardiac structure and function. Journal of Molecular and Cellular Cardiology, 2007. **42**(2): pp. 441-448.

[65] Potapova, I.A., et al., Mesenchymal stem cells support migration, extracellular matrix invasion, proliferation, and survival of endothelial cells in vitro. Stem Cells, 2007. **25**(7): pp. 1761-1768.

[66] Haznedaroglu, I.C. and Beyazit, Y., Review: Pathobiological aspects of the local bone marrow renin-angiotensin system: a review. Journal of Renin-Angiotensin-Aldosterone System, 2010. **11**(4): pp. 205-213.

[67] Taylor, A.A., Siragy, H., and Nesbitt, S., Angiotensin receptor blockers: pharmacology, efficacy, and safety. The Journal of Clinical Hypertension, 2011. **13**(9): pp. 677-686.

[68] Cleland, J.G., et al., Clinical trials update from the American Heart Association: REPAIR-AMI, ASTAMI, JELIS, MEGA, REVIVE-II, SURVIVE, and PROACTIVE. European Journal of Heart Failure, 2006. **8**(1): pp. 105-110.

[69] Ebrahimian, T.G., et al., Dual effect of angiotensin-converting enzyme inhibition on angiogenesis in type 1 diabetic mice. Arteriosclerosis, Thrombosis, and Vascular Biology, 2005. **25**(1): pp. 65-70.

[70] Huynh, K., et al., Cardiac-specific IGF-1 receptor transgenic expression protects against cardiac fibrosis and diastolic dysfunction in a mouse model of diabetic cardiomyopathy. Diabetes, 2010. **59**(6): pp. 1512-1520.

[71] O'Sullivan, J.F., et al., Potent long-term cardioprotective effects of single low-dose insulin-like growth factor-1 treatment postmyocardial infarction. Circulation: Cardiovascular Interventions, 2011. **4**(4): pp. 327-335.

[72] Huang, Y.-L., et al., Bone marrow stromal cell transplantation combined with angiotensin-converting enzyme inhibitor treatment in rat with acute myocardial infarction and the role of insulin-like growth factor-1. Cytotherapy, 2012. **14**(5): pp. 563-569.

[73] Numasawa, Y., et al., Treatment of human mesenchymal stem cells with angiotensin receptor blocker improved efficiency of cardiomyogenic transdifferentiation and improved cardiac function via angiogenesis. Stem Cells, 2011. **29**(9): pp. 1405-1414.

Chapter 10

Renin-Angiotensin System MicroRNAs, Special Focus on the Brain

Jose Gerardo-Aviles, Shelley Allen and Patrick Gavin Kehoe

Additional information is available at the end of the chapter

http://dx.doi.org/10.5772/67080

Abstract

MicroRNAs (miRNAs) are post-transcriptional regulators of gene expression with important roles in cancer, cardiovascular and neurological disorders. Present in the brain, they play numerous regulatory roles shaping the proteome in an orchestrated manner with other non-coding RNAs. An independent brain-specific renin-angiotensin system (RAS) exists that is subject to miRNA remodelling. The brain RAS regulates cerebral blood flow and electrolytic balance and is involved in neurotransmitter signalling and cognitive processes. Circulating microRNAs allow interaction between systemic and local RAS in the heart and the brain. Their screening and manipulation may be valuable towards understanding pathophysiology and development of treatments for various systemic and central nervous system diseases.

Keywords: non-coding RNAs, microRNAs, brain renin-angiotensin system, cerebrovascular disease, circulating microRNAs, biomarkers

1. Introduction

High blood pressure, leading to cardiovascular and cerebrovascular disorders, is the principal cause of morbidity and mortality worldwide [1–3]. The renin-angiotensin system (RAS) is a major regulator of cardiovascular function and pharmaceutical compounds targeting the RAS are frontline treatments to control high blood pressure [4, 5]. In addition, lifestyle risk factors such as obesity, insulin resistance, high alcohol and salt intake and ageing promote the development of hypertension through epigenetic mechanisms [6–9]. These mechanisms have attracted attention because of their reversibility by environmental and lifestyle modi-

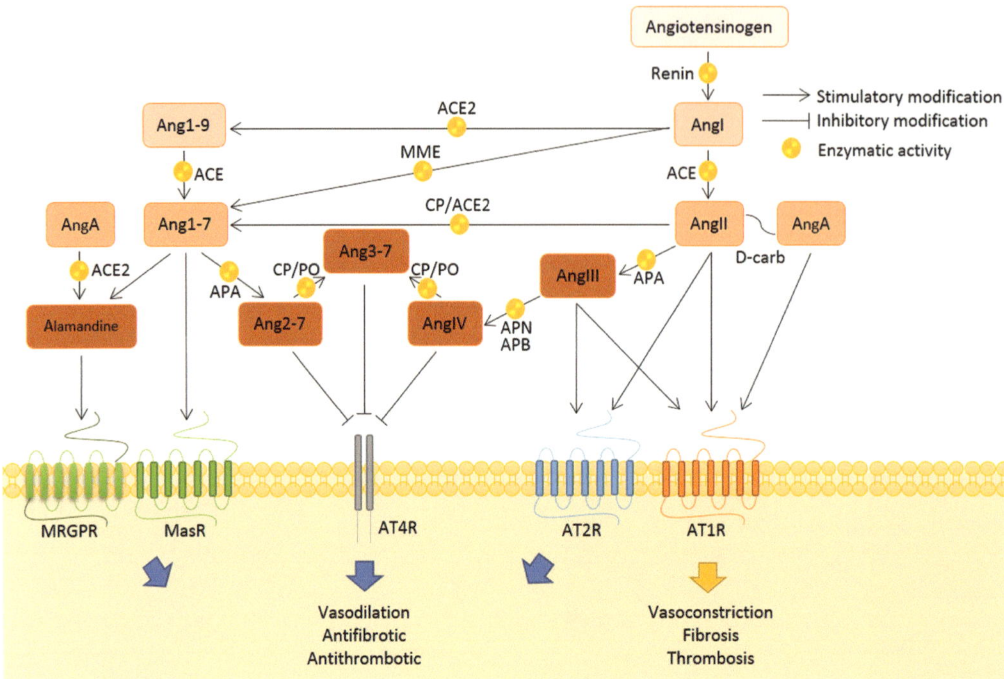

Figure 1. The renin-angiotensin system (RAS) and its components. This schematic depicts angiotensin ligands, receptors and the main enzymes involved; other peptidases and cathepsins also participate although to a lesser extent. All of the components of the RAS are present in the brain. RAS has two main axes: the pressor axis (tending towards an increase in blood pressure) comprising Ang II, ACE and AT1Rs and the counter-regulatory axis comprising Ang(1–7), ACE2 and MasR. Angiotensinogen is a substrate for renin to produce angiotensin I (Ang I), which is the inactive precursor of all angiotensin peptides. Conversion of Ang I to its most active ligand in the pressor axis, angiotensin II (Ang II), results from ACE-mediated hydrolysis [22]. Ang II is then sequentially converted to angiotensin III (Ang III) and angiotensin IV (Ang IV) by aminopeptidase A (APA) and aminopeptidase N (APN) respectively, which can be further cleaved by carboxypeptidase P (CP) and prolyl oligopeptidase (PO) to form angiotensin 3–7 (Ang3–7). Alternatively, Ang II can be converted, via the counter-regulatory axis to angiotensin 1–7 (Ang1–7) by carboxypeptidase P (CP) or ACE2, while both angiotensin A and Ang1–7 can be converted to alamandine by an ACE-mediated decarboxylation reaction [22–27]. Notably, angiotensin ligands acting on AT4R (also called insulin-regulated aminopeptidase (IRAP)) can have agonist or antagonist effects depending on whether or not they bind in the IRAP peptidase domain.

fications, making them important in the detection and treatment of multifactorial diseases such as hypertension [7, 10].

Some of those epigenetic modifications are mediated by miRNAs, defined as single-stranded, non-coding RNA sequences approximately 21–23 nucleotides in length, expressed under physiological and pathological conditions [11, 12]. Deletion of complexes involved in miRNA biogenesis resulted in deleterious and non-viable phenotypes, highlighting their necessary involvement in the cellular development and differentiation [13, 14]. To date, 28,645 miRNAs have been reported in miRbase, a widely used resource for miRNA cataloging and nomenclature [15]. As epigenetic regulators of gene expression, functions of miRNAs include RNA degradation, inhibition of protein expression, regulation of methylation and histone modification on DNA [12, 14, 16]. miRNAs perform these functions by complementary base pairing to the target mRNAs through a seed-pairing region of 6–8 nucleotides at the 5′ end of the miRNA. They also interact with other non-coding RNAs and mediate proteome remodelling. Non-coding RNAs represent 98% of the genome, comprising transfer and ribosomal RNA, small nuclear (snRNA) and nucleolar RNA (snoRNA), small interference RNA (siRNA), Piwi-interacting RNA (piRNA) and long non-coding RNAs (lncRNA) [14, 17, 18].

Dysregulation of miRNAs is associated with cancer, cardiovascular and neurodegenerative disorders. The RAS, with important signalling roles in numerous organs and regulatory pathways and being subject to miRNA-mediated remodelling, is a potential factor in many disorders. Thus, the presence of miRNAs that have the capacity to shift the balance between prominent and deleterious functions of the RAS to beneficial roles is interesting, particularly new advances in methods that allow the detection of circulating miRNAs. Exosomes and their role in cellular transport provide a source for miRNA profiling and the presence of miRNAs in the peripheral circulation suggests that they work in an autocrine, paracrine and also endocrine manner, allowing widespread distribution of miRNAs through the entire body. Therefore, screening of miRNA in biological fluids like a serum and cerebrospinal fluid is relevant for an understanding of normal function as well as pathophysiology with a view to potential novel treatments for the disease.

The discovery of local independent but interacting RAS systems, including the brain, which also interacts with systemic RAS [3], has helped to change the original view that the RAS was solely an endocrine system important in regulating blood pressure, electrolytic homeostasis, vascular injury and repair [19]. The brain RAS discussed here (**Figure 1**) is multifunctional including regulation of cerebral blood flow, electrolyte balance, neurotransmitters, learning and memory, many of which may be associated with certain neurological disorders [20, 21].

2. Biogenesis and function of miRNAs

Canonical miRNA biogenesis starts with transcription of the primary miRNA sequence by RNA polymerase II and III [14]. Approximately half (52%) of human miRNAs are located in intergenic regions, 40% in intronic and 8% in exonic [28]. Intergenic miRNAs are independently expressed through promoter elements; yet related miRNAs that often have overlapping targets can be located on different chromosomes and expressed under different conditions. Intronic and exonic miRNAs that are clustered within 50 kilobases from each other show similar expression, while those spaced further apart tend not to [29]. However, there are some exceptions. Some miRNAs separated by more than 50 kilobases retain high correlation, likely as a result of co-expression [30]. The differential localization and expression of miRNAs suggest an evolutionary response to environmental insults and specific cell responses, a theory supported by observed higher numbers of miRNAs expressed in organisms of higher complexity [31–33].

Figure 2A–F summarizes the process of miRNA biogenesis. Primary miRNAs are cleaved in the nucleus by a nuclear microprocessor complex comprised of the RNase III endoribonuclease DROSHA and its double-stranded RNA-binding protein DGCR8—DiGeorge Critical

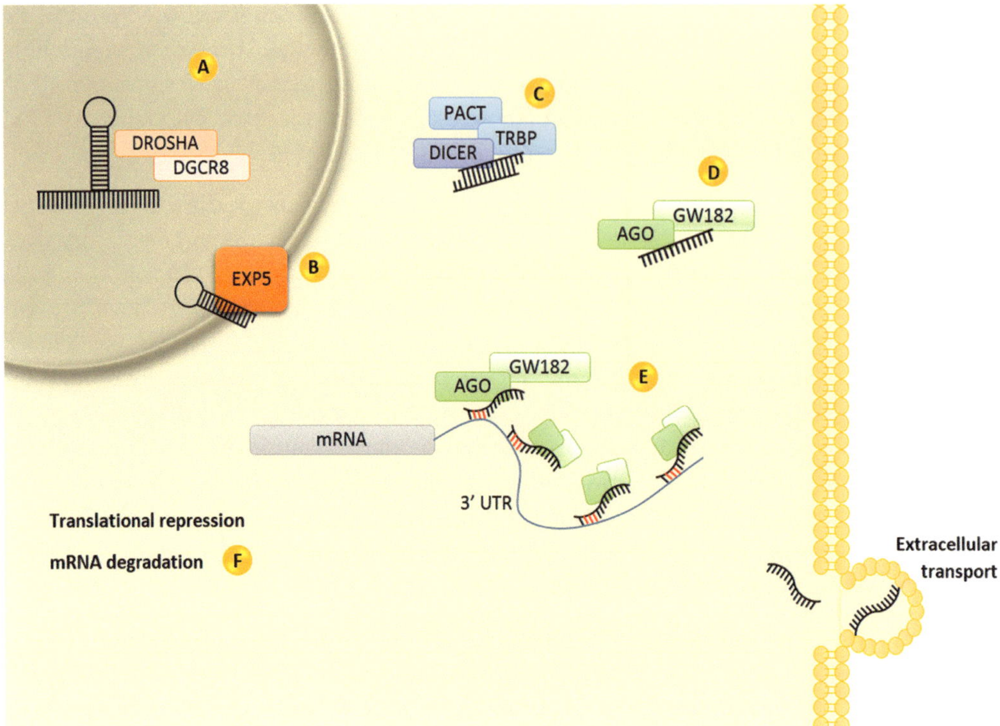

Figure 2. MicroRNA biogenesis and function. (A) Primary miRNAs are cleaved in the nucleus by the RNase III endoribonuclease DROSHA and DGCR8. (B) Once the primary miRNA is cleaved, the nuclear transport receptor exportin 5 binds the 3′ overhang structure of the pre-miRNA to export it to the cytoplasm. (C) The RNase III enzyme Dicer and TRBP and PACT target the pre-miRNA through the 3′ overhang, converting it into mature miRNA, liberating a duplex nucleotide structure with two nucleotides protruding at the 3′ end. (D) The guide strand is loaded into the RNA-induced silencing complex (RISC), and the passenger strand is degraded by RNases. (E) Complementary pairing with the seed region to mRNAs determines target binding and guides argonaute proteins to stop translation. Accumulation of untranslated mRNA in the cytoplasm allows recruitment of members of the GW182 protein family. (F) Deadenylase complexes cause destabilization of the transcript and further degradation by RNase activity.

Region 8, **Figure 2A** [34]. This cleavage by DROSHA/DGCR8 produces a 60 nucleotide stem-loop structure with a 3′ overhang, the pre-miRNA [11, 34, 35]. The primary miRNA can also be further subjected to RNA editing by ADARs (adenosine deaminases acting on RNA) that modify adenosine to inosine producing miRNA isoforms called isomiRs [36].

Exportin 5 allows export of the pre-miRNA to the cytoplasm, **Figure 2B** [36], where Dicer and substrate stabilizing binding partners, TRBP (trans-activation response RNA-binding protein) and PACT (protein activator of RNA-activated protein kinase) facilitate conversion into mature miRNA, **Figure 2C** [12, 14]. Two strands result from the unwinding of the duplex, the guide (3p) and passenger (5p) strands. Most of miRNA effects are mediated by the 3′ form; the 5′ form comprises <10% of all miRNA reads in humans [36]. The guide strand is loaded into the RNA-induced silencing complex (RISC) and the passenger strand is degraded by RNases, **Figure 2D**. IsomiRs can also be produced at this step by trimming and capping of the mature miRNA.

Non-canonical miRNA biogenesis is independent of DROSHA/DGCR8 processing in the nucleus. Such biogenesis arises if an intron is spliced lacking the sequences ordinarily flanking the stem region of a primary miRNA and it is of sufficient size to generate a pre-miRNA and it can be exported to the cytoplasm and further processed as a pre-miRNA to form a mirtron. Alongside mirtrons, other RNA sequences derived from transfer RNA and small nucleolar RNA are loaded into an RISC complex and act as miRNAs [13, 14, 29].

The RISC is a ribonucleoprotein complex that mediates mRNA degradation, destabilization or translational inhibition, whatever the biogenesis mechanism and comprises the miRNA guide strand and argonaute proteins, **Figure 2E**. The complementary base pairing of the miRNA seed region (2nd to 8th position on the 5′ end) to mRNAs determines target binding and guides argonaute proteins [28, 37, 38]. miRNA levels are dependent on argonaute proteins [39, 40] that are also present in the nucleus and currently, only miRNA-29b has been shown to translocate and localize in the nucleus [14, 39, 41]. In humans, argonaute 2 (also called eukaryotic translation initiation factor 2C) cleaves target mRNAs [29] but can also block other translation initiator factors and ribosomal subunits [42].

After pairing of the miRNA seed region, protein translation can be inhibited, **Figure 2E**. Accumulation of untranslated mRNA in the cytoplasm allows argonaute 2 to recruit members of the GW182 protein family, which are enriched in cytoplasmic areas called processing bodies (p-bodies) [42]. Here, the mRNA is destabilized by deadenylase complexes and further degraded by RNases [43–45]. Finally, the effect miRNAs have on protein or mRNA levels depends on the position where the miRNA binds and five different classes of miRNA binding have been determined [12, 46, 47]. Most miRNA effects are mediated by binding at the 3′ UTR of mRNA and further processing as described previously, non-canonical binding sites represent <1% [48].

3. MicroRNAs as autocrine, paracrine and endocrine molecules

miRNAs not only shape the intracellular proteome within specific cell types in response to microenvironment stimuli and cues, but can also mediate intercellular effects by means of nanotubes, exosomes and binding proteins, all mechanisms of intercellular communication [49]. Moreover, extracellular vesicles, including exosomes, microvesicles and apoptotic bodies, also participate in paracrine and endocrine signalling, as well as an intercellular transfer of miRNAs [50–52]. Exosomes, in particular, which are nanovesicles derived from endosomes are involved in cell-to-cell communication [53], contain significant amounts of miRNAs and are resistant to changes in temperature, pH and the effect of RNases making them reliable sources for screening [51, 54, 55]. miRNAs are transported by RNA-binding proteins and are taken up into intraluminal vesicles during the formation of multivesicular bodies in endosomes [56]. Upon fusion of the endosome to the plasma membrane, the intraluminal vesicles are released as exosomes and due to their lipid composition and size, they can easily transfer genetic material across lipid membranes [55, 56]. Several miRNAs are transferred in vivo and in vitro between fibroblasts, cardiomyocytes, human umbilical endothelial cells, mesenchymal stem cells, cardiac and cerebral endothelial cells [57, 58], while atheroprotective communication has been found between endothelial and smooth muscle cells through miRNAs [59].

miRNA transfer both propagates deleterious effects and helps recover cells from insults and prevent apoptosis. For example, miR-133 is increased in people with cardiovascular disease and is transferred through exosomes from multipotent mesenchymal stromal cells to astrocytes and neurons that promote recovery after stroke [60–63]. Furthermore, remote ischaemic conditioning, a technique of small cycles of ischaemia/reperfusion in distal extremities, was protective for cardiac and cerebrovascular effects in animal experiments and human clinical trials, with effects mediated by miRNAs such as miR-1 [64–69].

Exosomal circulating miRNAs have many properties that arguably make them ideal biomarkers, including their presence in peripheral blood, detection in many biological fluids, their stability in RNase-rich body fluids and their tissue-specific expression patterns. These have been described in cardio-cerebrovascular disorders, diabetes, dyslipidemia and neurodegenerative disorders [1, 70–76]. Furthermore, human exosomes can be used therapeutically as a gene delivery vector to provide cells with heterologous miRNAs [53].

4. Regulation of RAS by associated microRNAs

Given that there is further discussion of the biochemical functions of the RAS in other chapters, the discussion henceforth will focus on some of the most important components of the brain RAS and the miRNAs targeting them.

Since the vital function of the brain results in high physiological demands (i.e. requiring 20% of total cardiac output and a 10-fold higher oxygen and energy demand than other tissues), it requires strict coordination between blood flow and neuronal activity, a phenomena known as functional hyperaemia [77]. Cerebral blood flow is regulated by vasomotor, metabolic and neurogenic mechanisms, but can be modulated by vasoconstrictors such as Ang II and endothelin, vasodilators such as bradykinin, adenosine and other angiotensin ligands, while blood vessel capacity may be reduced or impeded by plaques of cholesterol, amyloid or fibrotic deposits.

Analysis by TargetScan [48], a software that predicts miRNA binding sites, suggests that 368 different miRNA families target RAS elements, the majority of which share transcripts. **Table 1** summarizes the total number of miRNAs and unique miRNAs with respect to RAS elements, as they have other targets outside the RAS. Angiotensin 4 receptor (also known as AT4R or IRAP) has 252 miRNA families associated with it, making it the highest amongst the RAS and approximately fivefold and threefold as many as that for arguably its better known receptors AT1R and AT2R. Notably, 88% of IRAP-associated miRNAs also regulate other RAS transcripts, suggesting its susceptibility to changes elsewhere in the RAS. In particular, IRAP has 28 miRNA families exclusively associated with it (also the most for RAS components), hinting at having high functional importance. Indeed, aminopeptidase B and dipeptidyl peptidase, necessary for Ang IV conversion, do not have exclusive miRNAs and thus may be subject to many regulatory effects.

A more in-depth examination of RAS-associated microRNAs, according to their functional impact in the RAS physiology is shown in **Table 2**. MiR-3163 targets the greatest number of RAS transcripts (N = 8) and may provide an over-arching level of regulation for the pathway

RAS element	Gene symbol	Total miRNA families	Unique miRNA families
Angiotensinogen	AGT	85	11
Angiotensin 1 receptor (AT1R)	AGTR1	46	1
Angiotensin 2 receptor (AT2R)	AGTR2	78	5
Angiotensin 4 receptor (AT4R/IRAP)	LNPEP	252	28
Mas receptor	MAS1	5	1
Angiotensin converting enzyme	ACE	59	4
Angiotensin converting enzyme 2	ACE2	54	4
Renin	REN	21	2
Neprilysin	MME	151	8
Aminopeptidase B	RNPEP	29	0
Aminopeptidase N	ANPEP	31	4
Aminopeptidase A	ENPEP	158	13
Dipeptidyl peptidase	DPP3	32	0

The total number of miRNAs represents miRNA families with binding sites at the 3'UTR region based on TargetScan [48]. Unique miRNAs are those considered solely with respect to other RAS elements.

Table 1. miRNA families targeting RAS elements.

as a whole, for example, in response to an external stimulus. miR-125-5p with five targets in common may function in a similar way, particularly since two of the targets are principal enzymes in RAS biochemistry. Yet, they make an ideal combination to block Ang II/AT1R and Ang IV/AT4R pathways and also shift the conversion of Ang I to Ang (1–7) via neprilysin and other peptidases to act on MasR.

In terms of RAS function, a group of microRNAs that can shift a predominant role of, for example, the Ang II/AT1R axis to opposing axes such as Ang(1–7)/MasR or Ang IV/AT4R could change cerebral blood flow, response to hypoxia and perhaps influence cognition and vice versa. Indeed, a panel of 17 miRNA families target aminopeptidase A and IRAP that could potentiate the formation of Ang IV (since aminopeptidase A converts Ang I and Ang II to Ang III, the Ang IV precursor for Ang IV). Thus, upregulation of those 17 miRNAs could modulate Ang III and IRAP to a greater extent than just one miRNA, such as miR-125. The net effect of reducing both ligand and receptor means that the function of the Ang IV/AT4R axis might be completely inhibited with likely deleterious effects on blood flow and cognitive performance. By contrast, downregulation of these miRNAs would increase the Ang IV/AT4R axis. The following section will discuss the effect of some specific miRNAs and their regulatory effects in RAS in the brain in health and in disease states.

RAS components	microRNA families in common	
ACE ACE2 ANPEP ENPEP LNPEP	1	**miR-125-5p**
ANPEP DPP3 ENPEP LNPEP	1	miR-670-3p
AGTR2 DPP3 LNPEP MME	1	miR-17-5p/20-5p/93-5p/106-5p/519-3p
ACE2 ENPEP LNPEP MME	3	miR-9-5p, miR-200-3p/429, miR-942-5p
AGTR2 LNPEP MAS1	1	miR-23-3p
ENPEP LNPEP MME	17	miR-26-5p, miR-30-5p, **miR-132-3p/212-3p**, miR-194-5p, miR-204-5p/211-5p, miR-216-5p, miR-376-3p, miR-376c-3p, miR-378-3p, miR-450b-5p, miR-518d-5p/519-5p, miR-522-3p, miR-580-3p, miR-653-5p, miR-1269, miR-3942-5p, miR-4766-3p
ACE2 ENPEP LNPEP	4	miR-374-5p/655-3p, miR-543, miR-4424, miR-1306-5p
ACE2 LNPEP MME	3	miR-374a-3p, miR-3194-3p, miR-5691
DPP3 LNPEP MME	5	miR-146-5p, miR-183-5p.1, miR-589-5p, miR-876-5p, miR-2355-5p
ACE2 DPP3 LNPEP	1	miR-329-3p/362-3p
ACE2 ENPEP MME	1	miR-140-3p.1
ENPEP LNPEP	17	miR-9-3p, miR-19-3p, miR-29-3p, miR-34b-5p/449c-5p, miR-105-5p, miR-122-5p, miR-144-3p, miR-320, miR-323-3p, miR-323b-3p, miR-382-3p, miR-494-3p, miR-514a-5p, miR-515-5p/519e-5p, miR-642a-5p, miR-3146, miR-5579-3p
DPP3 ENPEP	1	let-7-5p/98-5p
MAS1	1	**miR-143-3p**
ENPEP	13	**miR-133**, miR-142-3p.2, miR-219-5p, miR-371a-3p, miR-409-5p, miR-451, miR-496.1, miR-508-3p, miR-526b-5p, miR-877-5p, miR-1185-5p, miR-5094
ACE AGTR1 DPP3	1	**miR-34-5p/449-5p**
AGTR1	1	**miR-1-3p/206**
AGT AGTR1 AGTR2 DPP3 ENPEP LNPEP MME RNPEP	1	miR-3163

From 164 combinations of overlapping targets and miRNAs in common, only 14 are included here, 12 which if increased would favour vasoconstriction and 2 would increase vasodilation. Others tend to influence multiple RAS pathways, an example, miR-3163, is given at the bottom of the table. miRNAs in bold are described further in the text.

Table 2. A summary of the subgroups of miRNAs according to their functional effect in the RAS.

5. miRNAs and RAS: cerebrovascular regulation and cognitive function

5.1. MiR-1/206

The miR-1/206 family has been suggested to exclusively target AT1R in the RAS; however, it has an estimate of 790 other transcripts regulating other systems [48]. MiR-1 and miR-206 are located in chromosomes 20 and 6, respectively and share homology in the seed region.

An evaluation of biochemical, cardiovascular and performance indexes of aerobic exercise activity showed that some miRNAs were significantly increased. Specific correlations were found between miR-1, miR-133a and miR-206 and performance parameters, with miR-206 having the strongest positive correlation [78]. MiR-1 was also found to be decreased 1.4-fold in post-mortem cardiac tissue from acute myocardial infarction patients [79]. In contrast, elevated plasma miR-1 levels were reported to predict heart failure after acute myocardial infarction although they returned to basal levels after medication [80].

In conditions of hypoxia such as infarcts, oxygen/glucose deprivation or with ischaemia/reperfusion intervals, miR-1 is highly expressed [79, 80]. Under less stressful and non-life-threatening situations, miR-206 is transcribed [78], both of them targeting AT1R to decrease Ang II-mediated vasoconstriction and in doing so increasing the supply of oxygen and glucose to cells to prevent apoptosis.

MiR-1 overexpression inhibits contractility and proliferation of human vascular smooth muscle cells (VSMCs) in vitro in a negative feedback loop [81, 82]. MiR-1 is downregulated in VSMCs from spontaneous hypertensive rats and its overexpression in vivo inhibits the proliferation of VSMCs by targeting insulin-like growth factor 1 (IGF1) [83]. By contrast, miR-1 upregulation enhances angiogenic differentiation of human cardiomyocyte progenitor cells [84]. The opposite effects of miRNA in different cell types may be explained by its cell-specific expression. Indeed, even if the miRNA is expressed under physiological conditions, variations to this will depend on local gene expression in a time- and cell type-dependent manner.

Evidence of peripheral and central roles for miRNAs was seen in a transgenic mouse model of cardiac-specific overexpression where miR-1 levels were increased not only in the heart but also in the hippocampus and peripheral blood. Furthermore, the mice showed cognitive impairment by downregulation of brain-derived neurotrophic factor (BDNF), a target of miR-1 [85], providing strong evidence for a role in endocrine signalling and association between vascular disorders and cognitive impairment. Nevertheless, it is unlikely that the response depends exclusively on miR-1 and it is not known as to whether the associations are primary or secondary in nature.

Collectively, miR-1 may serve to support protective mechanisms to adapt to adverse hypoxic insults and remodel the proteome as a result. Indeed, as mentioned above, remote ischaemic conditioning showed a high correlation between ischaemia/reperfusion intervals and the levels of miR-1 in rats independent of BDNF mRNA and protein levels [69]. Hence, the miR-1/206 family is likely important in cardioprotection, prevention of stroke and consequently cognitive impairment. Already it is used in screening for myocardial infarction, monitoring and response to therapy and also has a tentative therapeutic use for increasing vasodilation and angiogenesis [86, 87].

However, a solitary miRNA or miRNA-target interaction, such as between miR-1/206 and AT1R, is unlikely to be able to explain a complete physiological response. Inherent properties between miRNA transcription, interactions between their targets, the timing of their expression and subcellular localization provide a more likely explanation. A panel of dysregulated miRNAs is likely to cause an imbalance in targets, proteins and pathways involved. Such a characteristic combination of altered miRNAs may be useful as diagnostic tools. For example, a diagnosis of cholangiocarcinoma can now be made with 100% accuracy in the presence of a 30-miRNA signature, three of them are useful for prognosis and monitoring and one of which has already entered a Phase I clinical trial as a potential treatment [88–91].

5.2. MiR-143

The Mas receptor (MasR) has the lowest number of associated miRNAs, implying steady and tightly regulated homeostatic expression, although other post-transcriptional modifications are also likely to be involved in its regulation. In addition, miR-143 is exclusive to MasR in the RAS and interestingly, it has been found to be dysregulated in vascular disorders [92]. MiR-143 is enriched in cardiac stem cells before becoming localized to smooth muscle cells, including neural vascular smooth muscle cells (VSMC) in mice and its expression was found to be dependent on heartbeat rate in zebrafish [93, 94]. In human peripheral blood mononuclear cells, miR-143 was upregulated in patients with essential hypertension and decreased in aortic aneurysms [95, 96]. Previous studies have focused on other targets of miR-143 in hypertension, yet the potential effect of miR-143 via the MasR remains elusive. Due to the small number of miRNAs attributed to the regulation of MasR, fluctuations in just one of them might have a significant effect on MasR protein levels.

5.3. MiR-132/212

Ang II regulated the miR-132/212 family in hypertensive rats and humans [97, 98] and this family has been attributed with both cardiovascular and brain-specific properties [99–103]. MiR-132/212 was initially thought to directly target AT1R with experimental studies demonstrating a prevalent effect in the RAS, but new advances and criteria in miRNAs have shown that the effect was due to various downstream second messengers of AT1R activation. miRNA-132/212 has multiple targets including Ang II and endothelin-1 (ET-1) signalling [99]. Thus, miRNA-132/212 might be relevant in hypoxic conditions to control the vasoconstrictor effects of Ang II and ET-1. Indeed, transplantation of pericyte progenitor cells from human adult vena safena (Bristol pericytes) induced pro-angiogenic activity in endothelial cells, mediated by pericyte-produced miR-132 in response to hypoxia and taken up by endothelial cells passing through exosomes [104–106].

MiR-132 expression is also regulated by CREB [107, 108], enhances the frequency and amplitude of excitatory potentials in neurons and increases dendritic length and arborization by targeting the brain-enriched GTPase-activating protein p250GAP [109, 110]. MiR-132 triggered marked increases in dendritic spine density, while either underexpression or overexpression of miR-132 caused cognitive impairment in supra-physiological conditions [100, 111]. Similarly, BDNF is regulated by CREB and a negative feedback interaction between the previously described miRNA-1/206 and miRNA-132/212 regulates BDNF expression in the brain [112]. Notably, miRNA-132/212 is also involved in the brain-immune axis and miR-132 mediates an anti-inflammatory effect by targeting acetylcholinesterase, thus increasing acetylcholine that reduces cytokine production [113, 114]. Furthermore, projections from basal forebrain neurons to cortical microvessels (nervi vasorum) and astrocytes containing primarily acetylcholine and nitric oxide synthase (NOS) have contributed to increased cerebral blood flow [77].

5.4. MiR-29

Another miRNA family dysregulated in cerebrovascular disorders and regulated by Ang II is miR-29 [74, 98]. The miR-29 family is linked to cardiac and vascular ageing and counteracts fibrosis by regulating extracellular matrix metallopeptidases [115]. Ang II increased miR-29b in cardiac fibroblasts with no effect in myocytes [116]. In the renal cortex of spontaneously hypertensive rats and in renal tubular epithelial cells, Ang II decreased the expression of miR-29b [117]. Notably, ET-1 decreased miR-29a expression in cardiac myocytes in vitro [118]. MiR-29b is increased in rat brain after focal ischaemia in vivo and in primary neurons exposed to oxygen/glucose deprivation in vitro [119]. Treatment of rats with peroxisome proliferator-activated receptor gamma (PPARγ) agonists protected against ischaemia-reperfusion injury by decreasing miR-29a and miR-29c levels; correspondingly, apoptosis was induced by overexpressing miR-29 [120]. However, mouse models of middle cerebral artery occlusion have inconsistently demonstrated increased and reduced miR-29 levels [119, 121–123]. These conflicting findings have a number of possible explanations including animal age and species, as well as techniques and biosamples used, or other factors discussed below.

Despite the inconsistent evidence, a meta-analysis of microRNAs induced by aerobic exercise in humans evaluated left ventricle hypertrophy and proposed miR-29 family to be antihypertrophic and miR-34 family to be prohypertrophic [124]. MiR-34 was increased in patients with cardiovascular disorders in response to stress [125], which promotes apoptosis and cardiac autophagy [102]. By contrast, myocardial hypertrophy induced by Ang II/AT1R activation in rats is antagonized by miR-34 and its inhibition stimulated Ang II signalling via atrial natriuretic peptide [126]. AT1R activation increased intracellular calcium levels producing vasoconstriction in vascular smooth muscle cells. In addition, in endothelial cells, elevation of intracellular calcium levels contributes to the inhibition of nitric oxide production by atrial natriuretic peptide [127].

5.5. MiR-34

MiR-34 is involved in cardiac and endothelial senescence, characterized by decreased production of the vasodilator nitric oxide by endothelial nitric oxide synthase, inflammation and resultant endothelial dysfunction [128]. MiR-34 promotes endothelial senescence by down-regulating the histone deacetylase sirtuin-1 [129] and regulates cardiac contractile function during ageing and after acute myocardial infarction, as a result of inducing DNA damage and telomere attrition [130]. Transplantation of bone marrow-derived mononuclear cells from patients with cardiovascular disease induced cell death, while inhibition of the elevated levels of miR-34a ex vivo improved the functional benefit of transplanted bone marrow-derived mononuclear cells in mice after acute myocardial infarction in vivo [131]. Inhibition of miR-34 also attenuated ischaemia-induced cardiac remodelling, atrial enlargement and improved systolic function [125, 132].

By contrast, miR-34 promoted differentiation of mouse embryonic neural stem cells to post-mitotic neurons by targeting sirtuin-1 [133]. Along with miR-132/212, miR-34 was upregulated in human epilepsy screenings and pilocarpine-induced status epilepticus in rats [134–139], suggesting neuronal activity-based regulation. MiR-34 expression in the amygdala is also linked to repression of stress-induced anxiety [140], modulates ageing and neurodegeneration in Drosophila [141] and is associated with cognitive impairment [142].

The miRNA families described are functionally relevant in the development of cardiovascular and cerebrovascular disorders, some of which appear to link cerebral ischaemia, endothelial dysfunction and cognitive impairment. Current therapy for cerebral ischaemia is limited to the use of recombinant tissue-plasminogen activator (tPA). Endogenous tPA is primarily expressed in endothelial cells and interactions between tPA and low-density lipoprotein receptor-related protein (LRP) are important for the hippocampal activity-dependent strengthening of synapses known as long-term potentiation (LTP) [143]. AT1R activation causes increased expression of tPA inhibitor (tPA-I), which binds to LRP and blocks its interaction with other ligands, including apolipoprotein E and alpha 2-macroglobulin [144]. Furthermore, tPA-I limits the maturation of proBDNF to BDNF and impedes protein synthesis-dependent late-phase LTP and hippocampal plasticity, mechanisms for learning and memory [145]. Chronic administration of tPA improved cognition in a APPswe/PS1 transgenic mice [146]. MiR-34 has two different binding sites at the 3'UTR of tPA-I, one of which has the highest probability of binding amongst the 108 miRNAs for this transcript. LRP1 is subject to regulation by 22 miRNAs, including miR-125 with one binding site and miR-212 with two binding sites [48].

There has been a recent consensus view on the roles of microRNAs, platelet and endothelial dysfunction in vascular disease and inflammation [147]. MiR-132/212 and miR-29 families target some proteins involved in endothelial dysfunction, such as the actin-related protein 2/3 complex, platelet-derived growth factor and aquaporin 4 [48]; the latter two are particularly relevant in the maintenance of blood-brain barrier (BBB) integrity [148, 149]. Factors involved in BBB disruption include chronic hypertension, ischaemia, trauma, infections and inflammation. Throughout the life course, these factors are likely to cause epigenetic modifications including miRNA fluctuations, leading to reduced protein translation and degradation of mRNA transcripts necessary for BBB integrity. BBB disruption is relevant in understanding the spectrum of clinical manifestations resulting from cerebrovascular disorders.

6. miRNAs challenges and considerations

More than 200 miRNAs have been found to be dysregulated in cerebrovascular disorders, with some inconsistency between studies [74–76, 150–152]. Inconsistencies likely relate partly to the size of the investigated cohorts, particularly since miRNAs may reflect the presence of comorbidities and hence statistical power and specificity would be lessened. Increasing the number of individuals and adding additional specificity (e.g. identifying disease-specific miRNAs as controls) might enable discrimination between the effects of dysregulated miRNAs. For instance, the ability to differentiate between changes in miRNAs associated with haemorrhagic and ischaemic cerebrovascular disorders and in the presence or absence of amyloid deposition or dementia, would be useful. Equally, changes in miRNA signatures could also explain pathophysiological processes in common, such as endothelial disruption and hypoxia due to hypoperfusion.

A second important factor in interpreting data across studies is that of methods used. miRNA detection with high sensitivity and specificity is demanding. The target sequence is present in the primary transcript, the precursor and the mature miRNA; some miRNAs within the same family differ by just a single nucleotide [153, 154]. Profiling can be achieved via three major methods: amplification using quantitative real-time polymerase chain reaction (qRT-PCR), hybridization based on microarrays and sequencing by next-generation sequencing (NGS) technologies [153, 155]. Due to the small size of miRNAs, guanidine-cytosine (GC) content and similar target sequence, hybridization-based methods lack specificity. NGS technologies have provided a considerable aid to advance the field of miRNA, elucidating new miRNAs and applying new criteria for the RNA sequences to be recognized as miRNAs. Studies evaluating sensitivity, specificity, quantification accuracy and reproducibility of different assays have shown that miRNA levels were dependent on the nature of the technique and also with differences between commercial kits [154, 156, 157]. Despite the advantages of NGS, a validation method is highly recommended for those dysregulated miRNAs in large-scale screenings. Although there is no specific consensus paper, qRT-PCR has been widely cited as the gold standard in miRNA research, providing specificity between isomiRs and using stem-loop primers for discrimination from primary miRNAs, pre-miRNAs and degraded mRNA [153, 158].

Another factor is the handling and sample source of miRNAs that are cell type specific and thus, the proportion of different cells contained in a sample can vary. In addition, blood contains high levels of RNase activity; while miRNAs are protected from RNase under normal conditions, their extraction causes immediate degradation if extracted and spiked back to plasma [153]. Other pre-analytic variables might also affect its profiling, such as centrifugation [159]. Collection and handling procedures are relevant to reliably detect dysregulated miRNAs. Exosomal RNA is protected by RNase A treatment and exosomes provide a consistent source of miRNA for disease biomarker detection [160]. Sources like formalin-fixed tissue have been found to be highly reliable [79, 153].

In studies of disease, the pathological stage of the disease, post-mortem status and the agonal state prior to death should also be considered as miRNAs measured could represent causal and/or responsive mechanisms. Thus, there is a need to discriminate between miRNAs produced under normal conditions in different cell types for effective comparisons with those regulated by an environmental insult (e.g. hypoxia), those regulated by the activation of a receptor (e.g. AT1R) or by a common downstream regulator (e.g. CREB). Indeed, during the natural history of a disease, microRNAs will likely fluctuate and their final signature might represent a retrospective picture of various protective mechanisms and aberrant dysregulations.

Finally, the effects of miRNAs on their targets should be viewed in the context of a whole functional analysis [161]. For instance, renin-sensitive microRNAs correlate with atherosclerosis plaque progression [162]. It is conceivable that only a specific combination of microRNAs produces a relevant physiological response. Several outcomes in miRNA research appear to be the result of well-defined miRNA-target-related effects. Nevertheless, the impact of a single miRNA via a specific target is related to the total number of different transcripts it targets and also by the number of other miRNAs that share the same target. It is reasonable to attribute a functional characteristic to a miRNA, based on the experimental outcome, such as in luciferase assays. However, luciferase assays are not able to differentiate between canonical and non-canonical binding sites, neither if the effects are a result of direct miRNA binding to the transcript or by modifying transcription factors.

Furthermore, the experimental outcome will depend on the mRNAs expressed in that cell at that time. For instance, 213 miRNAs can bind at the 3'UTR of the anti-apoptotic protein BCL-2, whereby one could assume that those 213 miRNAs are pro-apoptotic by downregulating BCL-2. However, one of those 213 miRNAs alone could have several hundred targets, some of which promote apoptosis and others favouring survival. Thus, examination of the complete array of targets is needed to provide a functional analysis including an assessment of overlapping targets between miRNAs [161, 163]. Another consideration is the probability rate by which a miRNA binds to the 3′ UTR. Agarwal et al. developed a score based on 14 features (total context score) to allow determination of the probability of miRNA binding and categorization of miRNAs into percentiles based on the total context score [48]. Finally, it is prudent to consider the number of copies of a miRNA expressed. Some miRNAs, such as miR-124 and miR-128, are highly expressed up to 30,000–50,000 copies per neuron, while others can be as low as 1–2 copies per neuron [29]. Therefore, the biological impact of miRNAs relies on the combinatorial signature, the number of miRNA copies expressed, their affinity for different transcripts and the existing mRNA environment accessible for remodelling.

7. Conclusions

In summary, miRNAs are essential for cell fate and differentiation and their effects depend on the mRNA environment expressed, which can be transient over time and subject to dysregulation that may lead to disease. As a highly dynamic and interactive process, epigenetics and particularly miRNAs play a significant role in cognition [164, 165]. Drosha and Dicer are expressed throughout the brain with a higher expression in the hippocampus and dentate gyrus [166]. Functional analysis through bioinformatics and the use of next-generation sequencing could reveal a miRNA signature that helps to explain the effects on pathways and the fluctuations seen over the development of a specific disease. This could allow identification of a small group of miRNAs that are determinant in the clinical manifestation and therefore potential targets for diagnosis and therapeutic intervention. These would have a great advantage as therapies due to their small size and lipidic transport across the BBB, direct intracellular interaction with the transcriptome and may be able to facilitate regeneration while obviating the consequence of a degenerative microenvironment.

Author details

Jose Gerardo-Aviles*, Shelley Allen and Patrick Gavin Kehoe

*Address all correspondence to: jose.gerardo-aviles@bristol.ac.uk

Dementia Research Group, Institute of Clinical Neurosciences, School of Clinical Sciences, University of Bristol, Southmead Hospital, Bristol, UK

References

[1] Romaine SP, Charchar FJ, Samani NJ, Tomaszewski M. Circulating microRNAs and hypertension-from new insights into blood pressure regulation to biomarkers of cardiovascular risk. Curr Opin Pharmacol. 2016;27:1-7. doi:10.1016/j.coph.2015.12.002

[2] Marques FZ, Booth SA, Charchar FJ. The emerging role of non-coding RNA in essential hypertension and blood pressure regulation. J Hum Hypertens. 2015;29(8):459-67. doi:10.1038/jhh.2014.99

[3] Re RN. Mechanisms of disease: local renin–angiotensin–aldosterone systems and the pathogenesis and treatment of cardiovascular disease. Nat Rev Cardiol. 2004;1(1):42-7. doi:10.1038/ncpcardio0012

[4] Turgut F, Balogun RA, Abdel-Rahman EM. Renin-angiotensin-aldosterone system blockade effects on the kidney in the elderly: benefits and limitations. Clin J Am Soc Nephrol: CJASN. 2010;5(7):1330-9. doi:10.2215/cjn.08611209

[5] Sibley S. Hypertension, obesity and the renin-angiotensin system: a tale of tight associations. Minnesota Medicine. 2003;86(1):46-8. Retrieved from https://www.ncbi.nlm.nih.gov/pubmed/12585560 [Accessed 2016-07-10].

[6] Batkai S, Thum T. MicroRNAs in hypertension: mechanisms and therapeutic targets. Curr Hypertens Rep. 2012;14(1):79-87. doi:10.1007/s11906-011-0235-6

[7] Friso S, Carvajal CA, Fardella CE, Olivieri O. Epigenetics and arterial hypertension: the challenge of emerging evidence. Transl Res. 2015;165(1):154-65. doi:10.1016/j.trsl.2014.06.007

[8] Munroe PB, Barnes MR, Caulfield MJ. Advances in blood pressure genomics. Circ Res. 2013;112(10):1365-79. doi:10.1161/CIRCRESAHA.112.300387

[9] Nazari-Jahantigh M, Wei Y, Schober A. The role of microRNAs in arterial remodelling. Thromb Haemost. 2012;107(4):611-8. doi:10.1160/TH11-12-0826

[10] Zhong X, Liao Y, Chen L, Liu G, Feng Y, Zeng T, et al. The MicroRNAs in the pathogenesis of metabolic memory. Endocrinology. 2015;156(9):3157-68. doi:10.1210/en.2015-1063

[11] Bartel DP. microRNAs genomics, biogenesis, mechanism and function. Cell. 2004;116:281-97. doi:10.1016/S0092-8674(04)00045-5

[12] Bartel DP. MicroRNAs: target recognition and regulatory functions. Cell. 2009;136(2):215-33. doi:10.1016/j.cell.2009.01.002

[13] Miyoshi K, Miyoshi T, Siomi H. Many ways to generate microRNA-like small RNAs: non-canonical pathways for microRNA production. Mol Genet Genomics. 2010;284(2):95-103. doi:10.1007/s00438-010-0556-1

[14] Winter J, Jung S, Keller S, Gregory RI, Diederichs S. Many roads to maturity microRNA biogenesis pathways and their regulation. Nat Cell Biol. 2009;11(3):228-34. doi:10.1038/ncb0309-228

[15] Kozomara A, Griffiths-Jones S. miRBase: annotating high confidence microRNAs using deep sequencing data. Nucleic Acids Res. 2014;42:D68-73. doi:10.1093/nar/gkt1181

[16] Zhou X, Yang P-C. MicroRNA: a small molecule with a big biological impact. MicroRNA. 2012;1(1):1. doi:10.2174/2211536611201010001

[17] Basak I, Patil KS, Alves G, Larsen JP, Moller SG. microRNAs as neuroregulators, biomarkers and therapeutic agents in neurodegenerative diseases. Cell Mol Life Sci. 2016;73(4):811-27. doi:10.1007/s00018-015-2093-x

[18] Pelechano V, Steinmetz LM. Gene regulation by antisense transcription. Nat Rev Genet. 2013;14(12):880-93. doi:10.1038/nrg3594

[19] Romero CA, Orias M, Weir MR. Novel RAAS agonists and antagonists: clinical applications and controversies. Nat Rev Endocrinol. 2015;11(4):242-52. doi:10.1038/nrendo.2015.6

[20] Wright JW, Kawas LH, Harding JW. The development of small molecule angiotensin IV analogs to treat Alzheimer's and Parkinson's diseases. Prog Neurobiol. 2015;125:26-46. doi:10.1016/j.pneurobio.2014.11.004

[21] Savaskan E. The role of the brain renin-angiotensin system in neurodegenerative disorders. Curr Alzheimer Res. 2005;2(1):29-35. doi:10.2174/1567205052772740

[22] Wright JW, Harding JW. Brain renin-angiotensin—a new look at an old system. Prog Neurobiol. 2011;95(1):49-67. doi:10.1016/j.pneurobio.2011.07.001

[23] Wright JW. Introduction: aminopeptidases and hypertension-mechanisms of action and therapeutic strategies. Heart Fail Rev. 2008;13(3):271-2. doi:10.1007/s10741-007-9076-4

[24] Wright JW, Kawas LH, Harding JW. A role for the brain RAS in Alzheimer's and Parkinson's diseases. Front Endocrinol. 2013;4:158. doi:10.3389/fendo.2013.00158

[25] Lautner RQ, Villela DC, Fraga-Silva RA, Silva N, Verano-Braga T, Costa-Fraga F, et al. Discovery and characterization of alamandine: a novel component of the renin-angiotensin system. Circ Res. 2013;112(8):1104-11. doi:10.1161/circresaha.113.301077

[26] Villela DC, Passos-Silva DG, Santos RA. Alamandine: a new member of the angiotensin family. Curr Opin Nephrol Hypertens. 2014;23(2):130-4. doi:10.1097/01.mnh.0000441052.44406.92

[27] Etelvino GM, Peluso AA, Santos RA. New components of the renin-angiotensin system: alamandine and the MAS-related G protein-coupled receptor D. Curr Hypertens Rep. 2014;16(6):433. doi:10.1007/s11906-014-0433-0

[28] Mohr AM, Mott JL. Overview of microRNA biology. Semin Liver Dis. 2015;35(1):3-11. doi:10.1055/s-0034-1397344

[29] O'Carroll D, Schaefer A. General principals of miRNA biogenesis and regulation in the brain. Neuropsychopharmacology. 2013;38(1):39-54. doi:10.1038/npp.2012.87

[30] Baskerville S, Bartel DP. Microarray profiling of microRNAs reveals frequent coexpression with neighboring miRNAs and host genes. RNA. 2005;11(3):241-7. doi:10.1261/rna.7240905

[31] Meunier J, Lemoine F, Soumillon M, Liechti A, Weier M, Guschanski K, et al. Birth and expression evolution of mammalian microRNA genes. Genome Res. 2013;23(1):34-45. doi:10.1101/gr.140269.112

[32] Berezikov E. Evolution of microRNA diversity and regulation in animals. Nat Rev Genet. 2011;12(12):846-60. doi:10.1038/nrg3079

[33] Guerra-Assunção JA, Enright AJ. Large-scale analysis of microRNA evolution. BMC Genomics. 2012;13(1):1. doi:10.1186/1471-2164-13-218

[34] Gregory RI, Yan KP, Amuthan G, Chendrimada T, Doratotaj B, Cooch N, et al. The microprocessor complex mediates the genesis of microRNAs. Nature. 2004;432(7014):235-40. doi:10.1038/nature03120

[35] Grimson A, Srivastava M, Fahey B, Woodcroft BJ, Chiang HR, King N, et al. Early origins and evolution of microRNAs and Piwi-interacting RNAs in animals. Nature. 2008;455(7217):1193-7. doi:10.1038/nature07415

[36] Ameres SL, Zamore PD. Diversifying microRNA sequence and function. Nat Rev Mol Cell Biol. 2013;14(8):475-88. doi:10.1038/nrm3611

[37] Czech B, Hannon GJ. Small RNA sorting: matchmaking for Argonautes. Nat Rev Genet. 2011;12(1):19-31. doi:10.1038/nrg2916

[38] Yoon JH, Abdelmohsen K, Gorospe M. Functional interactions among microRNAs and long noncoding RNAs. Semin Cell Dev Biol. 2014;34:9-14. doi:10.1016/j.semcdb.2014.05.015

[39] Kai ZS, Pasquinelli AE. MicroRNA assassins: factors that regulate the disappearance of miRNAs. Nat Struct Mol Biol. 2010;17(1):5-10. doi:10.1038/nsmb.1762

[40] Diederichs S, Haber DA. Dual role for argonautes in microRNA processing and posttranscriptional regulation of microRNA expression. Cell. 2007;131:1097-108. doi:10.1016/j.cell.2007.10.032

[41] Salmanidis M, Pillman K, Goodall G, Bracken C. Direct transcriptional regulation by nuclear microRNAs. Int J Biochem Cell Biol. 2014;54:304-11. doi:10.1016/j.biocel.2014.03.010

[42] Liu J, Valencia-Sanchez MA, Hannon GJ, Parker R. MicroRNA-dependent localization of targeted mRNAs to mammalian P-bodies. Nat Cell Biol. 2005;7(7):719-23. doi:10.1038/ncb1274

[43] Braun JE, Huntzinger E, Fauser M, Izaurralde E. GW182 proteins directly recruit cytoplasmic deadenylase complexes to miRNA targets. Mol Cell. 2011;44(1):120-33. doi:10.1016/j.molcel.2011.09.007

[44] Chekulaeva M, Mathys H, Zipprich JT, Attig J, Colic M, Parker R, et al. miRNA repression involves GW182-mediated recruitment of CCR4-NOT through conserved W-containing motifs. Nat Struct Mol Biol. 2011;18(11):1218-26. doi:10.1038/nsmb.2166

[45] Fabian MR, Cieplak MK, Frank F, Morita M, Green J, Srikumar T, et al. miRNA-mediated deadenylation is orchestrated by GW182 through two conserved motifs that interact with CCR4-NOT. Nat Struct Mol Biol. 2011;18(11):1211-7. doi:10.1038/nsmb.2149

[46] Friedman RC, Farh KK, Burge CB, Bartel DP. Most mammalian mRNAs are conserved targets of microRNAs. Genome Res. 2009;19(1):92-105. doi:10.1101/gr.082701.108

[47] Shin C, Nam JW, Farh KK, Chiang HR, Shkumatava A, Bartel DP. Expanding the microRNA targeting code: functional sites with centered pairing. Mol Cell. 2010;38(6):789-802. doi:10.1016/j.molcel.2010.06.005

[48] Agarwal V, Bell GW, Nam JW, Bartel DP. Predicting effective microRNA target sites in mammalian mRNAs. 2015;4:e05005. doi:10.7554/eLife.05005

[49] Belting M, Wittrup A. Nanotubes, exosomes and nucleic acid-binding peptides provide novel mechanisms of intercellular communication in eukaryotic cells: implications in health and disease. J Cell Biol. 2008;183(7):1187-91. doi:10.1083/jcb.200810038

[50] Paschon V, Takada SH, Ikebara JM, Sousa E, Raeisossadati R, Ulrich H, et al. Interplay between exosomes, microRNAs and toll-like receptors in brain disorders. Mol Neurobiol. 2016;53(3):2016-28. doi:10.1007/s12035-015-9142-1

[51] Chen X, Liang H, Zhang J, Zen K, Zhang CY. Horizontal transfer of microRNAs: molecular mechanisms and clinical applications. Protein Cell. 2012;3(1):28-37. doi:10.1007/s13238-012-2003-z

[52] Valadi H, Ekstrom K, Bossios A, Sjostrand M, Lee JJ, Lotvall JO. Exosome-mediated transfer of mRNAs and microRNAs is a novel mechanism of genetic exchange between cells. Nat Cell Biol. 2007;9(6):654-9. doi:10.1038/ncb1596

[53] Wahlgren J, De LKT, Brisslert M, Vaziri Sani F, Telemo E, Sunnerhagen P, et al. Plasma exosomes can deliver exogenous short interfering RNA to monocytes and lymphocytes. Nucleic Acids Res. 2012;40(17):e130. doi:10.1093/nar/gks463

[54] Vlassov AV, Magdaleno S, Setterquist R, Conrad R. Exosomes: current knowledge of their composition, biological functions and diagnostic and therapeutic potentials. Biochim Biophys Acta. 2012;1820(7):940-8. doi:10.1016/j.bbagen.2012.03.017

[55] Zhang J, Li S, Li L, Li M, Guo C, Yao J, et al. Exosome and exosomal microRNA: trafficking, sorting and function. Genom Proteom Bioinform. 2015;13(1):17-24. doi:10.1016/j.gpb.2015.02.001

[56] Janas T, Janas MM, Sapon K, Janas T. Mechanisms of RNA loading into exosomes. FEBS Lett. 2015;589(13):1391-8. doi:10.1016/j.febslet.2015.04.036

[57] Das S, Halushka MK. Extracellular vesicle microRNA transfer in cardiovascular disease. Cardiovasc Pathol. 2015;24(4):199-206. doi:10.1016/j.carpath.2015.04.007

[58] Sahoo S, Losordo DW. Exosomes and cardiac repair after myocardial infarction. Circ Res. 2014;114(2):333-44. doi:10.1161/CIRCRESAHA.114.300639

[59] Hergenreider E, Heydt S, Treguer K, Boettger T, Horrevoets AJ, Zeiher AM, et al. Atheroprotective communication between endothelial cells and smooth muscle cells through miRNAs. Nat Cell Biol. 2012;14(3):249-56. doi:10.1038/ncb2441

[60] Kuwabara Y, Ono K, Horie T, Nishi H, Nagao K, Kinoshita M, et al. Increased microRNA-1 and microRNA-133a levels in serum of patients with cardiovascular disease indicate myocardial damage. Circ Cardiovasc Genet. 2011;4(4):446-54. doi:10.1161/circgenetics.110.958975

[61] Xin H, Li Y, Buller B, Katakowski M, Zhang Y, Wang X, et al. Exosome-mediated transfer of miR-133b from multipotent mesenchymal stromal cells to neural cells contributes to neurite outgrowth. Stem Cells (Dayton, Ohio). 2012;30(7):1556-64. doi:10.1002/stem.1129

[62] Xin H, Li Y, Liu Z, Wang X, Shang X, Cui Y, et al. MiR-133b promotes neural plasticity and functional recovery after treatment of stroke with multipotent mesenchymal stromal cells in rats via transfer of exosome-enriched extracellular particles. Stem Cells. 2013;31(12):2737-46. doi:10.1002/stem.1409

[63] Wang F, Long G, Zhao C, Li H, Chaugai S, Wang Y, et al. Plasma microRNA-133a is a new marker for both acute myocardial infarction and underlying coronary artery stenosis. J Transl Med. 2013;11:222. doi:10.1186/1479-5876-11-222

[64] Hess DC, Blauenfeldt RA Andersen G, Hougaard KD, Hoda MN, Ding Y, et al. Remote ischaemic conditioning—a new paradigm of self-protection in the brain. Nat Rev Neurol. 2015;11:698-710. doi:10.1038/nrneurol.2015.223

[65] Hausenloy DJ, Candilio L, Evans R, Ariti C, Jenkins DP, Kolvekar S, et al. Remote ischemic preconditioning and outcomes of cardiac surgery. N Engl J Med. 2015;373:1408-17. doi:10.1056/NEJMoa1413534

[66] Hausenloy DJ, Yellon DM. The therapeutic potential of ischemic conditioning: an update. Nat Rev Cardiol. 2011;8(11):619-29. doi:10.1038/nrcardio.2011.85

[67] Li J, Rohailla S, Gelber N, Rutka J, Sabah N, Gladstone RA, et al. MicroRNA-144 is a circulating effector of remote ischemic preconditioning. Basic Res Cardiol. 2014;109(5):423. doi:10.1007/s00395-014-0423-z

[68] Hu Q, Luo W, Huang L, Huang R, Chen R. Apoptosis-related microRNA changes in the right atrium induced by remote ischemic perconditioning during valve replacement surgery. Sci Rep. 2015;6:18959. doi:10.1038/srep18959

[69] Brandenburger T, Grievink H, Heinen N, Barthel F, Huhn R, Stachuletz F, et al. Effects of remote ischemic preconditioning and myocardial ischemia on microRNA-1 expression in the rat heart in vivo. Shock. 2014;42(3):234-8. doi:10.1097/shk.0000000000000201

[70] Kinet V, Halkein J, Dirkx E, Windt LJ. Cardiovascular extracellular microRNAs: emerging diagnostic markers and mechanisms of cell-to-cell RNA communication. Front Genet. 2013;4:214. doi:10.3389/fgene.2013.00214

[71] Fang L, Ellims AH, Moore XL, White DA, Taylor AJ, Chin-Dusting J, et al. Circulating microRNAs as biomarkers for diffuse myocardial fibrosis in patients with hypertrophic cardiomyopathy. J Transl Med. 2015;13:314. doi:10.1186/s12967-015-0672-0

[72] Grasso M, Piscopo P, Confaloni A, Denti MA. Circulating miRNAs as biomarkers for neurodegenerative disorders. Molecules. 2014;19(5):6891-910. doi:10.3390/molecules19056891

[73] Guay C, Regazzi R. Circulating microRNAs as novel biomarkers for diabetes mellitus. Nat Rev Endocrinol. 2013;9(9):513-21. doi:10.1038/nrendo.2013.86

[74] Li M, Zhang J. Circulating microRNAs: potential and emerging biomarkers for diagnosis of cardiovascular and cerebrovascular diseases. Biomed Res Int. 2015;2015:730535. doi:10.1155/2015/730535

[75] Li WY, Jin J, Chen J, Guo Y, Tang J, Tan S. Circulating microRNAs as potential non-invasive biomarkers for the early detection of hypertension-related stroke. J Hum Hypertens. 2014;28(5):288-91. doi:10.1038/jhh.2013.94

[76] Wang W, Sun G, Zhang L, Shi L, Zeng Y. Circulating microRNAs as novel potential biomarkers for early diagnosis of acute stroke in humans. J Stroke Cerebrovasc Dis. 2014;23(10):2607-13. doi:10.1016/j.jstrokecerebrovasdis.2014.06.002

[77] Cipolla MJ. The cerebral circulation. In: Control of Cerebral Blood Flow, Chapter 5. San Rafael (CA): Morgan & Claypool Life Sciences; 2009.

[78] Mooren FC, Viereck J, Kruger K, Thum T. Circulating microRNAs as potential biomarkers of aerobic exercise capacity. Am J Physiol Heart Circ Physiol. 2014;306(4):H557-63. doi:10.1152/ajpheart.00711.2013

[79] Kakimoto Y, Kamiguchi H, Ochiai E, Satoh F, Osawa M. MicroRNA stability in postmortem FFPE tissues: quantitative analysis using autoptic samples from acute myocardial infarction patients. PLoS One. 2015;10(6):e0129338. doi:10.1371/journal.pone.0129338

[80] Zhang R, Niu H, Ban T, Xu L, Li Y, Wang N, et al. Elevated plasma microRNA-1 predicts heart failure after acute myocardial infarction. Int J Cardiol. 2013;166(1):259-60. doi:10.1016/j.ijcard.2012.09.108

[81] Chen J, Yin H, Jiang Y, Radhakrishnan SK, Huang ZP, Li J, et al. Induction of microRNA-1 by myocardin in smooth muscle cells inhibits cell proliferation. Arterioscler Thromb Vasc Biol. 2011;31(2):368-75. doi:10.1161/atvbaha.110.218149

[82] Jiang Y, Yin H, Zheng XL. MicroRNA-1 inhibits myocardin-induced contractility of human vascular smooth muscle cells. J Cell Physiol. 2010;225(2):506-11. doi:10.1002/jcp.22230

[83] Liu K, Ying Z, Qi X, Shi Y, Tang Q. MicroRNA-1 regulates the proliferation of vascular smooth muscle cells by targeting insulin-like growth factor 1. Int J Mol Med. 2015;36(3):817-24. doi:10.3892/ijmm.2015.2277

[84] van Mil A, Vrijsen KR, Goumans MJ, Metz CH, Doevendans PA, Sluijter JP. MicroRNA-1 enhances the angiogenic differentiation of human cardiomyocyte progenitor cells. J Mol Med. 2013;91(8):1001-12. doi:10.1007/s00109-013-1017-1

[85] Ma JC, Duan MJ, Sun LL, Yan ML, Liu T, Wang Q, et al. Cardiac over-expression of microRNA-1 induces impairment of cognition in mice. Neuroscience. 2015;299:66-78. doi:10.1016/j.neuroscience.2015.04.061

[86] Cheng C, Wang Q, You W, Chen M, Xia J. MiRNAs as biomarkers of myocardial infarction: a meta-analysis. PLoS One. 2014;9(2):e88566. doi:10.1371/journal.pone.0088566

[87] Li C, Pei F, Zhu X, Duan DD, Zeng C. Circulating microRNAs as novel and sensitive biomarkers of acute myocardial Infarction. Clin Biochem. 2012;45(10-11):727-32. doi:10.1016/j.clinbiochem.2012.04.013

[88] Simonson B, Das S. MicroRNA therapeutics: the next magic bullet? Mini Rev Med Chem. 2015;15(6):467-74. doi:10.2174/1389557515666150324123208

[89] Li XJ, Ren ZJ, Tang JH. MicroRNA-34a: a potential therapeutic target in human cancer. Cell Death Dis. 2014;5(7). doi:10.1038/cddis.2014.270

[90] Misso G, Martino MTD, Rosa GD, Farooqi AA, Lombardi A, Campani V, et al. Mir-34: a new weapon against cancer? Mol Ther Nucleic Acids. 2014;3(9):e194. doi:10.1038/mtna.2014.47

[91] Zhang MY, Li SH, Huang GL, Lin GH, Shuang ZY, Lao XM, et al. Identification of a novel microRNA signature associated with intrahepatic cholangiocarcinoma (ICC) patient prognosis. BMC Cancer. 2015;15:64. doi:10.1186/s12885-015-1067-6

[92] Zhao W, Zhao SP, Zhao YH. MicroRNA-143/-145 in cardiovascular diseases. Biomed Res Int. 2015;2015:531740. doi:10.1155/2015/531740

[93] Cordes KR, Sheehy NT, White MP, Berry EC, Morton SU, Muth AN, et al. miR-145 and miR-143 regulate smooth muscle cell fate and plasticity. Nature. 2009;460(7256):705-10. doi:10.1038/nature08195

[94] Miyasaka KY, Kida YS, Banjo T, Ueki Y, Nagayama K, Matsumoto T, et al. Heartbeat regulates cardiogenesis by suppressing retinoic acid signaling via expression of miR-143. Mech Dev. 2011;128(1-2):18-28. doi:10.1016/j.mod.2010.09.002

[95] Elia L, Quintavalle M, Zhang J, Contu R, Cossu L, Latronico MVG, et al. The knockout of miR-143 and -145 alters smooth muscle cell maintenance and vascular homeostasis in mice: correlates with human disease. Cell Death Differ. 2009;16(12):1590-8. doi:10.1038/cdd.2009.153

[96] Kontaraki JE, Marketou ME, Zacharis EA, Parthenakis FI, Vardas PE. Differential expression of vascular smooth muscle-modulating microRNAs in human peripheral blood mononuclear cells: novel targets in essential hypertension. J Hum Hypertens 2013;28(8):510-6. doi:10.1038/jhh.2013.117

[97] Eskildsen TV, Jeppesen PL, Schneider M, Nossent AY, Sandberg MB, Hansen PB, et al. Angiotensin II regulates microRNA-132/-212 in hypertensive rats and humans. Int J Mol Sci. 2013;14(6):11190-207. doi:10.3390/ijms140611190

[98] Obama T, Eguchi S. MicroRNA as a novel component of the tissue renin angiotensin system. J Mol Cell Cardiol. 2014;75:98-9. doi:10.1016/j.yjmcc.2014.07.004

[99] Eskildsen TV, Schneider M, Sandberg MB, Skov V, Bronnum H, Thomassen M, et al. The microRNA-132/212 family fine-tunes multiple targets in Angiotensin II signalling in cardiac fibroblasts. J Renin Angiotensin Aldosterone Syst. 2015;16(4):1288-97. doi:10.1177/1470320314539367

[100] Hansen KF, Karelina K, Sakamoto K, Wayman GA, Impey S, Obrietan K. miRNA-132: a dynamic regulator of cognitive capacity. Brain Struct Funct. 2013;218(3):817-31. doi:10.1007/s00429-012-0431-4

[101] Kumarswamy R, Volkmann I, Beermann J, Napp LC, Jabs O, Bhayadia R, et al. Vascular importance of the miR-212/132 cluster. Eur Heart J. 2014;35(45):3224-31. doi:10.1093/eurheartj/ehu344

[102] Pacurari M, Tchounwou PB. Role of microRNAs in renin-angiotensin-aldosterone system-mediated cardiovascular inflammation and remodeling. Int J Inflam. 2015;2015:101527. doi:10.1155/2015/101527

[103] Wanet A, Tacheny A, Arnould T, Renard P. miR-212/132 expression and functions: within and beyond the neuronal compartment. Nucleic Acids Res. 2012;40(11):4742-53. doi:10.1093/nar/gks151

[104] Emanueli C, Shearn AI, Angelini GD, Sahoo S. Exosomes and exosomal miRNAs in cardiovascular protection and repair. Vascul Pharmacol. 2015;71:24-30. doi:10.1016/j.vph.2015.02.008

[105] Campagnolo P, Cesselli D, Zen AAH, Beltrami AP, Kränkel N, Katare R, et al. Human adult vena saphena contains perivascular progenitor cells endowed with clonogenic and proangiogenic potential. Circulation. 2010;121:1735-45. doi:10.1161/CIRCULATIONAHA.109.899252

[106] Katare R, Riu F, Mitchell K, Gubernator M, Campagnolo P, Cui Y, et al. Transplantation of human pericyte progenitor cells improves the repair of infarcted heart through activation of an angiogenic program involving micro-RNA-132. Circ Res. 2011;109:894-906. doi:10.1161/CIRCRESAHA.111.251546

[107] Remenyi J, Hunter CJ, Cole C, Ando H, Impey S, Monk CE, et al. Regulation of the miR-212/132 locus by MSK1 and CREB in response to neurotrophins. Biochem J. 2010;428(2):281-91. doi:10.1042/BJ20100024

[108] Nudelman AS, DiRocco DP, Lambert TJ, Garelick MG, Le J, Nathanson NM, et al. Neuronal activity rapidly induces transcription of the CREB-regulated microRNA-132, in vivo. Hippocampus. 2010;20(4):492-8. doi:10.1002/hipo.20646

[109] Edbauer D, Neilson JR, Foster KA, Wang CF, Seeburg DP, Batterton MN, et al. Regulation of synaptic structure and function by FMRP-associated microRNAs miR-125b and miR-132. Neuron. 2010;65(3):373-84. doi:10.1016/j.neuron.2010.01.005

[110] Wayman GA, Davare M, Ando H, Fortin D, Varlamova O, Cheng HY, et al. An activity-regulated microRNA controls dendritic plasticity by down-regulating p250GAP. Proc Natl Acad Sci U S A. 2008;105(26):9093-8. doi:10.1073/pnas.0803072105

[111] Hansen KF, Sakamoto K, Wayman GA, Impey S, Obrietan K. Transgenic miR132 alters neuronal spine density and impairs novel object recognition memory. PLoS One. 2010;5(11):e15497. doi:10.1371/journal.pone.0015497

[112] Keifer J, Zheng Z, Ambigapathy G. A microRNA-BDNF negative feedback signaling loop in brain: implications for Alzheimer's Disease. MicroRNA. 2015;4:101-8. doi:10.2174/2211536604666150813152620

[113] O'Neill LA. Boosting the brain's ability to block inflammation via microRNA-132. Immunity. 2009;31(6):854-5. doi:10.1016/j.immuni.2009.11.004

[114] Shaked I, Meerson A, Wolf Y, Avni R, Greenberg D, Gilboa-Geffen A, et al. MicroRNA-132 potentiates cholinergic anti-inflammatory signaling by targeting acetylcholinesterase. Immunity. 2009;31(6):965-73. doi:10.1016/j.immuni.2009.09.019

[115] Seeger T, Boon RA. MicroRNAs in cardiovascular ageing. J Physiol. 2016;594(8):2085-94. doi:10.1113/JP270557

[116] Jeppesen PL, Christensen GL, Schneider M, Nossent AY, Jensen HB, Andersen DC, et al. Angiotensin II type 1 receptor signalling regulates microRNA differentially in cardiac fibroblasts and myocytes. Br J Pharmacol. 2011;164(2):394-404. doi:10.1111/j.1476-5381.2011.01375.x

[117] Pan J, Zhang J, Zhang X, Zhou X, Lu S, Huang X, et al. Role of microRNA-29b in angiotensin II-induced epithelial-mesenchymal transition in renal tubular epithelial cells. Int J Mol Med. 2014;34(5):1381-7. doi:10.3892/ijmm.2014.1935

[118] Li M, Wang N, Zhang J, He HP, Gong HQ, Zhang R, et al. MicroRNA-29a-3p attenuates ET-1-induced hypertrophic responses in H9c2 cardiomyocytes. Gene. 2016;585(1):44-50. doi:10.1016/j.gene.2016.03.015

[119] Shi G, Liu Y, Liu T, Yan W, Liu X, Wang Y, et al. Upregulated miR-29b promotes neuronal cell death by inhibiting Bcl2L2 after ischemic brain injury. Exp Brain Res. 2012;216(2):225-30. doi:10.1007/s00221-011-2925-3

[120] Ye Y, Hu Z, Lin Y, Zhang C, Perez-Polo JR. Downregulation of microRNA-29 by antisense inhibitors and a PPAR-gamma agonist protects against myocardial ischaemia-reperfusion injury. Cardiovasc Res. 2010;87(3):535-44. doi:10.1093/cvr/cvq053

[121] Pandi G, Nakka VP, Dharap A, Roopra A, Vemuganti R. MicroRNA miR-29c down-regulation leading to de-repression of its target DNA methyltransferase 3a promotes ischemic brain damage. PLoS One. 2013;8(3):e58039. doi:10.1371/journal.pone.0058039

[122] Kole AJ, Swahari V, Hammond SM, Deshmukh M. miR-29b is activated during neuronal maturation and targets BH3-only genes to restrict apoptosis. Genes Dev. 2011;25(2):125-30. doi:10.1101/gad.1975411

[123] Huang LG, Li JP, Pang XM, Chen CY, Xiang HY, Feng LB, et al. MicroRNA-29c Correlates with Neuroprotection Induced by FNS by Targeting Both Birc2 and Bak1 in Rat Brain after Stroke. CNS Neurosci Ther. 2015;21(6):496-503. doi:10.1111/cns.12383

[124] Fernandes T, Barauna VG, Negrao CE, Phillips MI, Oliveira EM. Aerobic exercise training promotes physiological cardiac remodelling involving a set of microRNAs. Am J Physiol Heart Circ Physiol. 2015;309(4):H543-52. doi:10.1152/ajpheart.00899.2014

[125] Harrison C. Cardiovascular disease: Inhibiting microRNA-34 benefits heart disease. Nat Rev Drug Discov. 2012;11(12):908. doi:10.1038/nrd3903

[126] Huang J, Sun W, Huang H, Ye J, Pan W, Zhong Y, et al. miR-34a modulates angiotensin II-induced myocardial hypertrophy by direct inhibition of ATG9A expression and autophagic activity. PLoS One. 2014;9(4):e94382. doi:10.1371/journal.pone.0094382

[127] Kiemer AK, Vollmar AM. Elevation of intracellular calcium levels contributes to the inhibition of nitric oxide production by atrial natriuretic peptide. Immunol Cell Biol. 2001;79(1):11-7. doi:10.1046/j.1440-1711.2001.00969.x

[128] Arunachalam G, Upadhyay R, Ding H, Triggle CR. MicroRNA signature and cardiovascular dysfunction. J Cardiovasc Pharmacol. 2015;65:419-29. doi:10.1097/FJC.0000000000000178

[129] Ito T, Yagi S, Yamakuchi M. MicroRNA-34a regulation of endothelial senescence. Biochem Biophys Res Commun. 2010;398(4):735-40. doi:10.1016/j.bbrc.2010.07.012

[130] Boon RA, Iekushi K, Lechner S, Seeger T, Fischer A, Heydt S, et al. MicroRNA-34a regulates cardiac ageing and function. Nature. 2013;495(7439):107-10. doi:10.1038/nature11919

[131] Xu Q, Seeger FH, Castillo J, Iekushi K, Boon RA, Farcas R, et al. Micro-RNA-34a contributes to the impaired function of bone marrow-derived mononuclear cells from patients with cardiovascular disease. J Am Coll Cardiol. 2012;59(23):2107-17. doi:10.1016/j.jacc.2012.02.033

[132] Bernardo BC, Gao XM, Winbanks CE, Boey EJ, Tham YK, Kiriazis H, et al. Therapeutic inhibition of the miR-34 family attenuates pathological cardiac remodeling and improves heart function. Proc Natl Acad Sci U S A. 2012;109(43):17615-20. doi:10.1073/pnas.1206432109

[133] Aranha MM, Santos DM, Sola S, Steer CJ, Rodrigues CM. miR-34a regulates mouse neural stem cell differentiation. PLoS One. 2011;6(8):e21396. doi:10.1371/journal.pone.0021396

[134] Dombkowski AA, Batista CE, Cukovic D, Carruthers NJ, Ranganathan R, Shukla U, et al. Cortical tubers: windows into dysregulation of epilepsy risk and synaptic signaling genes by microRNAs. Cerebral Cortex. 2016;26(3):1059-71. doi:10.1093/cercor/bhu276

[135] Gorter JA, Iyer A, White I, Colzi A, van Vliet EA, Sisodiya S, et al. Hippocampal subregion-specific microRNA expression during epileptogenesis in experimental temporal lobe epilepsy. Neurobiol Dis. 2014;62:508-20. doi:10.1016/j.nbd.2013.10.026

[136] Guo J, Wang H, Wang Q, Chen Y, Chen S. Expression of p-CREB and activity-dependent miR-132 in temporal lobe epilepsy. Int J Clin Exp Med. 2014;7(5):1297-306. doi:1940-5901/IJCEM0000469

[137] Peng J, Omran A, Ashhab MU, Kong H, Gan N, He F, et al. Expression patterns of miR-124, miR-134, miR-132 and miR-21 in an immature rat model and children with mesial temporal lobe epilepsy. J Mol Neurosci. 2013;50(2):291-7. doi:10.1007/s12031-013-9953-3

[138] Song YJ, Tian XB, Zhang S, Zhang YX, Li X, Li D, et al. Temporal lobe epilepsy induces differential expression of hippocampal miRNAs including let-7e and miR-23a/b. Brain Res. 2011;1387:134-40. doi:10.1016/j.brainres.2011.02.073

[139] Hu K, Xie Y-Y, Zhang C, Ouyang D-S, Long H-Y, Sun D-N, et al. MicroRNA expression profile of the hippocampus in a rat model of temporal lobe epilepsy and miR-34a-targeted neuroprotection against hippocampal neurone cell apoptosis post-status epilepticus. BMC Neurosci. 2012;13(1):1. doi:10.1186/1471-2202-13-115

[140] Haramati S, Navon I, Issler O, Ezra-Nevo G, Gil S, Zwang R, et al. MicroRNA as repressors of stress-induced anxiety: the case of amygdalar miR-34. J Neurosci. 2011;31(40):14191-203. doi:10.1523/jneurosci.1673-11.2011

[141] Liu N, Landreh M, Cao K, Abe M, Hendriks GJ, Kennerdell JR, et al. The microRNA miR-34 modulates ageing and neurodegeneration in Drosophila. Nature. 2012;482(7386):519-23. doi:10.1038/nature10810

[142] Choi SE, Kemper JK. Regulation of SIRT1 by microRNAs. Mol Cells. 2013;36(5):385-92. doi:10.1007/s10059-013-0297-1

[143] Zhuo M, Holtzman DM, Li Y, Osaka H, DeMaro J, Jacquin M, et al. Role of tissue plasminogen activator receptor LRP in hippocampal long-term potentiation. J Neurosci. 2000;20(2):542-9. Retrieved from http://www.jneurosci.org/content/20/2/542.full.pdf+html [Accessed 2016-08-15].

[144] Orth K, Madison EL, Gething M-J, Sambrook JF, Herz J. Complexes of tissue-type plasminogen-activator and its serpin inhibitor plasminogen activator inhibitor type 1 are internalized by means of the low density lipoprotein receptor-related protein/a2-macroglobulin receptor. Cell Biol. 1992;89:7422-6. Retrieved from https://www.ncbi.nlm.nih.gov/pmc/articles/PMC49722/pdf/pnas01090-0144.pdf [Accessed 2016-08-15].

[145] Bodiga VL, Bodiga S. Renin angiotensin system in cognitive function and dementia. Asian J Neurosci. 2013;2013:1-18. doi:10.1155/2013/102602

[146] ElAli A, Bordeleau M, Thériault P, Filali M, Lampron A, Rivest S. Tissue-plasminogen activator attenuates Alzheimer's disease-related pathology development in APPswe/PS1 mice. Neuropsychopharmacology. 2015;41(5):1297-307. doi:10.1038/npp.2015.279

[147] Cabrera-Fuentes HA, Alba-Alba C, Aragones J, Bernhagen J, Boisvert WA, Botker HE, et al. Meeting report from the 2nd International Symposium on New Frontiers in Cardiovascular Research. Protecting the cardiovascular system from ischemia: between bench and bedside. Basic Res Cardiol. 2016;111(1):7. doi:10.1007/s00395-015-0527-0

[148] Sweeney MD, Ayyadurai S, Zlokovic BV. Pericytes of the neurovascular unit: key functions and signaling pathways. Nat Neurosci. 2016;19(6):771-83. doi:10.1038/nn.4288

[149] Zhao Z, Nelson AR, Betsholtz C, Zlokovic BV. Establishment and dysfunction of the blood-brain barrier. Cell. 2015;163(5):1064-78. doi:10.1016/j.cell.2015.10.067

[150] Saugstad JA. Non-coding RNAs in stroke and neuroprotection. Front Neurol. 2015;6:50. doi:10.3389/fneur.2015.00050

[151] van Empel VP, De Windt LJ, da Costa Martins PA. Circulating miRNAs: reflecting or affecting cardiovascular disease? Curr Hypertens Rep. 2012;14(6):498-509. doi:10.1007/s11906-012-0310-7

[152] Yin KJ, Hamblin M, Chen YE. Non-coding RNAs in cerebral endothelial pathophysiology: emerging roles in stroke. Neurochem Int. 2014;77:9-16. doi:10.1016/j.neuint.2014.03.013

[153] Pritchard CC, Cheng HH, Tewari M. MicroRNA profiling: approaches and considerations. Nat Rev Genet. 2012;13(5):358-69. doi:10.1038/nrg3198

[154] Benes V, Castoldi M. Expression profiling of microRNA using real-time quantitative PCR, how to use it and what is available. Methods. 2010;50(4):244-9. doi:10.1016/j.ymeth.2010.01.026

[155] van Rooij E. The art of microRNA research. Circ Res. 2011;108(2):219-34. doi:10.1161/CIRCRESAHA.110.227496

[156] Mestdagh P, Hartmann N, Baeriswyl L, Andreasen D, Bernard N, Chen C, et al. Evaluation of quantitative miRNA expression platforms in the microRNA quality control (miRQC) study. Nat Methods. 2014;11(8):809-15. doi:10.1038/nmeth.3014

[157] Redshaw N, Wilkes T, Whale A, Cowen S, Huggett J, Foy CA. A comparison of miRNA isolation and RT-qPCR technologies and their effects on quantification accuracy and repeatability. Biotechniques. 2013;54(3):155-64. doi:10.2144/000114002

[158] Hunt EA, Broyles D, Head T, Deo SK. MicroRNA detection: current technology and research strategies. Annu Rev Anal Chem. 2015;8:217-37. doi:10.1146/annurev-anchem-071114-040343

[159] Zheng XH, Cui C, Zhou XX, Zeng YX, Jia WH. Centrifugation: an important pre-analytic procedure that influences plasma microRNA quantification during blood processing. Chin J Cancer. 2013;32(12):667-72. doi:10.5732/cjc.012.10271

[160] Cheng L, Sharples RA, Scicluna BJ, Hill AF. Exosomes provide a protective and enriched source of miRNA for biomarker profiling compared to intracellular and cell-free blood. J Extracell Vesicles. 2014;3:23743. doi:10.3402/jev.v3.23743

[161] Garzon R, Marcucci G, Croce CM. Targeting microRNAs in cancer: rationale, strategies and challenges. Nat Rev Drug Discov. 2010;9(10):775-89. doi:10.1038/nrd3179

[162] Deiuliis J, Mihai G, Zhang J, Taslim C, Varghese JJ, Maiseyeu A, et al. Renin-sensitive microRNAs correlate with atherosclerosis plaque progression. J Hum Hypertens. 2013;28(4):251-8. doi:10.1038/jhh.2013.97

[163] Thomas M, Lieberman J, Lal A. Desperately seeking microRNA targets. Nat Struct Mol Biol. 2010;17(10):1169-74. doi:10.1038/nsmb.1921

[164] Day JJ, Sweatt JD. Epigenetic mechanisms in cognition. Neuron. 2011;70(5):813-29. doi:10.1016/j.neuron.2011.05.019

[165] Landry CD, Kandel ER, Rajasethupathy P. New mechanisms in memory storage: piRNAs and epigenetics. Trends Neurosci. 2013;36(9):535-42. doi:10.1016/j.tins.2013.05.004

[166] Boissonneault V, Plante I, Rivest S, Provost P. MicroRNA-298 and microRNA-328 regulate expression of mouse β-amyloid precursor protein-converting enzyme 1. J Biological Chem. 2009;284(4):1971-81. doi:10.1074/jbc.M807530200

Chapter 11

Renin-Angiotensin System and Renal Allograft Long-Term Outcome: A Review

Rosa M. Viero and Luis Gustavo Modelli de Andrade

Additional information is available at the end of the chapter

http://dx.doi.org/10.5772/67082

Abstract

Recent developments in immunosuppressive therapy have reduced the loss of allografts from acute rejection, with a significant improvement in the one-year allograft survival. However, the introduction of more potent and selective new drug, had no effect on the development of chronic allograft dysfunction and the long-term outcome remains unchanged. Several and repeated different types of allograft insults such as delayed graft function, rejection episodes, drug nephrotoxicity, hypertension, dislipidemia determines a progressive damage with graft failure within a decade. There is no established maintenance immunosuppressive therapy that decreases chronic allograft dysfunction. The renin-angiotensin system is an important mediator in the pathogenesis of chronic progressive kidney diseases. Although the pathogenesis of chronic allograft nephropathy (CAN) is poorly understood, a reduced nephron function with hemodynamic changes associated with a cascade of inflammatory mediators, result in a chronic inflammatory process, progressive fibrosis and tissue remodeling. Recent evidence has shown beneficial effects of renin-angiotensin system blockade in the posttransplant with a decrease of blood pressure, proteinuria and inflammatory process.

Keywords: renal transplant, chronic allograft nephropathy, renin-angiotensin system, allograft survival

1. Introduction

The renin-angiotensin system (RAS) was described in the 1980s, and since then studies have focused on its role in the hemodynamic control [1]. The RAS is classically associated with blood pressure regulation and electrolyte balance. The system main peptide angiotensin II acts through two major receptors termed type 1 and type 2. They are widely distributed in the tissues, and have different functions; hemodynamic changes such as vasoconstriction and cellular proliferation are related to type 1 receptor and vasodilation and anti-cellular proliferation to type 2 [2].

All components of the RAS, including the receptors, are present very early in the human development (24–35 days of gestation), suggesting a role for angiotensin II in the organogenesis [3].

The RAS components are present in many tissues, and there are evidences for a tecidual angiotensin II biosynthesis with high concentrations in the kidneys (intrarenal RAS) [4, 5]. They are synthesized by different cells and interact locally with autocrine and paracrine effects. It has been suggested that the plasma RAS is important for acute regulatory mechanisms, whereas the tissue RAS may be more involved in chronic cardiovascular and renal regulation [6, 7].

Therefore, RAS maintains hemodynamic homeostasis and controls tecidual growth.

Pathologic consequences can result in overactivity of this cascade with an involvement of the RAS in several renal diseases. Regardless of the initial type of injury, all chronic renal diseases develop glomerular and vascular sclerosis, tubular atrophy and interstitial fibrosis, with progressive nephron loss and chronic renal failure. Adaptative changes in the remaining nephrons after initial injury cause more scarring and nephron loss, thus perpetuating a vicious cycle that results in the end-stage kidney. Chronic RAS activation is involved in these maladaptive mechanisms of progressive renal damage. Angiotensin II-mediated effects such as haemodynamics changes, glomerular and tubular hypertrophy and hyperplasia, infiltration of mononuclear cells and fibrogenesis were observed [8].

The system hyperactivity leads to progressive lesions presenting an important role in the pathophysiology of chronic cardiovascular and renal diseases. The RAS activation has been demonstrated in various kidney diseases, in both experimental and clinical studies [9, 10]. The system blockade, with inhibitors of angiotensin converting enzyme (ACE) of angiotensin II and angiotensin II-receptor blockers, shows large benefits in the treatment of chronic kidney diseases [11].

Thus, the classical approach of Angiotensin II as a vasoactive agent that participates in the systemic hemodynamic changes was expanded to recognize its role as a growth factor that modulates cell proliferation, synthesis and degradation of extracellular matrix.

A significant complication on renal transplantation is the chronic and progressive allograft dysfunction that develops months or years after transplantation. Recent advances with new immunosuppressive drugs did not improve the long-term allograft survival. Despite the well established knowledge of the ability of renin-angiotensin system blockade to control blood pressure and urinary protein excretion, the use of RAS inhibitors and blockers in renal transplant has been limited [12, 13].

We review our own observations and recent reports from the literature about the important role of RAS in the pathogenesis of chronic inflammatory process and local tecidual growth, in the chronic allograft dysfunction.

2. Case description

LAR, a 20-year-old woman with chronic renal failure due to focal and segmental glomerulosclerosis (FSGS) was admitted at the Clinical Hospital of Faculdade de Medicina de Botucatu

(UNESP) to receive a renal transplant. She underwent an HLA—haploidentical living donor transplant from a 50-year-old woman in 17 March 1993. Panel reactivity (PRA) against HLA class I and II antibodies was negative. Induction therapy has not been done. Maintenance therapy was performed with a triple immune suppressive regimen with prednisone (1 mg/kg/day), azathioprine (4 mg/kg/day) and cyclosporin (8 mg/kg/day). In the early follow-up, without a significant ischemic exposure, the patient had an episode of acute cellular rejection that was adequately treated. At hospital discharge her serum creatinine level was 1.2 mg/dl (eGFR = 60 ml/min) which remained up to 1 year post transplant. The patient started presenting mild proteinuria (0.28 g/24 h) and progressive deterioration of renal function over the years reaching creatinine of 1.8 mg/dl (eGFR = 39 mL/min) after 14 years of transplant (**Figure 1**). Immunosuppression at that time consisted of azathioprine (1.5 mg/kg/day), prednisone (10 mg) and cyclosporin in order to reach a serum level of 100–150 ng/ml. The renal biopsy diagnosis at this time (February 2007) was "chronic allograft nephropathy (CAN)" characterized by mild interstitial fibrosis and tubular atrophy, and intense arteriolar hyalin deposits observed in more than one arteriole, some with circumferential involvement (Banff grade I). A mild mononuclear inflammatory infiltrate was observed in scarred areas. The glomeruli and the small arteries were unremarkable (**Figures 2** and **3**). Tests for C1q, C3, IgG, IgA, IgM and C4d were all negative by immunofluorescence. Losartan was introduced (50 mg/day) and there was a gradual improvement of renal function over time (**Figures 1** and **4**).

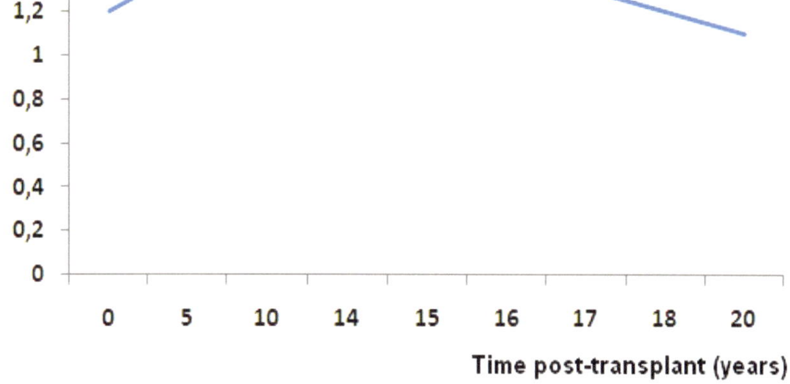

Figure 1. Serum creatinine levels after transplantation. Renal biopsy with chronic allograft nephropathy (CAN) and introduction of losartan 14 years after transplant.

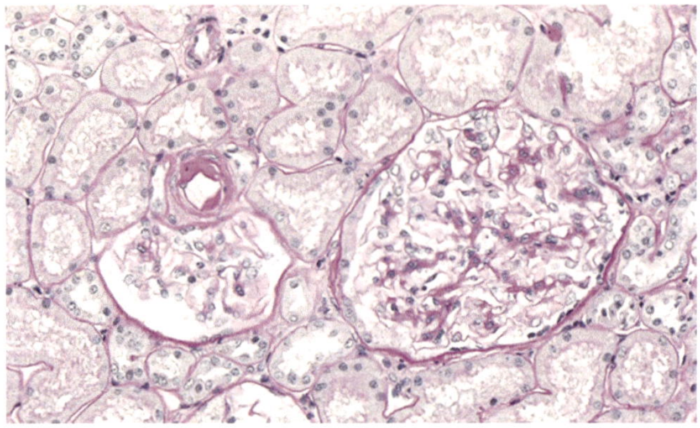

Figure 2. Renal allograft biopsy with arteriolar hyalin deposits. PAS-200×.

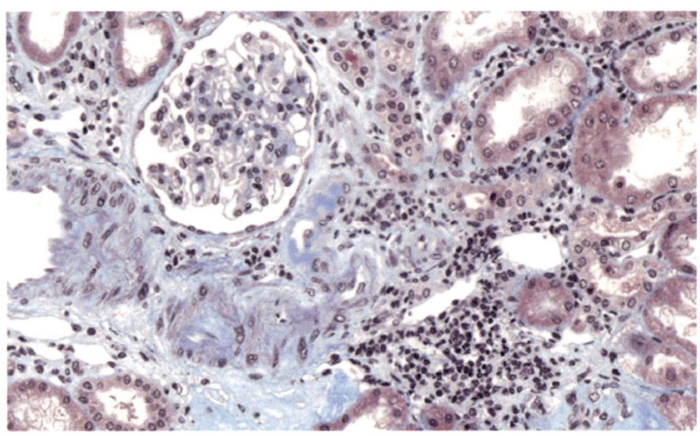

Figure 3. Renal allograft biopsy with focal area with tubulointerstitial fibrosis, tubular atrophy and mononuclear infiltrate. Arteriolar hyalinosis. Masson Trichrome-200×.

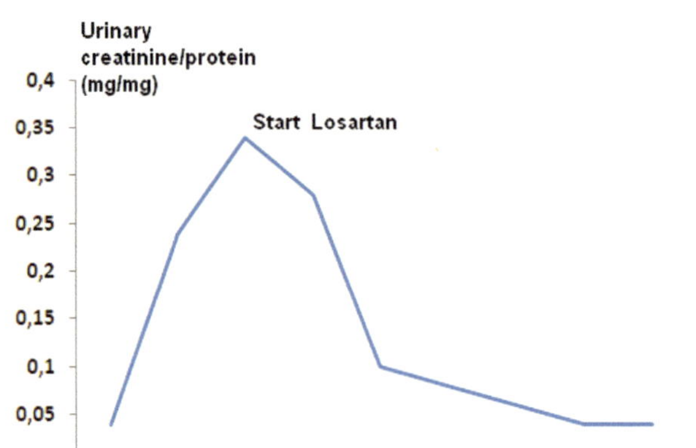

Figure 4. Proteinuria after transplantation. Renal biopsy with chronic allograft nephropathy (CAN) and introduction of losartan 14 years after transplant.

http://dx.doi.org/10.5772/67082

3. Case discussion and review of the literature

In our case, a young woman that received a successful renal transplant 14 years ago, now exhibited clinical evidences of chronic and slow progressive kidney injury manifested mainly by deterioration of renal function.

There were no morphological evidences of recurrence of her native kidney disease, the focal and segmental glomerulosclerosis (FSGS). The recurrent rate of primary FSGS is very high but, usually manifests with nephrotic syndrome much earlier in the posttransplant and have a lower graft survival. The degree of proteinuria of this patient was very mild and started after a long period of well functioning allograft.

There was also no morphological evidences of chronic rejection. Chronic allograft glomerulopathy and arteriopathy, Banff's morphological criteria for chronic rejection, were absent and C4d was negative.

Our diagnosis of renal biopsy was chronic allograft nephropathy.

3.1. Chronic allograft nephropathy and chronic allograft dysfunction

Chronic allograft nephropathy (CAN) is the major cause of late allograft loss. This is a heterogeneous and complex process caused by immunologic and non-immunologic factors including glomerular hyperfiltration, hypertension, dyslipidemia, delayed graft function, drug toxicity and recurrent or the novo nephropathy. Clinically, there is a gradual and progressive deterioration of renal function in association with hypertension and proteinuria [14, 15].

Similar to what occurs in the native chronic renal diseases, repeated injury of the renal allograft determines activation of adaptative mechanisms to maintain homeostasis, but also induces a reparative process with deposition of large quantities of an extra cellular matrix with formation of a connective scar. CAN is characterized histologically by glomerulosclerosis, arterial fibroelastic intimal hyperplasia, tubular atrophy and interstitial fibrosis. The extension of tubulointerstitial fibrosis correlates closely to the extent of renal allograft dysfunction [16–18].

However, CAN is a generic and a misleading term used for all causes of chronic allograft dysfunction with fibrosis, inhibiting the accurate diagnosis and appropriate therapy. These non-specific morphological findings make it difficult to recognize the causes. The 8th Banff Conference [19] proposed replacing CAN for an appropriate classification of chronic allograft dysfunction that enables the diagnosis of specific causes of chronic allograft dysfunction in order to treat adequately. Protection against complications and pathogenetic investigations of late graft deterioration have become important. Nevertheless, chronic allograft dysfunction remains an unresolved problem.

Thus, what should be a more specific diagnosis for our patient?

Histologic findings showed a non-specific parenchymal scarring characterized by interstitial fibrosis and tubular atrophy associated to arteriolosclerosis and a mononuclear inflammatory infiltrate.

Although the biopsy showed a mononuclear inflammatory infiltrate, there were no clinical and morphological criteria for late acute rejection; the inflammatory cells were observed only in areas of fibrosis and the decline of renal function was gradual over the years.

On the other hand, serology tests and stains for infectious agents were negative.

However, the presence of inflammatory cells even in the scarred areas of CAN should be considered a risk factor for a progressive lost of renal function decreasing the allograft survival [18, 20, 21]. The persistence of chronic active inflammation may be responsible for the progression of CAN [20].

In addition, long-term administration of the calcineurin inhibitors such as cyclosporin and tacrolimus, produce many allograft side-effects. The most important histological lesion in cyclosporine nephrotoxicity is the structural changes with hyalin deposits in the arterioles that is present in the patient biopsy [22]. On the other hand, these drugs induce hyperlipidaemia and hypertension, important risk factors for CAN development [23, 24]. There is also an interaction between cyclosporine-induced nephrotoxicity and the activation of the RAS. Shang et al. [25] reported an increased expression of renin and angiotensin II in the allograft with a diagnosis of cyclosporin nephrotoxicity, that was significantly higher in specimens with CAN than in those without CAN. The authors concluded that tissue RAS has an important role in the development of adverse effects of cyclosporin on the kidney.

Although the arteriolar hyalin deposits are mostly subendothelial, this morphological finding in the patient's biopsy are highly suggestive of cyclosporine nephotoxicity as a cause of CAN in our patient.

Although the main problem of this patient was renal insufficiency, she presented a mild proteinuria at the normal limit. We do not identify significant glomerular changes in the biopsy. Proteinuria and nephrotic syndrome is a frequent finding in CAN. The glomeruli displayed a spectrum of lesions, mostly non-specific glomerular changes, including global and segmental sclerosis, collapse of the glomerular capillaries and focal and segmental mesangial sclerosis. The degree of proteinuria closely correlated with the severity of renal injury in the CAN [26].

Several studies have suggested an implication of RAS in the pathogenesis of progressive allograft dysfunction and renin-angiotensin system inhibition provide an important strategy for therapeutic intervention [14, 16].

3.2. Renin-angiotensin system and chronic inflammatory process

Besides the action in the circulation, RAS components have an important role in the inflammatory process, acting directly or indirectly by various mechanisms. Increases vascular permeability by mechanical action in the vessels, cell skeletal rearrangement and release of mediators such as prostaglandins and leukotrienes [27].

It stimulates the synthesis and release of cytokines and chemokines such as *interleukin-6* (IL-6), *interleukin-8* (IL-8), *regulated upon activation normal T cell expressed and secreted*

http://dx.doi.org/10.5772/67082

(RANTES), *macrophage inflammatory protein-1 and 2* (MIP-1; MIP-2), *chemokine monocyte chemoattractant protein-1* (MCP-1) and adhesion molecules represented by the *integrins, selectins, intercellular adhesion molecule-1* (ICAM-1) and *vascular cell adhesion molecule-1* (VCAM-1). The stimulation for these mediator substances results in increased influx of cells to the tissue with proliferation and activation of mononuclear cells, mainly macrophages. Mononuclear cell infiltration and proliferation determine continuing tissue destruction and healing by fibrosis [27, 28].

Several studies have also demonstrated the role of angiotensin II in tissue repair by inducing growth factors such as *transforming growth factor β1* (TGFβ1), *platelet-derived growth factor* (PDGF), *fibroblastic growth factor* (FGF), *vascular endothelial growth factor* (VEGF), *tumor necrosis factor α* (TNFα) and *plasminogen activator inhibitor-1* (PAI-1) [10–12]. Excess extracellular matrix deposition is due to the increased synthesis by the activation of growth factors and by decreased degradation by inhibition of metalloproteinases. TGFβ1 is an important growth factor modulated by RAS activation, with a close connection with this system. It is involved with complex effects on cell growth and differentiation, expression of extracellular matrix, angiogenesis and tissue repair [29–31].

It has been demonstrated increased gene expression of components of the RAS and growth factors into tubular cells and interstitial fibroblasts. These data indicate local activation of the system that correlated with mediators associated with deposition of a matrix in areas of chronic injury and fibrosis [32, 33].

The interaction of RAS with other vasoactive systems such as aldosterone, nitric oxide, endothelin and kinins can enhance its vasoconstrictor and reparative action but also can stimulate anti-inflammatory effects [11].

3.3. Renin-angiotensin system and chronic allograft nephropathy

Several studies have demonstrated the participation of RAS in the development of lesions in CAN. After transplantation, the system is activated locally [34]. Recent evidences have shown RAS stimulating the secretion of cytokines and growth factors, especially TGFβ1, with increased extracellular matrix deposition [16].

The system determines vasoconstriction of the efferent arterioles increasing glomerular intracapillary pressure and filtration, with consequent proteinuria. Stimulates mesangial cell proliferation with matrix synthesis evolving with glomerular sclerosis. Determines hypoperfusion of the peritubular capillaries and hypoxia in the tubulointerstitial compartment. Proteinuria determines tubular cells injury, stimulates the system locally, which together with the chronic hypoxia leads to apoptosis and epithelial-mesenchymal transdifferentiation with extracellular matrix deposition. Stimulates fibroblast proliferation, transformation into myofibroblasts with deposition of matrix in the tubulointerstitial compartment. It is involved in intimal proliferation of vessels forming a neointima [16].

The studies have focused primarily the correlation of allograft survival with the system blockade by converting enzyme inhibitors and/or angiotensin II receptors blockers. Angiotensin converting enzyme inhibitors and/or angiotensin receptors blockers therapies are useful in the treatment of hypertension, improvement of the renal function, reduction of erythrocytosis and proteinuria in the posttransplant [35].

Yamada et al. [36] demonstrated that inhibition of angiotensin II converting enzyme determined in transplant patients increased response of plasma renin activity and increased urinary excretion of TGFβ1 in patients who developed chronic allograft nephropathy. The authors suggest that urinary TGFβ1 excretion clinically predicts the future development of chronic allograft dysfunction.

TGFβ1 levels in plasma and urine were increased in overt chronic allograft nephropathy [37, 38]. And a significant correlation between tecidual TGFβ1 and renal interstitial fibrosis has been reported [39].

Montanaro et al. [40] showed a reduction in proteinuria and increased creatinine clearance in patients treated with angiotensin converting enzyme and angiotensin II AT1 receptor blocker. This study suggested that RAS blockade has renoprotective effects when used in patients with good stable renal function and mild proteinuria, and prevent chronic allograft nephropathy.

Artz et al. [41] found that patients who were taking angiotensin converting enzyme inhibitors had overall less severe CAN and longer graft survival. Renal graft survival after treatment with RAS blockade was 6.3 years as opposed to 1.8 years in untreated patients.

Possible mechanisms of the renoprotective effects of angiotensin converting enzyme (ACE) inhibitors and angiotensin receptor blockers (ARB) include a reduction of intraglomerular capillary pressure due to efferent arteriolar vasodilation and a decreased production and/or expression of TGFβ1 [37]. A reduction of the plasminogen activator inhibitor (*PAI-1*) has also been associated with the rate of CAN progression [42].

Zaltzman et al. [43] studying a group of 40 patients with biopsy-proven CAN that were treated with RAS blockade demonstrated a slow decline in the renal function and 83% of graft survival at 5 years.

Moscoso-Solorzano et al. [44] showed a synergistic effect between ACE inhibition and mycophenolate mofetil (MMF), maintaining serum creatinine stable and decreasing and limiting the progression of proteinuria, as well as histological lesions. The death-censored graft survival analysis was much better for the group treated with ACE inhibition alone, following the group treated with ACE inhibition in combination with MMF.

Heinze et al. [45] studying 2031 patients, found a marked improvement in 10-year graft survival in patients on ACE inhibition or angiotensin II receptor blockers. Ten-year patient survival rates were 74% in the ACEI/ARB group and only 53% in the non-treated group. Ten-year graft survival was 59% in ACEI/ARB patients and 41% in non-users group.

Based on these important findings in the Heinze'study [45], Opelz et al. [46] conducted a similar analysis in 17,209 kidney transplant recipients; 33.5% of the patients were on treatment with an ACEI or ARB after 1 year of transplantation. The graft and patient survivals at 6 year were not significantly different between the patients with or without ACEI/ARB treatment.

http://dx.doi.org/10.5772/67082

The different methods to enrolled the patients in the groups that received or not the ACEI/ARB treatment can explain the contrasting results. They did not confirm the higher graft and patient survival rates reported by Heinze et al. [45] and do not recommend a widespread use of ACEI/ARB therapy.

A prospective study of 14 renal transplant patients with CAN, showed that treatment with losartan significantly decreased plasma levels of TGFβ1 by more than 50%. It was observed a significant correlation between the increase of circulating angiotensin II after 2 weeks of treatment and the decrease of plasma TGFβ1 at the end of the study period. The results suggest that the receptor blockade plays a role in the synthesis of TGFβ1 [37].

Some authors have studied gene expression of RAS components and inflammatory mediators in renal biopsies of patients with CAN.

Oka et al. [47] showed an increase in the number of renin positive cells in juxtaglomerular apparatus in CAN. Becker et al. [48] studied the correlation between the AT2 receptor mRNA with the expression of the matrix-modulating genes and histological evidence of chronic rejection. AT2 receptor correlated with TGFβ1, metalloproteinases and inhibitors of metalloproteinases, indicating that the AT2 receptor participates in the modulation of extracellular matrix. Mas et al. [49] also found a correlation between the expression of angiotensinogen and TGFβ1 in the allografts of patients with various degrees of CAN. Some authors [50] observed in CAN correlation between the expression of RAS components and TGFβ1 in the allograft with mRNA levels in the urine. Significant correlation has been observed between TGFβ1 mRNA in the allograft and interstitial fibrosis [39].

In experimental animals, the RAS blockade prevents the increase in mRNA levels of cytokines and growth factors in the allograft, decreases the infiltration of mononuclear cells and attenuates the renal lesions in the chronic rejection models [51–54]. Noris et al. [51] have shown in an experimental study of chronic nephropathy with established lesions decreased MCP-1 expression and inflammatory infiltrate with stabilization of glomerular injury and renal function recovery in animals treated with angiotensin converting enzyme.

There are also some studies investigating the role of RAS gene polymorphisms in the renal transplantation. Circulating and tecidual RAS activity are under genetic control. Genomic variants of the angiotensinogen, ACE, AT1 and AT2 receptors genes have been described. Some authors studied the impact of the various genotypes on renal allograft function. This is a further support about the importance of the RAS in the progression of non-immunological injuries leading to chronic kidney graft failure [55, 56].

In conclusion, the introduction of losartan in the patient under discussion resulted in a significant improvement of renal function.

RAS blockade, with inhibitors of angiotensin converting enzyme of angiotensin II and angiotensin II receptor blockers, shows large benefits in the treatment of chronic kidney diseases. The beneficial effects of RAS blockade in the renal transplant are due to hemodynamic changes lowering blood pressure and reduction of the inflammatory infiltrate ameliorating the renal function. However, there are insufficient data to determine the effect on patient or graft survival.

On the other hand, evidences indicate the existence of an ACE-independent alternative pathway for generation of angiotensin II that is not affected by ACE inhibitors [57]. This explains the different results among the various studies.

While ACE inhibition and angiotensin receptor blockers can reduce progression of chronic renal diseases in humans, they do not achieve full renoprotection, and patients may still progress to end stage renal disease. These findings are consistent with human studies showing that ACE inhibitors slow, but do not halt renal fibrosis. Larger randomized studies are required to assess whether or not angiotensin converting enzyme inhibition and angiotensin II receptor antagonist therapies have beneficial effects after kidney transplantation [16, 58].

Acknowledgements

Financial support by Fundação de Amparo à Pesquisa do Estado de São Paulo/State of São Paulo Research Foundation (FAPESP).

Author details

Rosa M. Viero[1]* and Luis Gustavo Modelli de Andrade[2]

*Address all correspondence to: viero@fmb.unesp.br

1 Department of Pathology, Botucatu Medical School, São Paulo State University (UNESP), Botucatu, São Paulo, Brazil

2 Department of Internal Medicine, Botucatu Medical School, São Paulo State University (UNESP), Botucatu, São Paulo, Brazil

References

[1] Basso N, Terragnoaa N. History about the discovery of the renin-angiotensin system. Hypertension 2001; **38**: 1246-1249.

[2] Kim S, Iwao H. Molecular and cellular mechanisms of angiotensin II-mediated cardiovascular and renal diseases. Pharmacol Rev 2000; **52**: 11-34.

[3] Schütz S, Le Moullec J-M, Corvol P, Gasc J-M. Early expression of all the components of the rennin-angiotensin-system in human development. Am J Pathol 1996; **149**(6): 2067-2079.

[4] Taugner R, Hackenthal E, Helmchen U, Ganten D, Kugler P, Marin-Grez M, Nobiling R, Unger T, Lockwald I, Keilbach R. The intrarenal rennin-angiotensin system. An immunocytochemical study on the localization of renin, angiotensinogen, converting enzyme, and the angiotensins in the kidney of mouse and rat. Klin Wochenschr 1982; **60**: 1218-1222.

[5] Navar LG, Lewis L, Hymel A, Braam B, Mitchell KD. Tubular fluid concentrations and kidney contents of angiotensin I and II in anesthetized rats. J Am Soc Nephrol 1994; **5**(4): 1153-1158.

[6] Paul M, Wagner J, Dzau VJ. Gene expression of the renin-angiotensin system in human tissues. Quantitative analysis by the polymerase chain reaction. J Clin Invest 1993; **91**: 2058-2064.

[7] Campbell DJ. Circulating and tissue angiotensin systems. J Clin Invest 1977; **79**: 1-6.

[8] Fogo AB. Mechanisms of progression of chronic kidney disease. Pediatr Nephrol 2007; **22**: 2011-2022.

[9] Lewis EJ, Hunsicker LG, Bain RP, Rohde RD: The effect of angiotensin-converting-enzyme inhibition on diabetic nephropathy. The Colaborative Study Group. N Engl J Med 1993; **329**: 1456-1462.

[10] Graciano ML, Cavaglieri RC, Dellê H, Dominguez WV, Casarini DE, Malheiros DMAC, Noronha IL. Intrarenal renin-angiotensin system is upregulated in experimental model of progressive renal disease induced by chronic inhibition of nitric oxide synthesis. J Am Soc Nephrol 2004; **15**: 1805-1815.

[11] Brewster UC, Perazella MA. The renin-angiotensin-aldosterone system and the kidney: Effects on kidney disease. Am J Med 2004; **116**: 263-272.

[12] Ponticelli C. Progression of renal damage in chronic rejection. Kidney Intern 2000; **57**(Suppl. 75): S-62-S70.

[13] Remuzzi G, Perico N. Routine renin-angiotensin system blockade in renal transplantation? Curr Opin Nephrol Hypert 2002, **11**(1): 1-10.

[14] Cornell LD, Colvin RB. Chronic allograft nephropathy. Curr Opin Nephrol Hypertens 2005; **14**: 229-234.

[15] Nankivell BJ, Borrows RJ, Fung CLS, O'Connell PJ, Allen RDM, Chapman JR. The natural history of chronic allograft nephropathy. N Eng J Med 2003; **349**: 2326-2333.

[16] Waller JR, Nicholson ML. Molecular mechanisms of renal allograft fibrosis. Brit J Surg 2001; 88: 1429-1441.

[17] Womer KL, Vella JP, Sayegh MH. Chronic allograft dysfunction: Mechanisms and new approaches to therapy. Sem Nephrol 2000; **20**(2): 126-147.

[18] Racusen LC, Regele H. The pathology of chronic allograft dysfunction. Kidney Intern 2010; **78**(Suppl. 119): S27–S32.

[19] Solez K, Colvin RB, Racusen LC, Sis B, Halloran PF, Birk PE, Campbell PM, Cascalho M, Collins AB, Demetris AJ, Drachenberg CB, Gibson IW, Grimm PC, Haas M, Lerut E, Liapis H, Mannon RB, Marcus PB, Mengel M, Mihatsch MJ, Nankivell BJ, Nickeleit V, Papadimitriou JC, Platt JL, Randhawa P, Roberts I, Salinas-Madrigal L, Salomon DR, Seron D, Sheaff M, Weening JJ. Banff'05 meeting report: Differential diagnosis of chronic

allograft injury and elimination of chronic allograft nephropathy ('CAN'). Am J Transpl 2007; **7**: 518-526.

[20] Shishido S, Asanuma H, Nakai H, Mori Y, Satoh H, Kamimaki I, Hataya H, Ikeda M, Honda M, Hasegawa A. The impact of repeated subclinical acute rejection on the progression of chronic allograft nephropathy. J Am Soc Nephrol 2003; **14**: 1046-1052.

[21] Divella C, Rossini M, Loverre A, Schena A, Maiorano A, Gesualdo V, Zaza G, Grandaliano G, Schena FP. Immunohistochemical characterization of glomerular and tubulointerstitial infiltrates in renal transplant patients with chronic allograft dyasfunction. Nephrol Dial Transplant 2010; **25**: 4071-4077.

[22] Arias M, Séron D, Moreso F, Bestard O, Praga M. Chronic renal allograft damage: Existing challenges. Transplantation 2011; **91**(9S): S4–S25.

[23] Satterthwaite R, Aswad S, Sunga V, Shidban H, Bogaard T, Asai P, Khetan U, Akra I, Mendez RG, Mendez R. Incidence of new-onset hypercholesterolemia in renal transplant patients treated with FK506 or cyclosporine. Transplantation 1998; **65**(3): 446-449.

[24] Copley JB, Staffeld C, Lindberg J, Hansen A, Bailey C, Anand R, Van Veldhuisen P. Cyclosporin to tacrolimus: Effect on hypertension and lipid profiles in renal allografts. Transplant Proc 1998; **30**(4): 1254-1256.

[25] Shang M-H, Yuan W-J, Zhang S-J, Fan Y, Zhang Z. Intrarenal activation of renin angiotensin system in the development of cyclosporine A induced chronic nephrotoxicity. Chin Med J 2008; **121**(11): 983-988.

[26] Yakupoglu U, Baranowska-Daca E, Rosen D, Barrios R, Suki WN, Truong LD. Posttransplant nephrotic syndrome: A comprehensive clinicopathologic study. Kidney Intern 2004; **65**: 2360-2370.

[27] Suzuki Y, Ruiz-Ortega M, Lorenzo O, Rupérez M, Esteban V, Egido J. Inflammation and angiotensin II. The Intern J Biochem Cell Biol 2003; **35**: 881-900.

[28] Cheng ZJ, Vapaatalo H, Mervaala E. Angiotensin II and vascular inflammation. Méd Sci Monit 2005; **11**(6): RA194-205.

[29] Fogo AB. Renal fibrosis and the renin-angiotensin system. Adv Nephrol Necker Hosp 2001; **31**: 69-87.

[30] Mezzano SA, Ruiz-Ortega M, Egido J. Angiotensin II and renal fibrosis. Hypertension 2001; **38**: 635-643.

[31] Gilbert RE, Wilkinson-Berka JL, Kelly DJ. Angiotensin and renal fibrosis. Contrib Nephrol 2001; **135**: 171-186.

[32] Campistol JM, Inigo P, Larios S, Bescos M, Oppenheimer F. Role of transforming growth factor-β-1 in the progression of chronic allograft nephropathy. Nephrol Dial Transplant 2001; **16**(Suppl. 1): 114-116.

[33] Wolf G. Lesão renal devido à ativação do sistema renina-angiotensina-aldosterona pela via do fator de crescimento transformador-β. Kidney Int 2007; 2 : 129-133.

[34] Rettig R, Buch M, Gerstberger R, Schnatterbeck P, Paul M. Effects of kidney transplantation on renin-angiotensin system of the recipients. Kidney Int 1994; **44** : 1536.

[35] Hiremath S, Fergusson D, Doucette S, Mulay AV, Knoll GA. Renin angiotensin system blockade in kidney transplantation: A systematic review of the evidence. Am J Transplant 2007; **7**(10): 2350.

[36] Yamada K, Hatakeyama E, Arita S, Sakamoto K, Kashiwabara H, Hamaguchi K. Prediction of chronic renal allograft dysfunction from evaluations of TGFβ1 and the renin-angiotensin system. Clin Exp Nephrol 2003; **7**: 238-242.

[37] Campistol JM, Iñigo P, Jimenez W, Lario S, Clesca PH, Oppenheimer F, Rivera F. Losartan decreases plasma levels of TGFβ1 in transplant patients with chronic allograft nephropathy. Kidney Int 1999; **56**(2): 714-719.

[38] Boratynska M. Urine excretion of transforming growth factor-β1 in chronic allograft nephropathy. Ann Transplant 1999; **4**: 23-28.

[39] Sharma VK, Bologa RM, Xu GP, Li B, Mouradian J, Wang J, Serur D, Rao V, Suthanthiran M. Intragraft TGFβ1 mRNA: A correlate of interstitial fibrosis and chronic allograft nephropathy. Kidney Int 1996; **49**(5): 1297-1303.

[40] Montanaro D, Gropuzzo M, Tulissi P, Vallone C, Boscutti G, Mioni R, Risaliti A, Baccarani U, Adani GL, Sainz M, Bresadola F, Mioni G. Renoprotective effect of early inhibition of the renin-angiotensin system in renal transplant recipients. Transplant Proc 2005; **37**: 991-993.

[41] Artz MA, Hilbrands LB, Borm G, Assmann KJM, Wetzels JFM. Blockade of the renin-angiotensin system increases graft survival in patients with chronic allograft nephropathy. Nephrol Dial Transplant 2004; **19**: 2852-2857.

[42] Lahlou A, Peraldi MN, Thervet E, Flahault A, Delarue F, Soubrier F, Rossert J, Hertig A, Rondeau E. Chronic graft dysfunction in renal transplant patients: Potential role of plasminogen activator inhibitor type 1. Transplantation 2002; **73**(8): 1290-1295.

[43] Zaltzman JS, Nash N, Chiu R, Prasad GVR. Renin-angiotensin system blockade in biopsy-proven allograft nephropathy. Transplant Proc 2003; **35**: 2415-2417.

[44] Moscoso-Solorzano GT, Mastroianni-Kirsztajn G, Ozaki KS, Franco MF, Pacheco-Silva A, Câmara NOS. Synergistic effect of mycophenolate mofetil and angiotensin-converting enzyme inhibitor in patients with chronic allograft nephropathy. Braz J Med Biol Res 2009; **42**: 445-452.

[45] Heinze G, Mitterbauer C, Regele H, Kramar R, Winkelmeier WC, Curran GC, Oberbauer R. Angiotensin-converting enzyme inhibitor or angiotensin II type 1 receptor antagonist therapy is associated with prolonged patient and graft survival after renal transplantation. J Am Soc Nephrol 2006; **17**: 889-899.

[46] Opelz G, Zeier M, Laux G, Morath C, Dohler B. No improvement of patient or graft survival in transplant recipients treated with angiotensin-converting enzyme inhibitors or angiotensin II type 1 receptor blockers: a collaborative transplant study report. J Am Soc Nephrol 2006; **17**: 3257-3262.

[47] Oka K, Moriyama T, Takahara S, Naruse M, namba Y, Ichimaru N, Kyo M, Kokado Y, Okuyama A, Ito T, Imai E, Aozasa K. Increased expression of renin in chronic allograft nephropathy. Transplant Proc 2005; **37**: 2131-2134.

[48] Becker BN, Jacobson LM, Hullett DA, Radke NA, Oberley TD, Brazy PC, Kirk AD. Type 2 angiotensin receptor expression in human renal allografts: An association with chronic allograft nephropathy. Clin Nephrol 2002; **57**: 19-26.

[49] Mas V, Alvarellos T, Giraudo C, Massari P, Boccardo G. Intragraft messenger RNA expression of angiotensinogen: Relationship with transforming growth factor beta-1 and chronic allograft nephropathy in kidney transplant patients. Transplantation 2002; **74**(5): 718-721.

[50] Mas V, Maluf D, Archer K, Yaneck K, Mas L, King A, Gibney E, Massey D, Cotterell A, Fisher R, Posner M. Establishing the molecular pathways involved in chronic allograft nephropathy for testing new noninvasive diagnostic markers. Transplantation 2007; **83**: 448-457.

[51] Noris M, Mister M, Pezzotta A, Azzollini N, Cassis P, Benigni A, Gagliardini E, Perico N, Remuzzi G. ACE inhibition limits chronic injury of kidney transplant even with treatment started when lesions are established. Kidney Int 2003; **64**: 2253-2261.

[52] Smit-van Oosten A, Henning RH, Goor HV. Strain differences in angiotensin-converting enzyme and angiotensin II type I receptor expression. Possible implications for experimental chronic renal transplant failure. J RAAS 2002; **3**(1): 46-53.

[53] Szabo A, Lutz J, Schleimer K, Antus B, Hamar P, Philipp T, Heemann U. Effect of angiotensin-converting enzyme inhibition on growth factor mRNA in chronic renal allograft rejection in the rat. Kidney Int 2000; **57**: 982-991.

[54] HS Ziai F, Nagano H, Kusaka M, Coito AJ, Troy JL, Nadeau KC, Rennke HG, Tilney NL, Brenner BM, Mackenzie. Renal allograft protection with losartan in Fisher→Lewis rats: Hemodynamics, macrophages, and cytokines. Kidney Int 2000; 57: 2618-2625.

[55] Barocci S, Ginevri F, Valente U, Torre F, Gusmano R, Nocera A. Correlation between angiotensin-converting enzyme gene insertion/deletion polymorphism and kidney graft long-term outcome in pediatric recipients. Transplantation 1999; **67**: 534-538.

[56] Hueso M, Alia P, Moreso F, Beltrán-Sastre V, Riera L, González C, Navarro MA, Grinyó JM, Navarro E, Séron D. Angiotensin-converting enzyme genotype and chronic allograft nephropathy in protocol biopsies. J Am Soc Nephrol 2004; **15**(8): 2229-2236.

[57] Hollenberg NK. Pharmacologic interruption of the renin-angiotensin system and the kidney: Differential responses to angiotensin-converting enzyme and renin inhibition. J Am Soc Nephrol 1999; **10**(Suppl): S239–S242.

[58] Campbell RC. The renin-angiotensin system: A 21st century perspective. J Am Soc Nephrol 2004; **15**: 1963-1964.

Chapter 12

Local Renin-Angiotensin System at Liver and Crosstalk with Hepatic Diseases

Eylem Taskin and Celal Guven

Additional information is available at the end of the chapter

http://dx.doi.org/10.5772/65919

Abstract

The systemic renin-angiotensin system mainly regulates blood pressure and maintains kidney function. Recent studies have realized that renin-angiotensin system (RAS) has been found in many tissues, such as heart, liver, and kidney. Although RAS in heart and kidney has been well documented, the RAS in the liver has been evaluated in a few studies. Therefore, this chapter will be assessed it. Based on findings, RAS in the liver has presented almost all of its components, such as angiotensin-I (Ang-I), angiotensin-II (Ang-II), angiotensin-converting enzyme (ACE), angiotensin type-1 receptor (AT1), angiotensin type-2 receptor (AT2), named as classical RAS. Expect these components, the local RAS has had alternative pathway components, including angiotensin-converting enzyme 2 (ACE2) and chymase. Classical RAS has an opposite effect of alternative RAS. Although these local RAS might not be such a crucial for the tissue, it could be a more vital function under pathophysiologic conditions. The chapter the local RAS in the liver the under both physiologic and pathophysiologic conditions is highlighted.

Keywords: angiotensin-II, angiotensin-converting enzyme 2, local renin-angiotensin system, liver pathologies

1. Introduction

Although early studies focused on the systemic renin-angiotensin system (RAS) which are important endocrine cascade to regulate the salt-water balance, scientists have recognized there is one more RAS, called as local or tissue RAS except for classical systemic effects [1]. The first recognition of local RAS has been reported that the in dog's brain the renin was found [2]. Then, various tissues, such as the heart, liver, kidney, vasculature, skeletal muscles, pancreas, retina, adipose, neuronal, and reproductive tissue, have been shown to present local RAS [2–6]. Though systemic RAS can have a role in the regulation of cardiovascular homeostasis, there is accumulating evidence to suggest that the local RAS may affect tissue angiogenesis, proliferation, cell growth, apoptosis, tissue inflammation, differentiation, hormonal secretion, fibrosis and/or dependent of systemic RAS. The local RAS has the paracrine effect in the tissue. Indeed, it does not have to come along with the systemic RAS [2, 5].

The liver is critical organ to maintain not only to glucose homeostasis [7] but also almost all of the body's metabolic activities. The liver tissue has a great regeneration capacity against to repair of liver injury also [8]. The organ has reported existing both of systemic and local RAS [7]. The chapter could, therefore, focus on the local RAS in liver. However, there are limited studies available to study on local RAS. So, the aim of the present chapter is to analyze and sum up the participation of local RAS on both physiology and pathophysiology of liver tissue.

2. The renin angiotensin system in liver

2.1. The component of local renin-angiotensin system in liver tissue

The component of local renin-angiotensin system in liver is divided two as a classical and alternative component of liver renin-angiotensin system.

2.1.1. The classical component of local renin-angiotensin system in liver tissue

Before starting to evaluate the physiological and pathophysiological importance of RAS, it should be given some recent findings about which component of RAS present in the liver tissue. Giving that the elements of the system are so important to bring out its effects on the target tissue, it is expressed that almost all of RAS components could present in the liver tissue, like other organ and tissue. One common consideration about RAS might be upregulation and/or disruptions of distributions of its components, including angiotensinogen, renin, ACE, Ang-II, and AT1 (**Figure 1**) [6]. One of the recent data shows that local RAS components were found at cholangiocytes [2]. Hepatic Kupffer cells [3] and nuclear region of hepatocytes [4] also locally produce angiotensin-II (Ang-II) [9].

Angiotensinogen, predominantly produced in the liver, is one of α2-globulin glycoproteins with 452 amino acids around 60 kDA [2]. Although angiotensinogen is well known to produce in the liver, local angiotensin synthesized was also reported in a few hepatocytes from and Kupffer cell in human tissue [8]. Although it is clear that the primary source of the precursor of angiotensinogen is the hepatocytes, Kupffer cells, and bile duct epithelium have produced to low level of angiotensinogen as well. Cirrhotic livers are reported to increase angiotensinogen and plasma renin level and activity in both humans and animal studies [6]. Depletion of angiotensin is emphasized to lead to hypotension, and kidney pathomorphological changes, decrease survival. The authors suggested that liver and brain angiotensin are enough to maintain blood pressure and prevent pathomorphological changes in the kidneys [10]. This information is emphasized that angiotensin produced from the liver is the primary source of the body.

Even though Ang-I production via renin has not been found in the liver tissue, some clues are indicated that *de novo* production of it might be found locally in hepatic-mesenteric vascular beds and circulation plasma as well [6].

http://dx.doi.org/10.5772/65919

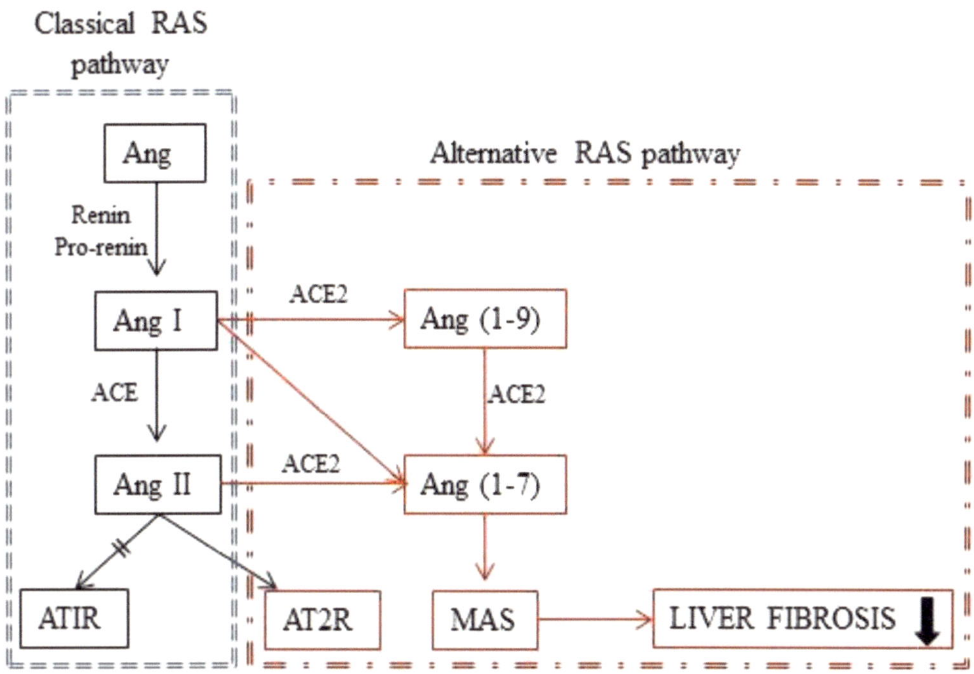

Figure 1. A schematic diagram of the classical and alternative renin-angiotensin system. ACE: angiotensin converting enzyme, ACE2: angiotensin-converting enzyme-2, Ang-I: angiotensin-II, Ang-II: angiotensin-II, Ang-1-7: angiotensin1-7, Ang-1-9: angiotensin1-9, AT1: angiotensin type-1receptor, AT2: angiotensin type-2 receptor, Mas: mas receptor. The figure was modified from Refs. [17, 18].

Renin is expressed at the liver as well [5–7]. It is surprising that renin expression in the female is higher than male in liver tissue of both mice and rats [7]. Furthermore, its expression was found at liver cells such as cholangiocytes, hepatocytes, and hepatic stellate cells (HSC) [9]. Renin receptor was reported to have low-level expression mRNA at liver and kidney, but the high level of the heart, brain, and placenta. Also, it was outlined that the animals have been reported to suffer from liver fibrosis, nephroangiosclerosis probably leads to the activation of ERK1/2 and enhancing of plasminogen activator inhibitor-1, cardiac, and aortic hypertrophy when prorenin transgene express at liver in the rats [11].

The expressions of ACE and AT1 are found at vascular endothelium, hepatocytes, and bile duct epithelial cells. This distribution could be changed under pathologic conditions. For example, in the fibrotic liver, fibrous septa, mesenchymal cells (HSCs and myofibroblasts), and Kupffer cells are also produced to ACE and AT1 [12]. AT1 is predominantly found in the liver. However, AT2 genes are found in a trace amount or not in the normal and pathologic liver as well. At the same time, it was reported so far that AT2 receptor gene expression was found from isolated human hepatocytes and stellate cells. This high expression of AT1 might be the elevation of the liver due to the participation of it in the inflammatory, proliferative process, and vascular effect in the liver. This info consists of fibrosis and the degree of portal hypertension to the AT1 expression on septal myofibroblast [6]. The receptor is pointed out to be at hepatocytes, HSCs, Kupffer cells, bile duct cells, myofibroblast, and vascular endothelial cells [12]. One of the previous studies is stated that ACE could present only liver at tissue-specific ACE knockdown animals, but not a gastrointestinal tract, heart, vascular or spleen. The only kidney might be seen ACE activity but at a trace level. Additionally hepatocytes, the testis is also found express of ACE at liver-specific ACE knockdown mice. Although there is no ACE found at vascular, blood pressure at liver-specific ACE knockdown mice is reported to be pretty standard. The authors implied that adequate ACE in the liver controls the essential kidney function for maintaining homeostasis, but there is no obligation to present of vascular ACE expression to regulate normal blood pressure. Indeed, adequate ACE in any organ is enough to maintain kidney function, resulting in mean blood pressure control [13].

Ang-II might be present in cholangiocytes and activated HSC which is also highly express active renin, ACE at *in vitro* and *in vivo* studies [14]. Some recent studies have been shown that AT1 could present in the liver [5]. Ang-II production from cholangiocytes probably increases at bile duct ligation (BDL). The expression of RAS component at different liver cell types might have both paracrine and autocrine impact on the target tissue. It seems that activation of cholangiocytes RAS could trigger the other cell type's RAS. This concept may help us to explain how to relate RAS at liver pathologies [14]. Many RAS components, such as renin, ACE, Ang-II, AT1, and ACE2 seem to be un-regulated under pathophysiological conditions [7]. But, Ang-II that can exist in the liver tissue could enhance at the pathophysiologic circumstance [6]. Ang-II relates to promoting some liver disease, i.e., liver fibrosis, and proliferation and activation of hepatic stellate cells. So, there is reported to have some prophylactic effects against to liver failure [7]. One of the previous studies noticed that active RAS blocking by either angiotensin-converting enzyme (ACE) or AT1 inhibition led to attenuate liver fibrosis by suppressing HCS and hepatic TGF-β1 in chronic liver injury [9]. The component of local RAS was found in the liver of obese and type-2 diabetes patients. The upregulation of angiotensinogen in liver was shown in type-2 diabetic patient with and without obesity. Its upregulation expression was also determined at hyperglycemia in obese Sprague-Dawley rats, but not in nondiabetic and diet-induce obese rats. Therefore, it is likely to diabetes than obesity much more related to hepatic angiotensinogen production. There is an active interaction determined between TNF-α and local RAS in liver. So, TNF-α increases ACE, angiotensinogen, and the expression of angiotensin AT1 mRNA in the liver. At this moment, the upregulation of local RAS may in the liver is associated with obesity and developing insulin resistance and liver fibrosis [14].

Recent studies have shown to the paradigm shift of RAS. Ang-II receptors and some proteins have been proved to interact with each other by using several methods. For example, it has been indicated that AT1-related protein probably acts a negative regulator, including its cell proliferation and vascular remodeling by enhancing AT1 internalization. Angiotensin type-2 receptor (AT2)-related protein has an adverse impact on the AT2 effect, e.g., growth. Furthermore, AT1 might form either homodimers or heterodimers with other partners, including AT2, bradykinin B2 receptor, epidermal growth factor (EGF) receptor, dopamine receptor, endothelin receptor type B and Mas receptor. This dimerization of Ang-II receptors is unknown neither physiologic nor pathophysiologic importance. Therefore, more new studies are needed to get a better understanding of the dimerization function under physiologic and pathophysiologic

http://dx.doi.org/10.5772/65919

conditions [15]. Also, there is indicated to be the active interaction between RAS components in the mammals. The interaction was shown when renin or Ang-II infusion at perfused mammalian liver enhances angiotensinogen release, and this effect does not link the glucocorticoid secretion. But glucocorticoid present is required to maintain angiotensinogen gene synthesis. It should not rule out that such a kind of studies were carried out by using at the supraphysiologic level of Ang-II. But, it also pointed out this positive interaction could be a more pathophysiologic circumstance, such as depletion of sodium and water and hemorrhage, too [16].

2.1.2. The alternative component of local renin-angiotensin system in liver tissue

Alternative pathway has been thought for a while (**Figure 1**). The alternative paths are ACE2 and chymase that are discuss in this chapter. ACE2 is found at heart, kidney, gastrointestinal tract as well as liver and lung. ACE2 is one of the type-I integral proteins, expressed fundamentally at the cell surface as an ectoenzyme. ACE2 has ectodomain at the membrane; however, metalloprotease ADAM17 is reported to modify to make an active soluble form of it. So, its soluble form could be detected in plasma and urine as well. Moreover, ACE2 is one of the members of the M2 zinc metalloproteinase family as well as somatic and testicular types of ACE. ACE2 has 805 amino acid residues and similarities with human ACE at 41%. Although somatic ACE has two active sites at N- and C-domains, ACE2 has only one active site. The other difference of ACE2 from ACE is a carboxypeptidase, but ACE is a peptidyl dipeptide. Moreover, ACE2 is reported not to blockage by using any ACEI, e.g., captopril, enalaprilat or lisinopril. ACE2 can cleave only one residue from C-terminus of Ang-I and Ang-II that have limited biological effects. The ACE2 effects on Ang-I and Ang-II could produce angiotensin-1-7 (Ang-1-7) and angiotensin-1-9 (Ang-1-9), respectively. But, in these two pathways Ang-1-7 is produced more likely by ACE2. That is why ACE2 could accept to provide Ang-1-7. Ang-1-7 interacts with AT2, BK2 and Mas receptors. Taking together this finding, ACE2-Ang-1-7-Mas axis could modulate the axis of ACE-Ang-II-AT1 [6]. Based on these findings, it is reported that Mas-binding Ang-1-7 produced by ACE2 is the fifth receptor of RAS. ACE2 was increased in liver injury and cirrhosis, resulting in enhancing Ang-1-7 at the plasma and tissue level. The local RAS elements are introduced to express from the cancerous tissue. Some evidence has been shown that RAS is related liver cancer. For example, ACE and AT1 antagonist drugs (captopril, irbesartan; respectively) give rise to minimize cancer growth, liver metastases and angiogenesis in colorectal cancer liver metastases animals [5]. It was shown that ACE, Ang-II and AT1, classic components of RAS, were high expression in rats with biliary fibrosis as well as ACE2 in liver, and plasma, Mas in liver, Ang-1-7 in plasma. This finding can be concluded that local RAS in the liver has both classical (ACE-Ang-II-AT1) and ACE2-Ang-1-7-Mas pathways that play important role in chronic injury. RAS pharmacologically inhibition by ACE and AT1 inhibitors is well established to have a therapeutic effect on many diseases including hypertension, heart failure or diabetes due to blocking Ang-II and AT1. Some recent evidence has been pointing out that these inhibitions have caused to elevate ACE2 and Ang-1-7. The most impressive result from these kinds of experiments is that there is no functional effect of ACE2 elevation in normal animals. Therefore, ACE2 elevation could conclude to be pivotal importance under the only pathophysiologic circumstance, but not a physiologic condition [6].

The other alternative Ang-II production process is via chymase. The enzyme, chymase, is a chymotrypsin-like, presents in the mast cell secretory granules. It is also produced as an inactive form and activated by dipeptidyl peptidase I (DPPI), a thiol proteinase, in the mast cell granules. The optimal pH for DPPI is at 6.0. But mast secretory granules have controlled at 5.5, and there is no chymase activity at 5.5. The optimal pH for chymase is around 7 and 9. As soon as the chymase is secreted into interstitial tissue at 7.4, it can reach to its optimal pH, resulting in gaining activation. The only mast cell-stimulated tissue can secrete it under inflammation circumstance because there may be found any chymase inhibitors in the regular target. Chymase can produce Ang-II from Ang-I. Additionally, chymase can activate TGF-β and metalloproteinase-9 (MMP-9) from their inactive forms. Both of them participate in tissue fibrosis and inflammation. It is stated that there might be a positive correlation between Ang-II and chymase in the human liver fibrosis due to finding a high level of both. Moreover, it is suggested that chymase and Ang-II levels could indicate fibrotic severity. So, chymase inhibition could alleviate the liver fibrosis in animal models. Therefore, new studies are required to clarify the interaction of chymase, Ang-II, and liver fibrosis [19].

2.2. Intracellular pathway of local renin-angiotensin system in liver

Ang-II is reported to cooperate with an intracellular signal pathway to amplify its effect. Therefore, in this section some recent information about the intracellular mediators of local RAS is given. One of these signal amplification pathways may be mitogen-activated protein kinases (MAPK), which are ERK1/2, JNK, and P38 MAPK. MAPK plays a crucial role in cellular differentiation, proliferation, migration, and fibrosis. ERK1/2 has some vital effects on cholangiocyte proliferation. Additionally, MAPK, Ang-II can activate nuclear factor-κB (NF-κB) [20]. Ang-II gives rise to trigger proliferation by stimulation of the cAMP signal pathway [9] as well. It is noticed that human fibrotic liver samples were found less AT1 expressing at hepatocytes, but high expressing in hepatic stellate cells (HSCs), vascular endothelium, and bile duct epithelium. The local RAS-induced HSC via AT1 and activation of NADPH oxidase results in fibrotic liver, and cholangiocyte proliferation by AT1 triggering a cAMP, PKA, ERK1/2, and pCREB-dependent signaling pathway [9]. Hepatic stellate cell (HSC) is the most effective cell type of liver to the deposit of connective tissue at respond of liver injury. Fifteen percentage of liver tissue composes of HSC. Both of Ang-II and renin are reported to increase liver cirrhosis patients. It is reported that Ang-II might relate to the development of the liver fibrosis by activation of HSC via TGF-β1 through AT1. This exacerbating effect of Ang-II on liver fibrosis probably mediates phosphorylation of c-Jun and p42/44 MAPK in AT1. Activated HCS produces Ang-II that led to fibrosis via NADPH oxidase. Also, a definite link is found between TGF-β1 and Ang-II for the development of liver fibrosis. Therefore, Ang-II may give rise to elevated TGF-β1, resulting in the production of collogen-1 via AT1 in the liver. There is a kind of positive feedback in the liver which is that TGF-β1 activates HSC, and HSC can produce much more TGF-β1 production [21].

Most of these injury factors are linked to oxidative stress based on reactive oxygen (ROS) and reactive nitrogen species. The ROS production is produced by some enzymes, for instance, mitochondrial leakage, tetrahydrobiopterin coenzyme oxidation, xanthine oxidase, endothelial nitric oxide synthase, nicotine adenine dinucleotide phosphate (NADPH) at both membrane and cytosolic compartment [2]. It might seem that oxidative stress is also critical pathways for RAS's effect, especially in development of pathologies [22]. HSC could also relate to oxidative stress by increasing AT1 and nonphagocytic NADPH oxidase enzyme system. NADPH oxidase is one of multicomponent enzyme systems, which is activated by rac1, p47phox, gp91phox, p22phox, nox1, p40phox, and p67phox. Ang-II triggers p47phox phosphorylation via AT1 on activated HSC to increase ROS production. One of the AT1 receptor antagonists, losartan, could block the ROS formation through NADPH oxidase inhibition [23]. This formed superoxide by NADPH oxidase could oxidize tetrahydrobiopterin (BH4) that is a cofactor of nitric oxide synthase (NOS). So, if BH4 is formed at high concentration, NOS enzyme could be dimerized and produces nitric oxide (NO). But, when the BH4 level is low, the balance between NOS and BH4 can shift to produce superoxide, resulting in decreasing NO production but increasing peroxynitrite (ONOO) formation. So, AT1-initiated oxidative stress could lead to inactivate NO, lipid oxidation, and activate redox-sensitive genes, e.g., proinflammatory cytokines, matrix metalloproteinases, chemotaxis, and adhesion molecules [15]. So, local RAS can produce ROS via Ang-II-AT1 axis [2].

Ang-II might relate to inducing tumor progress interaction with HSC in liver. Ang-II activates cAMP but not IP3. But many studies have shown that AT1 activates IP3, diacylglycerol, and reactive oxygen species. The activation of cAMP by Ang-II was also shown in renal mesangial cells. Moreover, PKA/ERK/CREB signaling pathway is reported to be an important intracellular component of the Ang-II effect on stimulated biliary proliferation. This notion was supported by attenuation of proliferation through inhibition PKA and ERK1/2. This intracellular pathway was present cholangiocytes that have shown own local RAS. Ang-II causes fibrosis by expresses of collagen 1A1 and fibronectin 1 in a primary rat cholangiocyte cell line, as well as IL6, which is one of the proliferative cytokines playing a role in biliary hyperplasia [9].

The other pathway might be Jak2/STAT for local RAS in the liver. Jak2 kinases are vital for the transcription of angiotensinogen mRNA *in vivo*. Ang-II stimulates STAT5B and co-activator of it, p300, in the liver. It is also stated that STAT3/p300/CBP pathway is critical for IL6 dependent activation of human angiotensinogen gene in HepG2 cells. NF-κB might involve Ang-II's inflammatory response, as well as IL-6, inducing the hepatic acute-phase reaction [24].

Ang-II has played an important role in the development of fibrosis, including liver, heart, lung, and pancreas. Some soluble factors such as cytokines, oxidative stress, chemokines, and growth factor increase ECM production [25]. TGF-β1 is one of the most profibrotic cytokines to accumulate some extracellular matrix (ECM) [15]. Local Ang-II predominantly induces of TGF-β [25]. Some of ECM element is noncollagenous glycoproteins, including hyaluronic acid (HA) and proteoglycan. Therefore, elevation of HA in plasma is given an important clue to assess the diagnosis of liver fibrosis. Ang-II is locally synthesized by activated HSC, moreover, and crucially involves the development of liver fibrosis. α-SMA is considered to be an important indicator for activation of HSC. It is reported that the positive effect of Ang-II is not only to activate and/or proliferate of HSC but also elevate fibrogenic cytokine, collagen deposition, and matrix synthesis. When RAS can block by using inhibitors for AT1 or ACE, Ang-II's fibrotic effects decrease. Local RAS plays a crucial role in the development of liver fibrosis

[15]. How local Ang-II can help established the fibrosis may be related to transforming growth factor-beta (TGF-β). More attention would give for the interaction of Ang-II and TGF-β. There are many TGF-β isoforms; however, TGF-β1 is the most investigated isoform. TGF-β associates the intracellular Smad signaling. Therefore, the TGF-β/Smad signaling is reported to play a crucial role to accumulate collagen, one of the major component proteins of the extracellular matrix (ECM), resulting in tissue fibrogenesis. Smad acts the most important transcriptional factor for TGF-β-mediated responses including fibrosis. Ang-II has been indicated to induce Smad2 and Smad4 signaling via AT1 for gene transcription, but the transcription is not strictly bound to TGF-β. Also, Smad7 has a function to counteract of the TGF-β pathway. Moreover, when Smad3 is decreased, or Smad7 expression is increased, tissue fibrosis from liver, skin, or kidney is indicated to diminish. Downregulation of CTGF is also prevented from developing fibrosis. CTGF is one of the crucial elements of fibrosis at a couple of organs. CTFG is a potent trigger of myofibroblasts and ECM synthesis and deposition. So, CTFG is upregulated by Ang-II by AT1, resulting in activation of Smad signaling and independent Rho/Rho kinase pathways of TGF-β. Based on these findings, both ACE and AT1 antagonists could alleviate CTGF expression and fibrosis as well. Also, the reverse can do the same effect on fibrosis [25]. Not only does TGF-β decrease the degradation of the matrix by metalloproteinase (MMP) but also synthesize connective tissue growth factor (CTGF), which is autoinduction of TGF-β. That is why Ang-II blockage by ACE or its receptor inhibition could reversed the tissue fibrogenesis in target tissue by modulation of TGF-β1 expression. Fibrosis is one of chronic and progressive processes mediated by the complex interaction between cell, ECM, cytokine, and growth factor. However, there is still no efficient and well-tolerated antifibrotic therapy due to lack of the main molecular pathways of it. The inhibition of Ang-II is reported to attenuate 40–60% TGF-β1 production, resulting in a reduction of hepatic fibrosis. Ang-II can stimulate Smad pathway also activate CTGF by TGF-β independently. The interaction of local Ang-II and TGF-β1 should, therefore, be elucidated in previous studies [25].

2.3. The function of local renin-angiotensin systems in the liver tissue

Locally formed angiotensin peptides have aggravated system's effects, notably cell growth, antiproliferation, apoptosis, production of reactive oxygen species (ROS), secretion of the hormone, proinflammatory and profibrogenesis. Till date, the importance of hepatic RAS under both physiologic and pathophysiologic condition has not been evaluated well yet, expect for heart and kidney [6]. However, the local RAS becomes so important to under pathophysiologic conditions in hepatic tissue based on the little present of RAS members compared to systemic RAS [12]. The local RAS plays a paracrine role in modulation of some processes, including inflammation, fibrosis, angiogenesis, cell proliferation, apoptosis, and survival under both physiological and pathophysiological circumstances. After recognition of an alternative RAS pathway (ACE2, Ang-1-7, etc.), it has to be changed to view its importance of tissue function. The task can be divided as its action on the systemic level including blood pressure control, tissue perfusion, and sodium and fluid balance, and on paracrine level including proliferation, inflammation, angiogenesis, apoptosis [17]. Consequently, local RAS might be amply of some diseases at liver since angiotensin-II gives rise to trigger oxidative stress. Moreover, the liver has an important role to detox of toxin which means that it may be very susceptibility to oxidative stress [22]. Recent data, from animal and human studies, suggest that the counteraction of local RAS would be of importance in modulating of liver diseases. The RAS not only can regulate blood pressure and volume, but also modulates inflammatory process [20]. The local RAS has importance under both physiologic and pathophysiologic conditions [6].

Local RAS plays a pivotal role for the tissue function both physiologic and pathophysiologic conditions based on paracrine and autocrine impacts of it [26]. RAS also modulate the body metabolic process [18]. Locally produced RAS has some specific role in apoptosis, angiogenesis and regulation of cell proliferation [27]. The RAS is thought to participate probably in liver regeneration and tumor as well [27]. Ang-II is important because of its effects including vasodilatation, antiproliferation, elevation of baroreflex sensitivity, facilitation of bradykinin activity at bradykinin receptor (BK2), inhibition of C-domain ACE activity and AT1 receptor antagonism, but some of them are counteract with Ang-II effects [6]. It is necessary to find the answer of the question why the local RAS has crucial regulation of tissues. One of the explanations of the issue is that the amount of local RAS components is independently controlled by its level in tissue [28]. It means that the mimetic or antagonist drugs could not be able to alter of the RAS members' concentration. The other possible explanation of it is that local Ang-II has a vital role in controlling of sympathetic neurotransmission and smooth muscle hyperplasia without effects of sodium balance which is under controlled by systemic Ang-II [28].

RAS was probably reported to be related to some hepatic pathogenesis, including hepatic stellate cell inflammation, proliferation, elevation of portal vein pressure, and hepatic fibrogenesis, as well [29]. RAS activation was reported in the patients with liver cirrhosis [30, 31], liver inflammation [12], nonalcoholic fatty liver disease [12], and fibrosis [4, 9]. RAS triggers oxidative stress at liver [32]. Moreover, blockage of RAS in the liver has improved for regeneration and inhibition of tumor progression [17]. There is an active interaction between the plasma ACE level and patient with liver fibrosis [29]. On the other hand, the local production of Ang-II might not be entirely blocked by ACE inhibitors due to that there are alternative pathways that are chymase [33].

Angiotensin-II, the most active member of RAS, has been indicated to have some pathologic effects, such as inflammation, oxidative stress, prothrombotic [18], cirrhosis [34], and acute liver injury [35]. Ang-II causes to contract vascular smooth cell and triggers nicotinamide adenine dinucleotide phosphate oxidase (NADPH), thereby elevation of superoxide radicals [20]. Interestingly, local RAS in liver and tumor necrosis factor-alpha (TNF-α) was suggested to have some interaction for developing insulin resistance and atherosclerosis by activation of plasminogen activator inhibitor-1 (PAI-1) production [14]. By better knowledge of inhibition, local RAS in the liver might be able to prevent at least of these kinds of diseases. Local RAS has a pivotal role under the pathophysiologic circumstance, resulting from tissue inflammation, trauma, hypoxia-ischemia, ischemia-reperfusion, hyperglycemia, hyperlipidemia, hyperhomocysteinemia, and hyperuricemia and autocrine/paracrine effect on the target organ [2]. One of the recent studies reported that RAS blockage by using ACE, captopril, inhibits the liver tumor growth in mice. Moreover, captopril was indicated to increase liver regeneration as well. How the captopril could enhance its recovery might be explained by increasing of HCS.

HCS can secrete MMP-9, resulting in accumulation of extracellular matrix. HCS could produce some terminating factors including IL-1, TGF-β at the late stages of liver regeneration [27].

In addition to other effects, Ang-II could modulate the immune system by releasing macrophage/monocyte chemoattractant protein (MCP)-1, MCP-2, granulocyte colony-stimulating factor as well as increasing macrophage infiltration. It might be thought that macrophage infiltration can fight microorganism and tumor cells. The macrophage's role in the late stage of tumor development is still needed to clarify. But some evidence is shown that macrophage infiltration might trigger cancer growth and metastasis. For instance, Kupffer cells could promote immune escape and facilitate metastatic colonies at a late stage of the disease. The macrophages could produce many cytokines to initiate angiogenesis, tumor growth, and metastasis. It is reported that Ang-II could stimulate macrophage infiltration and angiogenesis through AT1 and VEGF in a melanoma model. There might be an active interaction between macrophage and Ang-II. Because macrophage could produce ACE for the synthesis of Ang-II [5]. Ang-II increases the production of TNF, IL-1β the infiltration of CD43+ inflammatory cells which are inflammatory proteins [36].

2.4. The crosstalk of local renin-angiotensin system and liver pathologies

This chapter's main aim is underlined of local RAS and its contribution of liver pathologies. But, it should be accepted that there is a limited study to evaluate or investigate this interaction. Analyzing the interaction might be difficult. Because local and systemic RAS are hard to distinguish from each other. Also, they both could involve in developing liver pathologies or changing of liver function for some cases. That is why it will be divided the subhead of each liver pathology.

There are many factors determined to cause to liver diseases, such as alcohol, viral hepatitis, drug abuse, and autoimmune hepatitis. Chronic damage to liver causes liver fibrosis, leading to liver cirrhosis. Liver fibrosis is also produced by type-2 diabetes, concerned with obesity and steatosis that is fat accumulating in the liver [18]. There are two main cell types to overcome that kind of pathologies, as well as healthy maintaining the liver function. One of these cells is Kupffer cells. The cells are a type of mobile macrophages bound to endothelial cells. The cells physiologically synthesize immune-suppressive cytokine such as IL-10 to block HSC activation and/or collagen production. When the liver is injured, Kupffer cells are activated and start to release inflammatory cytokines, associating with apoptosis. But, the others such as IL6 or IL-1ß could involve liver fibrosis by increasing ECM, collagen-I, some fibrogenic cytokines such as TGF-ß1. The second type of cells is hepatic stellate (HSC), perivascular mesenchymal cells that are located in Disse space at the liver. The task of HCS is to metabolize vitamin-A, synthesize cytokines, growth, and inflammatory factors. That is why the cell plays a vital role in development of liver fibrosis and also participate liver inflammation [18]. High activation of ACE and angiotensin-II type-1 (AT1) receptor suggests at the liver disease. Furthermore, AT1 at liver plays a role in HSC activation by phosphorylation of Janus kinase-2 [37]. Besides, AT1 knockout mice were shown to decrease hepatic fibrosis. Also, Ang-II stimulates to the hepatic stellate cell for production more Ang-II [32]. When Kupffer cells are triggered by oxidative stress to produce proinflammatory cytokine after liver degenerations, resulting in also activation of HSC subsequently to synthesize collagen. After activation of

HSC, the cells moves to the degenerative area, then transform into interstitial myofibroblast. The myofibroblast can also produce cytokines, chemokines, matrix metalloproteinases, and tissue inhibitors of metalloproteinase (TIMPs). Local Ang-II has also affected on endothelial function. The endothelial cells have many tasks for regulation vascular tone, coagulation, cell growth, and leukocytes migration. All of the function of the endothelial cell requires a balance between vasodilatation such as nitric oxide and vasoconstriction such as Ang-II. Endothelial cell is very sensitive to the cell redox state [18].

2.4.1. The local renin-angiotensin system in liver and portal hypertension

Portal hypertension is one of the complications of cirrhosis having high of morbidity and mortality rates. Portal hypertension is interacted with RAS and sympathetic system, resulting in retention of water and salt then ascites [38]. If portal hypertension could be decreased, the complications of it could be declined as well. One of the drugs causing to reduce portal pressure is RAS inhibitors. Based on the suggestion, cirrhosis might cause vasodilation at the systemic and splanchnic vessel, so RAS could be activated to make up for the hypotension, resulting from Ang-II production. Elevated Ang-II gives rise to high-intrahepatic resistance both static and dynamic ways, and portal venous inflow through sodium and water retention. Ang-II also increases aldosterone production which has been thought to participate in developing inflammation, oxidative stress, endothelial dysfunction, insulin resistance, and fibrosis. But, there is still more evaluation for analyzing of the beneficial effect of RAS inhibitions on the patient with portal hypertension-induced by cirrhosis. Not only does Ang-II cause vasoconstriction in the hepatic microvasculature, but also endothelin, thromboxane-A2, leukotrienes, and norepinephrine also cause the vasocontraction. Therefore, it might be suggested that nitric oxide (NO) could not have efficient enough to overcome of that vasoconstriction. NO impairment could, therefore, help to progressive of liver dysfunction. So, the blockage of RAS may have a therapeutic effect on the early stage of cirrhosis. The local RAS might have some contributions to developing portal hypertension and virtually cirrhosis [39].

2.4.2. The local renin-angiotensin system in liver and hepatocellular carcinoma

Hepatocellular carcinoma (HCC) has been reported to be the most prevalent type of cancer throughout worldwide [30], being the fifth most predominant tumor case [17]. The patient with HCC has been informed to have only 5 years survival due to metastasis and recurrence based on angiogenesis [30]. HCC is one of the most severe complications of cirrhosis [6]. Although liver is one of the few tissues having regeneration, liver resection can perform at HCC and colorectal cancer (CRC) liver metastases patients for removing tumorous part of tissue [17]. CRC is the second leading cause of death at both genders, most of which are related to liver metastasis by 70% of CRC patients [17]. Liver resection is maybe best treatment for these diseases [17]. Also, some patients are indicated to die after liver resection operation due to metastasis of liver from the inside or outside tissue. This tumor recurrence is suggested based on some factor elevation including growth, angiogenic factor, and also modulation of extracellular matrix [17].

It is speculated that RAS might participate in liver regeneration and tumor modification by tumor proliferation and apoptosis, angiogenesis, and ECM remodeling [17]. RAS might participate in the development of this carcinoma due to its angiogenic and proliferative effects. Moreover, Ang-II could enhance vascular endothelial growth factor (VEGF), the most efficient angiogenic factor, which is decline by ACEI in mice with tumor [6]. Therefore, studies are indicated to be interaction Ang-II and vessel cancer growth. ACE having a homolog of ACE can convert to Ang-1-9 and Ang-1-7 from Ang-I and Ang-II, respectively. Elevated ACE2 is reported to block cell invasion, angiogenesis, VEGF in non-small cell cancer cell line. The activation of VEGF by Ang-II is thought to be concerned with VEGF/eNOS pathway and inflammation as well. So, it is well documented that RAS plays a role in cancer progression or metastasis. Moreover, the alternation of RAS element in the local cancer tissue might be related to cancer severity. RAS could be elevated in the patient with cirrhosis, found a high level of both Ang-II and Ang-1-7. Ang-1-7 is a potent antifibrosis. Ang-II can trigger VEGF in dose and time-dependent manner, also HSC for contraction and proliferation. One of the studies was shown that AT1 inhibition markedly declines liver fibrosis and VEGF expression. So, they pointed out that the interaction of Ang-II-VEGF is so important for the development of liver fibrosis and HCS activation. HCC patients were shown to have low expression of ACE2, although Ang-II, ang-1-7 and VEGF were high levels in the patient [30].

In addition to VEGF, Ang-II's angiogenic effect might be concerned with epidermal growth factor, angiopoietin 2, basic fibroblast growth factor, and an insulin-like growth factor that plays a major role in both liver regeneration and tumor growth. Moreover, both systems are reported to associate with liver regeneration. Although ACE-Ang-II-AT1 axis might be enhanced at early stages of its restoration, ACE2-Ang-1-7-Mas axis could be activated at the later stages of the recovery. RAS expression was reported to be cancer specific alternation. For examples, CRC metastases were indicated to elevate AT2, ACE, and Mas expressions, but decrease AT1 and angiotensinogen expressions. Moreover, AT1 was speculated to be healthy tissue cells, including Kupffer as well as the tumor and stromal infiltrating cell. But, the other RAS receptors, e.g., Mas, were found an only tumorous liver tissue. The other example was indicated that ACE localization was suggested to be hepatic endothelial cells, apical and cytoplasm of cancer and vascular cell because of neovascularization and cancer cell homeostasis. Also the other CRC metastases from colorectal adenoma, sarcomas prostate cancer was also speculated to be the crucial importance of RAS. So, pharmacological blockage of RAS by ACE or AT1 antagonist gives rise to decline the growth of cancer. ACE antagonist was probably decreased the severity of tumors in some kinds of tumor, e.g., prostate, breast, and CRC. The other view was pointed out that cancer growth could be a decline in AT1 knockdown mice based on attenuation of VEGF, angiogenesis. This finding was suggested that AT1 plays an important role. Also, the drop of AT1 might cause to enhance alternative RAS pathway action (ACE2, Mas). The other explanation of these was that when AT1 was chronically blockaded by the drug, it might be shifted a balance to AT2 which is well known to have a different effect from AT1. Although AT1 has mitogenic and angiogenic effects, AT2 triggers apoptosis and inhibits proliferation. AT2's effect on VEGF is the double direction. AT2 is reported to activate VEGF; it is also shown to antagonize VEGF as well. The other aspect should also be considered that AT2 could modulate NO and BK pathways in which both has participated angiogenesis. Moreover, the other candidate for angiogenesis process could be proliferator-activated receptor-γ (PPAR-γ) because plenty of AT1 antagonists enhanced PPAR-γ attenuation of cancer proliferation. Why many of studies have focused on the regulation of angiogenesis by RAS is related to how to regulate tumor growth. But it should be noticed that Ang-II could be produced by another enzyme, chymase which also enhance Ang-1-7. Thus, ACE inhibitors can just block one way, resulting in one alternative pathway still efficient for its production. The other important point is that the alternative RAS pathway could syntheses Ang-1-7as well. Ang-1-7 has been reported to reduce metastases in mice since it led to diminish in cyclooxygenase-2. Elevation of cyclooxygenase-2 is related to cancer growth, inflammation, angiogenesis, thanks to enhancing prostaglandin E2, D2, and thromboxane A2. Ang-1-7 could also moderate thromboxane A2 as well as prostaglandins. ACE inhibition increases not only Ang-1-7 levels but also BK levels. However, the elevation of BK is not beneficial effect on the tumorous cell due to stimulation of cancer growth by angiogenesis and inflammation [17].

2.4.3. The local renin-angiotensin system in liver and cholangiocarcinoma

Cholangiocarcinoma (CCA) is one of the uncommon malignant tumors. This tumor type is also related to local RAS. According to a recent study, the development of CCA is associated with inflammation and biliary duct cell injury due to obstruction of bile flow rate. Cytokines productions in the biliary tissue by inflammation process are responsible for the malignant transformation. Locally produced Ang-II is reported to involve to the proliferation and activation of CCA cells which express Ang-I as a growth factor in local effect (autocrine and paracrine). The local effect of Ang-II could modulate the balance between intrahepatic proliferation and fibrosis. Moreover, the patient with CCA was found to high ACE level. That is why it will be vital to understand the interaction of CCA and RAS in developing new strategies for cancer therapy to improve the patient's life and life quality as well [40].

2.4.4. The local renin-angiotensin system in liver and cancer growth

Cancer growth and metastasis are well documented to related angiogenesis. The new vessel growth is associated with Ang-II and VEGF/VEGF-A, especially useful in vascular endothelial cells. Ang-II's new vessel formative effect is through AT1. Its angiogenic effect of Ang-II is consisted within several cancer models. For instance, VEGF is shown to secrete through Ang-II-AT1 in ovarian cancer cells. Also, ACE inhibitors are reported to decline the neovasculature in cancer tissue. VEGF is defined to use similar pathways in many tissues. After VEGF overexpression in cancerous tissue, the fibrin at extravascular is accumulated, but the extracellular matrix is degraded. Then, the endothelial cell can migrate into the stroma, forming enlarged but thinned vessel-walled, named as mother vessel. After this stage, the vascular development is reported to differ from each tissue and many daughter vessels from mother vessel could be developed branches and caused to disrupt vessel organization, including muscular arteries and veins and produced glomeruli bodies, a kind of disorganized tangle vessel (**Figure 2**). Ang-II is indicated to enhance vascular permeability by increasing some permeability factors such as prostaglandins, nitric oxide, NF-κB, VEGF, and endothelin [5].

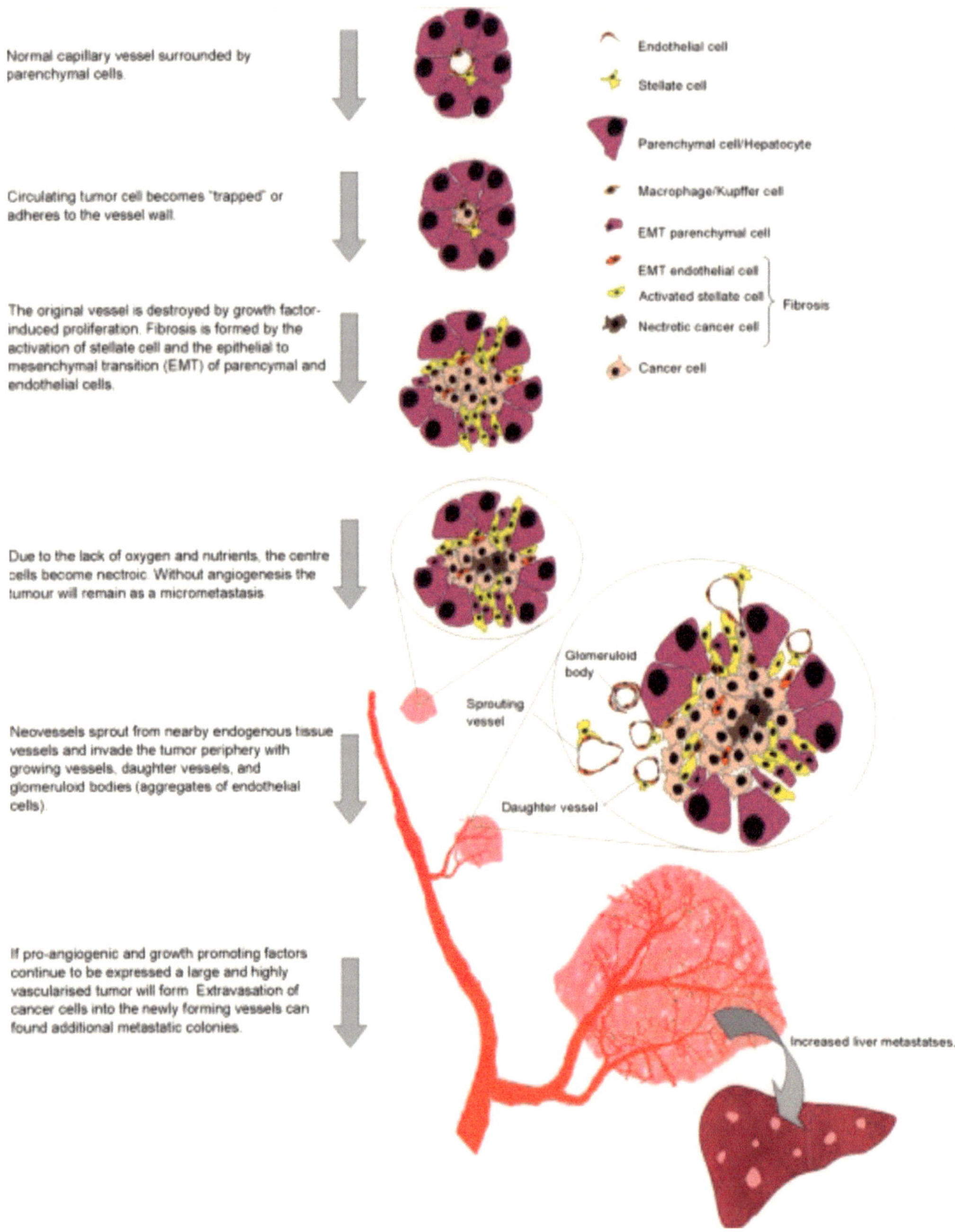

Figure 2. The development of cancer angiogenesis, growth and metastasis [5].

2.4.5. *The local renin-angiotensin system in liver and cholangiopathy*

Primary sclerosing cholangitis (PCS), an ischemic cholangiopathy, might be related to local RAS within the portal tract. Ang-II production may increase in portal tract due to biliary epithelial stimuli, including infections, drugs, and toxins. The other possibility of activation of RAS in it-portal tract relies on localized biliary tract ischemia such as microvascular thrombosis; immune-mediated endothelial is or toxic injury to arterioles. Local RAS in the liver has suggested that Ang-II could modify bile secretion by elevation of the production of bile acid independent bile flow and by the nonvascular effect of Ang-II on hepatocytes or biliary epithelial. Elevation of Ang-II production can trigger some responses, such as inflammatory cytokines releasing from mesenchymal cells, biliary epithelia, and vascular endothelial, inflammatory cells influx, and the activation of portal tract mesenchymal cells with fibrogenesis. There is a vicious cycle with lymphocytic obliteration and occlusion of the peribiliary plexus and hepatic artery microvasculature, and biliary tract ischemia. These alternations give rise to enhance portal tract edema and venous pressure, promote cholestasis as well [41].

2.4.6. *The local renin-angiotensin system in liver and insulin resistance*

The liver is well known to regulate blood glucose that is why insulin could block glucose production on hepatocytes and indirectly decreasing lipolysis in the adipose tissue, and free fatty acids. When insulin resistance is developed it enhances gluconeogenesis and lipolysis to elevate glucose and free fatty acids in circulation. Therefore, liver tissue plays pivotal role in developing insulin resistance [2]. Metabolic syndrome, in other words insulin resistance [12], is a complex disease related to obesity, dyslipidemia, hyperglycemia, and hypertension as well. Metabolic syndrome is one of the risk factors for developing type-2 diabetes and cardiovascular diseases [42]. Therefore, this kind of illness might also be related to insulin resistance.

Ang-II involves the development of the insulin resistance [15]. Ang-II declines the insulin-stimulated tyrosine phosphorylation and thus to block the interaction between phosphatidylinositol-3-kinase and insulin receptor substrate (IRS-1) and downregulation insulin receptor signal. Hence, Ang-II increases liver glycogenolysis and thus increases gluconeogenesis. Taking together, these findings indicated that Ang-II could impair insulin metabolic effects, thus participating in developing insulin resistance. Also, Ang-II led not only to decrease lipid storage capacity and triglyceride at adipose tissue but also increase the accumulation of triglyceride in liver tissue. These effects might have a well-established pivotal contributing to developing insulin resistance as well. So, ACE inhibition is reported to improve the insulin sensitivity [43].

The local RAS in the liver might link to improve the insulin resistance related to plasminogen activator inhibitor (PAI)-1 in liver tissue. Furthermore, PAI-1 might be activated by TGF-β. Takeshita et al. also found that TNF-α increased PAI-1 both mRNA and protein productions in hepatocytes. They reported of TNF-α could trigger the protein kinase C (PKC), p38 mitogen-activated protein, kinase/extracellular signal-regulated kinase (ERK), protein tyrosine kinase, and NF-κB pathways to induce PAI-1 production in the liver. Ang-II activates PKC and NF-κB by 1,2-diacylglycerol production in primary rat hepatocytes. At this moment, the local RAS inhibition by AT1 antagonist could abolish TNF-α-induced PAI-1 protein and mRNA in liver [14]. The studies are suggested that both classical and alternative RAS pathways might involve developing insulin resistance. The classical pathway is ACE-Ang-II-AT1. So, one of the previous studies was shown that AT1 inhibition could improve the oral glucose test without alteration of the plasma insulin level in diabetic animals. Indeed, Ang-II-AT1 axis probably has a significant role in developing insulin resistance. Therefore, insulin sensitive tissue, primarily skeletal muscles could be increased glucose uptake by AT1 inhibition. This elevation is, however, thought in partly to relate to the elevated insulin-mediated IRS1-IP3-GLUT4 axis. On the contrary, it is suggested that angiotensin receptor blocker could increase insulin secretion at animals with type-II diabetes. Additionally, it is reported to enhance glucose uptake at adipose tissue, one of the sensitive insulin organs, at AT2-knockdown animals [44]. Alternative RAS pathways, ACE2/An-1-7/Mas axis, might be the high beneficial effect on diabetes based on enhancing glucose reuptake, diminishing glycogen production, and insulin resistance in hepatocytes via Akt/PI3K/IRS-1/JNK insulin signaling. Also, Ang-1-7 declines inflammation factors from adipose tissue in obese animal [18].

Giving that there might be a relationship aldosterone and insulin, systemic RAS could, also, participate in developing insulin resistance. Because aldosterone could cause insulin resistance based on its hypokalaemia effect on pancreatic beta cells, and also its direct action on insulin receptor, elevation gluconeogenesis at the liver, and sodium-glucose cotransporters. The other possible effect of aldosterone is suggested to enhance oxidative stress and inflammation in pancreatic beta cells and cause insulin resistance in adipocytes tissue. Interestingly, aldosterone is emphasized to affect insulin metabolism in liver, cardiovascular, renal, adipose, and muscle tissues. Insulin enhances angiotensinogen expression in the liver [45].

2.4.7. The local renin-angiotensin system in liver and liver cirrhosis

The role of RAS in liver cirrhosis was shown to enhance intrahepatic pressure via AT1 by experimental and human cirrhosis. Ang-II gives rise to contract and proliferates of HSC. There has been indicated that an increase of intracellular calcium ion due to the production of ROS, release of proinflammatory cytokine and chemokines lead to activate Kupffer cells. These cytokines, thus, could destroy hepatocytes and modulate extracellular matrix remodeling. Moreover, TGF-β could transform from HSC to myofibroblast, so it plays a crucial effect on the development of fibrosis. Kupffer cells are part of the reticuloendothelial system (80–90%) and thus are a primary source of cytokines. These cytokines might activate HSC, resulting in the production of ECM components, such as TGF-β, fibronectin. Ang-II is reported to develop fibrosis by proinflammatory cytokine. Also, Ang-II triggers to the mononuclear cell to synthesize more cytokines, especially TGF-β. Moreover, Kupffer cells have shown to express some RAS components, including renin, ACE, and AT1 [34].

2.4.8. The local renin-angiotensin system in liver and ischemia/reperfusion injury

Local RAS is reported to play a vital role in I/R injury in the liver. Angiotensinogen, renin, and ACE were indicated to involve in I/R injury in the liver. So, ACE inhibition could have a positive impact on I/R injury due to liver transplantation. Also, ACE might participate to inflammation, fibrosis, and anoxemia of local tissue. ACE2 is newly discovered homology of ACE and can transform Ang-II to Ang1-7 which can antagonize Ang-II's vasocontraction effects. When ACE2 is a knockdown, resulting in markedly elevating of Ang-II's expression therefore, it is suggested that ACE2 and ACE can antagonize each other. But this correlation between ACE2 and ACE has not been found at liver transplantation yet. It might be due to complication factors interaction of liver transportation, and therefore more studies need to evaluate to reveal this complicated interaction in liver pathologies. But, up to now we know that ACE2 plays a negative role in RAS. Furthermore, local ACE2 is thought to relate to tissue hypoxia as well. In parallel, the expression and activity of local ACE2 are found to significantly elevated in the lighting biliary tract in rats and human hepatic cirrhosis and other chronic hepatic injuries. The hypoxia is believed to have significant contribution in the increase of ACE2 expression, and upregulation of its may participate some protective mechanisms against hypoxia conditions. However, healthy liver tissue just is of a trace expression of ACE and ACE2, but their mRNA and protein expressions have been elevated in the transplanted liver of rats. ACE might relate to inflammation due to Ang-II which increases the production of TNF, CINC-1, and ICAM-1 in tissue via AT1. So, ACE inhibition reduces I/R injury after experimental liver transplantation by the inflammatory promotion process. Also, it is reported that renin expression elevated fivefold after reperfusion following the I/R model by clamping the portal vein. According to the findings authors concluded that renin significantly enhanced at the initial stage of liver transportation, resulting in elevation of Ang-I. These elevations lead to increase ACE expression, eventually increasing Ang-II which gave rise to diminish blood supply in transplanted liver and aggravates the liver hypoxia, combine with inflammation [46].

2.4.9. The local renin-angiotensin system in liver and liver fibrosis

There are many pathologies of liver to cause liver fibrosis, such as alcohol, nonalcoholic fatty liver, chronic hepatitis B, and C. Liver fibrosis's characterization is related to accumulate matrix proteins in the tissue, including elastin, collagen, basement glycoproteins, proteoglycans, hyaluronan, and finally changing of the matrix composition. Under normal physiologic conditions, Disse space in the liver just has proteoglycan, nonfibril forming collagens, such as type IV, VI, and XIV and also glycoprotein, i.e., fibronectin, laminin, and tenascin. But, under the pathophysiologic conditions, these spaces have some alternation with enhancing fibronectin and tenascin, then the accumulation of Type I, Type III collagen, elastin, and laminin. Thereby, liver parenchyma has to be remodeled to accumulate bands of scar tissue. HSC in the liver is a perivascular mesenchymal cell, the chiefly fibrogenic cell-type. One of its primary functions is retinoid (vitamin A) storages under normal physiologic conditions. However, HSC shifts into interstitial myofibroblast which can produce ECM components, profibrotic and proinflammatory cytokines and chemokines under the pathophysiologic condition, such as liver fibrosis. The activation of HSC can be triggered by responding to paracrine trigger from its surrounding cell-like hepatocytes and Kupffer cells as well as alternation of ECM. These process can be maintained by some factors and autocrine profibrogenic triggers, i.e., TGF-β 1 and platelet-derived growth factor. Nowadays, a well-established pivotal participant of both inflammatory cells and activated HSCs is Ang-II [6]. Ang-II can start a proliferation of myofibroblast and stellate cells, resulting in initiate inflammatory cell and release some profibrotic molecules, i.e., TGF-β, CTGF, and IL-1β. Both human and animal studies reported that overexpression of some component of RAS was found at fibrotic liver which is related to between Ang-II and TGF-β1 [47]. It suggests that inhibition of hepatic RAS has a beneficial effect on suppressing steatosis and fibrosis [12]. Therefore, increasing of Ang-II levels in liver tissue is tightly associated with fibrosis [32].

There is some evidence indicated that both classic and alternative RAS might play a role in the development of liver fibrosis. ACE-Ang-II-AT1 axis, classic RAS, is reported to be most important for developing liver fibrosis (**Figure 3**). There is an exciting agreement that the drugs of ACE and AT1 inhibitors have been succeeding to heal of liver fibrosis by downregulation of some keys cytokines and inflammatory elements. The infusion of Ang-II is reported to cause bile duct epithelial cell proliferation, and exacerbation of liver fibrosis in rats with the bile duct ligation, resulting in to have the contribution of both local and systemic RAS. Also, Ang-II has a potential effect on cell growth and fibrosis which is critical processes of inflammation and wound healing as well. This process is activated HCSs by Ang-II though AT1. Moreover, when Ang-II incubates with activated HCS, it is shown to enhance intracellular calcium concentration, cell contraction, cellular proliferation via mitogen-activated protein kinase pathways. Ang-II in human HSCs causes profibrogenic effects on ROS generation via NADPH oxidase. NADPH oxidase is also expressed in Kupffer cells, sinusoidal endothelial cells that have to participate in developing fibrosis by ROS production as well. Hepatic fibrosis also related to the local RAS's effect on extracellular matrix (ECM) which has a balance between ECM output and degradation by two enzymes. The name of these two enzymes is matrix metalloproteinases (MMP) and tissue inhibitors of metalloproteinases (TIMP), which produce and degrade ECM, respectively. The balance equals to 1:1. The Ang-II can run to balance favor of TIMP1 in HSCs via AT1, induction of protein kinase C. ACE or AT1 inhibitors, therefore, can make a balance again between these two enzymes in animal models of fibrosis. The other profibrotic effects of Ang-II depend on amplification of inflammatory response, inducing acute-phase reactants, ROS, releasing of inflammatory and fibrotic cytokines including IL6, IL1, TGF-β, TNF-α chronic, and ECM deposition in liver injury. It has also induced monocyte chemoattractant protein-1 (MCP-1) and IL-8 from HCS. MCP-1 triggers leucocytes for fortification and activation. MCP-1 could be upregulated its genes by Rho intracellular pathways via Ang-II and AT1 axis. Ang-II can upregulate genes by activator protein-1 (AP-1), signal transducer, and activator of transcription (STAT) and NF-κB, which have proinflammatory efficiency, e.g., IL-6. Ang-II and NF-κB are reported to have a kind of positive feedback interaction on triggering the transcription of angiotensinogen via AT1. Kupffer cells might participate in this proinflammatory effect of Ang-II by AT1. In other words, activated Kupffer cells by Ang-II in the alcoholic liver disease generate TGF-β and TNF-α. That is why these proinflammatory effects of the Kupffer cell could be declined by AT1 but not ACE inhibitors. This finding suggested that AT1 in Kupffer cell is a pivotal role in Ang-II's inflammatory effect [6]. Human studies of fibrotic treatment are reported to have difficulties based on the requirement of taking multiple biopsies from the patient. This brings an enormous ethic problem and also makes the patient suffering from pain. This cannot be acceptable for anyone. The other difficulties of human studies is related to the illness progression very slow in the most disease, e.g., hepatitis-C, nonalcoholic liver disease. This slow progression makes it difficult to determine of therapeutic beneficial of treatment. It may overcome when the studies are planned for tracking patient for many years [6].

Fibrosis is a complicated process including collagen-I accumulation, epithelial to mesenchymal transition (EMT). EMT triggered by TGF-ß1 is a kind of structural and cellular alteration leading to separate cells, lose cell polarity, and gain cell adhesion, resulting in facilitating cell

http://dx.doi.org/10.5772/65919

motility. Responding to EMT, the extracellular matrix could be exposed to change for allowing cell motility and express some growth factors, e.g., VEGF. Ang-II elevates TGF-ß1 level, α-smooth muscle actin and decreases E-cadherin. The fibrosis development after hepatic bile duct ligation is reported to participate in both Ang-II and Ang-1-7. According to these findings, although Ang-II levels increase in the first week after bile ligation, Ang-1-7 levels enhance after 3 weeks of bile ligation. It also emphasized that Ang-II tends to back to its normal level after 1 week, but Ang-1-7 maintained its priority after 2 weeks [5]. On the basis of these findings, it will be concluded that classical pathways of RAS, ACE-Ang-II-AT1 has involved in the development of liver fibrosis more than alternative RAS pathway, ACE2-Ang-1-7-Mas (**Figure 2**).

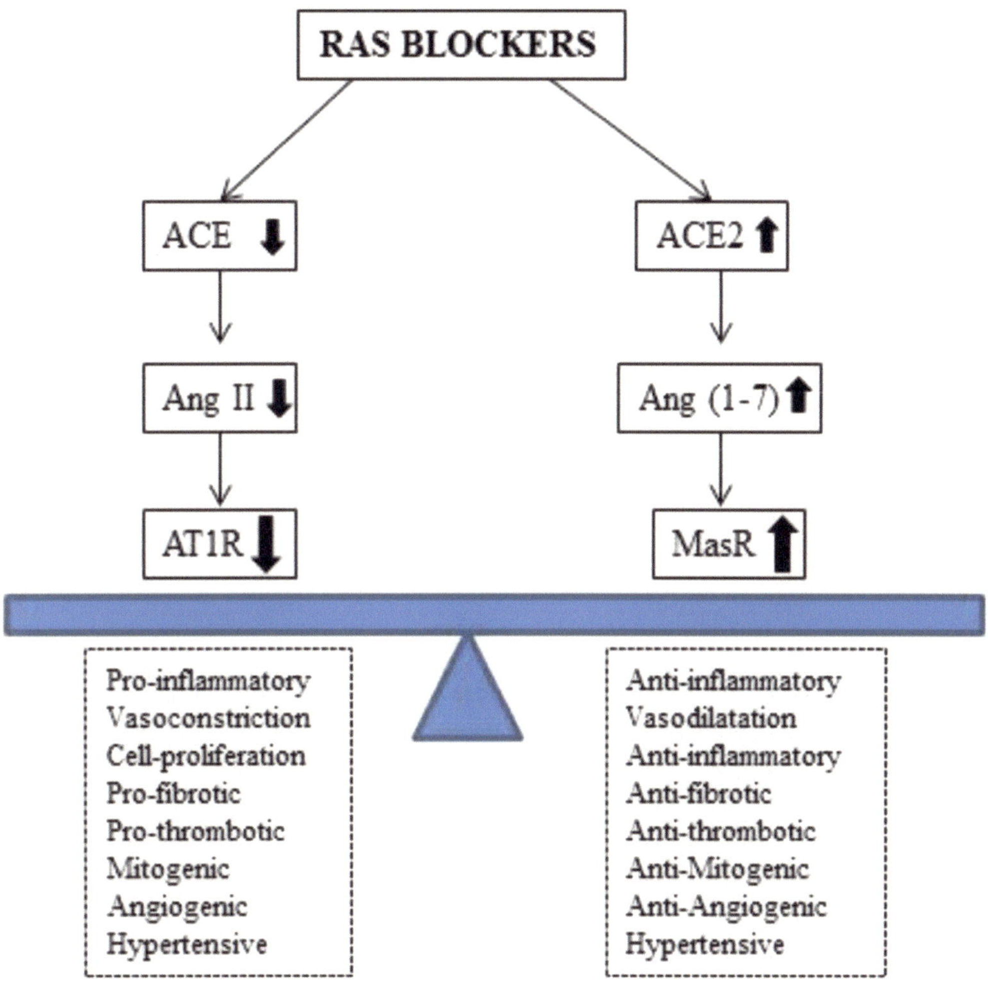

Figure 3. The effect of classical and alternative renin-angiotensin system and the effect on renin angiotensin system blockers. The figure was modified from Refs. [6, 18].

2.4.10. The local renin-angiotensin system in liver and nonalcoholic fatty liver disease

Nonalcoholic fatty liver disease (NAFLD) is a predominantly chronic hepatic disease in developed countries, and its prevalence is around 10–24% in the countries. The disease is linked to some illness, including obesity, hyperlipidemia, hypertension, type-2 diabetes, and insulin resistance (IR) [12], thus hepatic function could be elevated by losing weight [48]. In particular, there is a significant interaction between NAFLD and IR, also named metabolic syndrome that has found approximately 95% NADFLD patient. NADFLD has reported elevating inflammation and oxidative stress, leading to release inflammatory cytokines and abnormal lipoprotein [12]. Because metabolic syndrome is related to accumulate enormous triglycerides in the tissue, it is shown that ACE antagonist by drugs could help to lose the weight in an obese patient [48]. Additionally, according to one of experimental study, the liver was indicated to gain weight when fed the high-fat diet for 12 weeks. In contrast, ACE inhibition by perindopril was shown to reduce the liver weight and food consume as well. The authors suggested that low-food intake might be concerned with Ang-II and corticotropin-releasing hormone (CRP), anorexic brain peptide. Ang-II receptors were reported to express at CRP-containing neurons. Thus, Ang-II is thought to decline CRP expression from the neurons. Local Ang-II could cause to release leptin from isolated adipocytes; ACEI could block the releasing of leptin. One of the novel results of authors was that ACE activity is high in rat with obese-induced by high-fatty acid diet. They thought that elevation of ACE in liver led to accumulate triglyceride. Also, they speculated to associate with elevation ACE and developing insulin resistance and type-2 diabetes. They implied when ACE could be pharmacologically antagonized; insulin signaling could be modified in the liver, resulting in triggering insulin receptor and enhancing glucose uptake by elevation bradykinin based on decline cleavage by ACE [48]. Indeed, liver function is also affected by systemic RAS.

Ang-II plays a significant role in the development of liver inflammation and fibrosis. So, when Ang-II is blocked by ACE and ACE antagonist drugs, it helps to modify some factors, e.g., decreasing cytokine production such as TNF-α, decreasing TGF-β, elevation of adiponectin, insulin, and insulin signaling at the cellular level as well as limiting the HSCs activity. HCS in the healthy liver has very low concentration of RAS elements, but the cell increases the RAS expression, e.g., ACE, AT1 under the pathophysiologic circumstance. After activation of HCS, the cell could produce Ang-II which led to trigger some fibrogenic effects, such as cell migration, proliferation, inflammatory cytokine, and collagen secretions through commonly AT1 [12]. Ang-II's fibrogenic effects in the liver, kidney, and also heart are concerned with TGF-β. Therefore, RAS inhibition is reported to the therapeutic effect on liver fibrosis and inflammation based on NAFLD. The oxidative stress levels are reported to relate to NAFLD and also IR severity. It is shown to enhance some factors, including TNF-α, TGF-β, plasminogen activator-1, IL6, and CRP at the patients with NAFLD [12].

Additionally, the liver might be affected by cardiorenal metabolic syndrome (CRS) and type-2 diabetes mellitus based on metabolic toxicities with the development of the nonalcoholic fatty liver disease or steatohepatitis. The liver tissue has occurred some cellular remodeling during those pathologies. In the beginning, hepatocytes increase the fat accumulation as a result of lipolysis, triglycerides, and free fatty acids. Accumulation of fat triggers oxidative stress and

ROS production. Two hypotheses have been proposed to elucidate nonalcoholic fatty liver disease progression. The first theory is associated with CRS causing to the development of steatosis. The second approach is associated with hepatocytes injury, inflammation, and fibrosis, which causes mostly oxidative stress, elevated cytokines synthesis. The development of fibrosis and accumulation of ECM predominantly rely on HCS activity, a sinusoidal pericyte cell. HCS led to accumulate type-I and type-III collagen around hepatic sinusoids, probably resulting in destroying the structural and function of sinusoidal and endothelial cell-hepatocytes. Local RAS in the liver has shown to play a major role in the development of liver fibrosis. That is why Ang-II blockage could be attenuate oxidative stress, steatosis, inflammation, and fibrosis[2]. Those studies were pointed out the role of systemic RAS in NADFLD. We can speculate that there is no available research directly indicated the local RAS in liver. While Ang-II could involve a kind of NADFLD, it still needs also to evaluate the role of local RAS in liver.

2.4.11. The local renin-angiotensin system in liver and acute liver failure

Paracetamol is one of the commonly utilized drugs as a painkiller and for decreasing fever when it is used at therapeutic doses. It caused hepatotoxicity when it overdoses, a worldwide problem, resulting in acute liver failure. The drug's metabolized process is mainly carried out at liver and converted to it nontoxic metabolites which extracted by urine. But, its small proportion usually less than 5% is also metabolized by the cytochrome P450 (CYP) enzyme system (generally CYP2E1), and converted to it highly reactive metabolite, named as N-acetyl-p-benzoquinone imine (NAPQI). Its reactive metabolite leads to a toxic effect through oxidative stress. NAPQI covalently binds intracellular proteins based on its reactive electrophilic property. Although NAPQI reacts with reduced glutathione (GSH) shifting to nontoxic metabolites at its therapeutic dose, it also reacts with GSH at high doses of paracetamol, but GSH could not have enough level of enormous reactive metabolites, resulting from oxidative stress and mitochondrial dysfunction. GSH is one of the vital antioxidant enzymes for suppressing of the oxidative compound. A decline of GSH could cause mitochondrial oxidative, depress mitochondrial respiration, and adenosine triphosphate deprivation, resulting in hepatocytes and sinusoidal endothelial cells necrosis. Ang-II is well documented to exaggerate oxidative stress. So, Ang-II blocked by aliskiren, renin inhibitors, is reported to decline acute toxicity of liver-induced by paracetamol by decreasing oxidative stress. Moreover, aliskiren is shown to reduce elevated TGF-α and downregulate activated Kupffer cells and HSCs at the acute liver injury induced by paracetamol [49].

3. Conclusion

After recognition of local RAS, the new insight of RAS is shifted to local or tissue due to its endocrine function. Systemic RAS may not play important role under pathophysiologic conditions but local RAS may play a crucial role under pathophysiologic conditions, especially independent and/or dependent systemic RAS. The studies have shown that local RAS in the liver has a crucial role not only in maintaining the physiologic functions but also in developing pathophysiology. There are limited studies available to evaluate local RAS under a pathophysiologic circumstance. The component of local RAS may present a small amount expression in the normal liver tissue. However, its component expressions are increased under a pathophysiologic condition, leading to enhance of importance and effects of RAS in the tissue. So, some pathophysiologic conditions have been indicated to relate to local RAS, such as liver fibrosis, portal hypertension, insulin resistance, liver cirrhosis, cancer growth, and metastasis. That is why the new studies are needed to evaluate the local RAS under a pathophysiologic condition.

Author details

Eylem Taskin[1]* and Celal Guven[2]

*Address all correspondence to: eylemtaskin@yahoo.com

1 School of Health, Physiotherapy and Rehabilitation, T.C. Istanbul Bilim University, Istanbul, Turkey

2 Biophysics Department, Medical Faculty, Adiyaman University, Adiyaman, Turkey

References

[1] Leung, P.S. and P.O. Carlsson, Tissue renin-angiotensin system: its expression, localization, regulation and potential role in the pancreas. J Mol Endocrinol, 2001. **26**(3): pp. 155-64.

[2] Hayden, M.R., et al., Possible mechanisms of local tissue renin-angiotensin system activation in the cardiorenal metabolic syndrome and type 2 diabetes mellitus. Cardiorenal Med, 2011. **1**(3): pp. 193-210.

[3] Emdin, M., et al., Biomarkers of activation of renin-angiotensin-aldosterone system in heart failure: how useful, how feasible? Clin Chim Acta, 2015. **443**: pp. 85-93.

[4] Zhang, X., et al., Tetramethylpyrazine inhibits angiotensin II-induced activation of hepatic stellate cells associated with interference of platelet-derived growth factor beta receptor pathways. FEBS J, 2014. **281**(12): pp. 2754-68.

[5] Ager, E.I., J. Neo, and C. Christophi, The renin-angiotensin system and malignancy. Carcinogenesis, 2008. **29**(9): pp. 1675-84.

[6] Warner, F.J., et al., Liver fibrosis: a balance of ACEs? Clin Sci (London), 2007. **113**(3): pp. 109-18.

[7] Cheng, Q. and P.S. Leung, An update on the islet renin-angiotensin system. Peptides, 2011. **32**(5): pp. 1087-95.

[8] Michalopoulos, G.K. and M.C. DeFrances, Liver regeneration. Science, 1997. **276**(5309): pp. 60-6.

[9] Afroze, S.H., et al., Activation of the renin-angiotensin system stimulates biliary hyperplasia during cholestasis induced by extrahepatic bile duct ligation. Am J Physiol Gastrointest Liver Physiol, 2015. **308**(8): pp. G691-701.

[10] Kang, N., et al., Reduced hypertension-induced end-organ damage in mice lacking cardiac and renal angiotensinogen synthesis. J Mol Med (Berl), 2002. **80**(6): pp. 359-66.

[11] Nguyen, G., C. Burckle, and J.D. Sraer, The renin receptor: the facts, the promise and the hope. Curr Opin Nephrol Hypertens, 2003. **12**(1): pp. 51-5.

[12] Orlic, L., et al., Nonalcoholic fatty liver disease and the renin-angiotensin system blockers in the patients with chronic kidney disease. Wien Klin Wochenschr, 2015. **127**(9-10): pp. 355-62.

[13] Cole, J.M., et al., New approaches to genetic manipulation of mice: tissue-specific expression of ACE. Am J Physiol Renal Physiol, 2003. **284**(4): pp. F599-607.

[14] Takeshita, Y., et al., Cross talk of tumor necrosis factor-alpha and the renin-angiotensin system in tumor necrosis factor-alpha-induced plasminogen activator inhibitor-1 production from hepatocytes. Eur J Pharmacol, 2008. **579**(1-3): pp. 426-32.

[15] Iwanami, J., et al., Inhibition of the renin-angiotensin system and target organ protection. Hypertens Res, 2009. **32**(4): pp. 229-37.

[16] Wong, M.K., W. Ge, and N.Y. Woo, Positive feedback of hepatic angiotensinogen expression in silver sea bream (*Sparus sarba*). Mol Cell Endocrinol, 2007. **263**(1-2): pp. 103-11.

[17] Koh, S.L., E.I. Ager, and C. Christophi, Liver regeneration and tumour stimulation: implications of the renin-angiotensin system. Liver Int, 2010. **30**(10): pp. 1414-26.

[18] Moreira de Macedo, S., et al., The role of renin-angiotensin system modulation on treatment and prevention of liver diseases. Peptides, 2014. **62**: pp. 189-96.

[19] Takai, S., D. Jin, and M. Miyazaki, New approaches to blockade of the renin-angiotensin-aldosterone system: chymase as an important target to prevent organ damage. J Pharmacol Sci, 2010. **113**(4): pp. 301-9.

[20] Peters, B.S., et al., The renin-angiotensin system as a primary cause of polyarteritis nodosa in rats. J Cell Mol Med, 2010. **14**(6A): pp. 1318-27.

[21] Pereira, R.M., et al., Renin-angiotensin system in the pathogenesis of liver fibrosis. World J Gastroenterol, 2009. **15**(21): pp. 2579-86.

[22] Taskin, E., et al., The cooperative effect of local angiotensin-II in liver with adriamycin hepatotoxicity on mitochondria. Med Sci Monit, 2016. **22**: pp. 1013-21.

[23] El-Ashmawy, N.E., et al., Antifibrotic effect of AT-1 blocker and statin in rats with hepatic fibrosis. Clin Exp Pharmacol Physiol, 2015. **42**(9): pp. 979-982

[24] Guo, Y., E. Mascareno, and M.A. Siddiqui, Distinct components of Janus kinase/signal transducer and activator of transcription signaling pathway mediate the regulation of systemic and tissue localized renin-angiotensin system. Mol Endocrinol, 2004. **18**(4): pp. 1033-41.

[25] Wengrower, D., et al., Losartan reduces trinitrobenzene sulphonic acid-induced colorectal fibrosis in rats. Can J Gastroenterol, 2012. **26**(1): pp. 33-9.

[26] Januel, E., et al., Impact of renin-angiotensin system blockade on clinical outcome in glioblastoma. Eur J Neurol, 2015. **22**(9): pp. 1304-9.

[27] Koh, S.L., et al., Blockade of the renin-angiotensin system improves the early stages of liver regeneration and liver function. J Surg Res, 2013. **179**(1): pp. 66-71.

[28] Swales, J.D. and N.J. Samani, Localisation and physiological effects of tissue renin-angiotensin systems. J Hum Hypertens, 1989. **3(**Suppl 1): pp. 71-7.

[29] Efe, C., et al., Angiotensin-converting enzyme for noninvasive assessment of liver fibrosis in autoimmune hepatitis. Eur J Gastroenterol Hepatol, 2015. **27**(6): pp. 649-54.

[30] Ye, G., et al., The association of renin-angiotensin system genes with the progression of hepatocellular carcinoma. Biochem Biophys Res Commun, 2015. **459**(1): pp. 18-23.

[31] Gao, N., et al., The inhibitory effect of angiotensin II on BKCa channels in podocytes via oxidative stress. Mol Cell Biochem, 2015. **398**(1-2): pp. 217-22.

[32] Goh, G.B., et al., Renin-angiotensin system and fibrosis in non-alcoholic fatty liver disease. Liver Int, 2015. **35**(3): pp. 979-85.

[33] Lee, H.A., et al., Tissue-specific upregulation of angiotensin-converting enzyme 1 in spontaneously hypertensive rats through histone code modifications. Hypertension, 2012. **59**(3): pp. 621-6.

[34] Leung, P.S., et al., Expression and localization of AT1 receptors in hepatic Kupffer cells: its potential role in regulating a fibrogenic response. Regul Pept, 2003. **116**(1-3): pp. 61-9.

[35] Chan, H., P.S. Leung, and M.S. Tam, Effect of angiotensin AT1 receptor antagonist on D-galactosamine-induced acute liver injury. Clin Exp Pharmacol Physiol, 2007. **34**(10): pp. 985-91.

[36] Beyazit, Y., et al., Elevated levels of circulating angiotensin converting enzyme in patients with hepatoportal sclerosis. Dig Dis Sci, 2011. **56**(7): pp. 2160-5.

[37] Magliano, D.C., et al., Short-term administration of GW501516 improves inflammatory state in white adipose tissue and liver damage in high-fructose-fed mice through modulation of the renin-angiotensin system. Endocrine, 2015. **50**(2): pp. 355-67.

[38] John, S. and P.J. Thuluvath, Hyponatremia in cirrhosis: pathophysiology and management. World J Gastroenterol, 2015. **21**(11): pp. 3197-205.

[39] Tandon, P., et al., Renin-angiotensin-aldosterone inhibitors in the reduction of portal pressure: a systematic review and meta-analysis. J Hepatol, 2010. **53**(2): pp. 273-82.

[40] Beyazit, Y., et al., Increased ACE in extrahepatic cholangiocarcinoma as a clue for activated RAS in biliary neoplasms. Clin Res Hepatol Gastroenterol, 2011. **35**(10): pp. 644-9.

[41] Patel, T., Aberrant local renin-angiotensin II responses in the pathogenesis of primary sclerosing cholangitis. Med Hypotheses, 2003. **61**(1): pp. 64-7.

[42] Jing, F., M. Mogi, and M. Horiuchi, Role of renin-angiotensin-aldosterone system in adipose tissue dysfunction. Mol Cell Endocrinol, 2013. **378**(1-2): pp. 23-8.

[43] Strazzullo, P. and F. Galletti, Impact of the renin-angiotensin system on lipid and carbohydrate metabolism. Curr Opin Nephrol Hypertens, 2004. **13**(3): pp. 325-32.

[44] Iwai, M. and M. Horiuchi, Role of renin-angiotensin system in adipose tissue dysfunction. Hypertens Res, 2009. **32**(6): pp. 425-7.

[45] Stiefel, P., et al., Role of the renin-angiotensin system and aldosterone on cardiometabolic syndrome. Int J Hypertens, 2011. **2011**: p. 685238.

[46] Xia, C.Y., et al., High expression of angiotensin-converting enzyme and angiotensin-converting enzyme 2 in preservation injury after liver transplantation in rats. Hepatol Res, 2009. **39**(11): pp. 1118-24.

[47] Speca, S., et al., Cellular and molecular mechanisms of intestinal fibrosis. World J Gastroenterol, 2012. **18**(28): pp. 3635-61.

[48] Velkoska, E., et al., Metabolic effects of low dose angiotensin converting enzyme inhibitor in dietary obesity in the rat. Nutr Metab Cardiovasc Dis, 2010. **20**(1): pp. 49-55.

[49] Karcioglu, S.S., et al., The role of RAAS inhibition by aliskiren on paracetamol-induced hepatotoxicity model in rats. J Cell Biochem, 2016. **117**(3): pp. 638-46.

Chapter 13

The Function of Renin and the Role of Food-Derived Peptides as Direct Renin Inhibitors

Anne Pihlanto and Sari Mäkinen

Additional information is available at the end of the chapter

http://dx.doi.org/10.5772/intechopen.69513

Abstract

Food proteins contain active peptide fragments encrypted within their structure that can exert beneficial effects on human health above and beyond their expected nutritional value. Among many types of food-derived peptides, peptides with antihypertensive activity have received the most significant attention due to the prevalence of hypertension and its associated complications with pharmacological interventions. One strategy for the selection of potential food-derived antihypertensive peptides is to search for *in vitro* renin inhibitory activity. Thus far, various food protein-derived peptides and protein hydrolysates have shown *in vitro* renin inhibitory capacity. Many of these peptides have induced antihypertensive effects when orally administered to spontaneously hypertensive rats, and also, antihypertensive effects in hypertensive humans have been reported. Indeed, the results indicate that antihypertensive food protein-derived peptides may be acting at the same time via multiple pathways at the protein level as well as at the gene level modulating the renin-angiotensin system. Important knowledge on structure-function parameters of peptides is increasing constantly, which can greatly enhance the production and processing of peptides with high physiological efficacy. By means of novel nutrigenomic approaches, it is possible and, in future, perhaps essential to investigate the impact of peptides on the expression of genes and hence endeavor to optimize the nutritional and health effects delivered by peptides. Novel technologies are available to standardize and stabilize the concentrations of active peptides in the products in down-stream processing. The existing data provide strong potential for developing new added-value products with scientifically approved health effects for consumers. This review provides an overview of food-derived peptides that may mediate the antihypertensive activities through inhibiting renin, one of the key enzymes in renin-angiotensin system, and reviews also the safety and applicability aspects of the these peptides.

Keywords: bioactive peptide, renin inhibition, antihypertensive, peptides

1. Introduction

Cardiovascular diseases (CVD) account approximately one third of the total deaths, totaling ≈17 million annually worldwide [78]. Hypertension is considered one of the key risk factors for the development of CVD such as coronary heart diseases, peripheral artery disease and stroke, and kidney disease. Hypertension is often termed as "silent killer" affecting 1 billion people worldwide and causes up to 9 million deaths every year. In addition to health burden, treatment and prevention of hypertension are also associated with substantial socioeconomic consequences. A range of synthetic drugs, such as direct vasodilators, diuretics, adrenergic inhibitors, and angiotensin converting enzyme inhibitors, are commonly used for the treatment of hypertension [50]. The estimated costs for treating hypertension and related diseases were $156 billion in the USA in 2011 and nearly €110 billion in Europe in 2006. Healthy lifestyle choices and early treatment for individuals with mild hypertension are of high importance for reducing the global healthcare costs [50].

In addition to nutritive value of food proteins, they can have various biological activities either intact or after released during processing or digestion. The active peptide fragments, bioactive peptides, can exert beneficial effects on human health in addition to nutritional value. These fragments can be released from various food proteins by gastrointestinal digestion or food processing. According to the Biopep and BioPD (bioactive peptide database) databases, more than 1200 different bioactive peptides have been recorded. These peptides have 2–20 amino acids and molecular masses of less than 6000 Da. Their bioactivity is mainly determined by their composition and amino acid sequence [17, 56, 64]. Especially, peptides with antihypertensive activity have received the significant attention due to the persistence of hypertension and its associated complications. Inhibition of angiotensin I converting enzyme (ACE) has been the main target of these peptides. ACE plays crucial role through renin-angiotensin system (RAS) in the regulation of blood pressure and electrolyte balance in human body. At present, the correlation between *in vitro* and *in vivo* antihypertensive activities appears to be weak [18, 23]. To develop effective antihypertensive peptides, it is important to understand the complex pathophysiology of hypertension and the potential targets where these bioactive peptides may exert their specific actions. This review provides an overview of food-derived peptides that may mediate the antihypertensive activities through inhibiting renin, one of the key enzymes in RAS.

2. Renin-angiotensin-aldosterone system

In cascade system of blood pressure regulation, the renin-angiotensin-aldosterone system (RAAS) plays a key role. The importance of RAAS in diseases such as hypertension, congestive heart failure, and chronic renal failure has been recognized; moreover, the inhibition of RAAS is an effective way to intervene with the pathogenesis of these disorders [11, 43]. Secretion of renin (EC 3.4.23.15) is the first step in RAAS pathway and, importantly, also the rate-limiting step of the RAAS by converting angiotensinogen (Ang) into inactive decapeptide angiotensin I (Ang I), which is converted at the endothelial surface of blood vessels by the enzyme ACE into angiotensin II (Ang II), the primary effector molecule of the RAAS. Therefore, physiological total renin activity, measured as plasma renin activity, can reliably indicate the risk of hypertension, and the inhibition of renin activity by natural products can be explored for the management of hypertension. Inhibition of renin could provide a more effective treatment for hypertension as it prevents the formation of Ang-I, which can be converted to angiotensin II (Ang-II), the vasoconstrictor compound, independent of ACE, by the enzyme chymase. In addition, unlike ACE which acts on a number of substrates, angiotensinogen is the only known substrate of renin. ACE inhibitors and AT1 receptor blockers (ARBs) are proven to be effective therapeutic agents in the treatment of CVD. However, both ACE inhibitors and ARBs lead to a substantial compensatory rise of circulating active renin and Ang peptides that may eventually limit their therapeutic potential [24, 67]. Moreover, the increased Ang I can be converted to Ang II by nonACE pathways, mediated by chymase and chymotrypsin-like enzyme. In addition to the side effects of ACE inhibitors, such as cough and angioedema, a meta-analysis of randomized controlled trials in 2010 suggested that ARBs are associated with a modestly increased risk of new cancer diagnosis, although conclusions about the exact risk of cancer associated with each particular drug have not been drawn [65]. Therefore, direct renin inhibition may be an alternative pharmacological approach to RAS inhibition.

The first-generation renin inhibitors were peptide analogs prosegment of renin or substrate analogs of the amino-terminal sequence of angiotensinogen containing the renin cleavage site and were synthesized already more than 30 years ago. The second generation inhibitors were peptidomimetic agents that are dipeptide inhibitors of the active site. However, the clinical use of these renin inhibitors is limited due to poor metabolic stability and oral bioavailability, short duration of action, weak antihypertensive activity, and high cost of synthesis [61, 66]. Pepstatin, a statine-containing hexapeptide, is the first reported renin inhibitor, but the inhibitory activity of pepstatin was remarkably lower against renin than against pepsin [20]. An endogenously expressed renin-binding protein (RnBP) has been reported to inhibit renin activity [68] based on the selective binding mediated by a leucine zipper (f195–216) in RnBP [33]. The primary RnBP sequence in the renin-binding region is a valuable information for designing potent renin-inhibiting peptides that may be identified and released from food proteins using bioinformatic tools. Aliskiren is the only commercial clinically proven synthetic renin inhibitor for managing hypertension; it has been approved for use in Europe and the United States from 2007 [34]. It has been found to be a more effective antihypertensive agent than ACE inhibitors [74], but recent clinical evidence suggests that Aliskiren may be harmful to patients with type 2 diabetes who are at risk of developing cardiovascular and renal diseases [54].

3. Structural characteristics of food protein-derived renin inhibitory peptides

To reduce the time and cost-intensive steps in the peptide discovery with the conventional pathway, it is important to understand the relationship between peptide structure and subsequent bioactivity. By utilizing the knowledge of structure activity relationship putatively, active peptide sequences can be released in a targeted manner. To date, the research has focused in production and characterization of bioactive peptides, and data concerning the structure-activity relationship are still quite limited.

Renin is a 335-amino acid, glycosylated aspartic protease belonging to pepsin-like family [14, 69]. In contrast to other aspartic proteases such as pepsin, which cleaves a wide variety of substrates, renin specificity is very restricted. The high specificity of renin catalysis is explained by the restricted three-dimensional space of the active site. The C- and N-terminal domains of renin form a deep cleft constructing the active site in which the inhibitors bind [34, 60]. Angiotensinogen is the highly specific physiological substrate of renin, but new renin inhibitors—among which the best known is nonpeptidic Aliskiren—have been developed based on the structural data of the active site [34]. Aliskiren is an orally active renin inhibitor with a very high binding affinity for renin [77], but it is a complicated molecule and thus, drugs simpler in structure and with high bioavailability are desirable in the drug market.

The structure of the active site of renin and the binding of Aliskiren is illustrated in **Figure 1** [58]. It is known that the binding to the catalytic aspartate residues is vital for all the protease inhibitors [9]. The active renin inhibitors seem to presuppose interactions with the aspartate residues of renin (Asp 32 or Asp 215) and the S3sp sub pocket unique for renin. Thus, it has been suggested that any new renin inhibitor should interact with these sites in the active site of renin [58].

Several renin inhibitor peptide sequences have been identified thus far (**Table 1**), however, quite little is known on detailed structure-activity relationship (SAR). Some general characteristics, such as hydrophobicity and molecular size of the peptide fractions, are suggested to correlate with the renin inhibitory activity, but the results are somewhat contradictory [2, 31, 36, 40, 44]. Taken together, the position of amino acid residues in the peptide sequence is more important for the renin inhibition capacity than the actual molecular size or total net charge.

The presence of N-terminal aliphatic (e.g., leucine, isoleucine, valine) and C-terminal bulky amino acid residues (e.g., phenylalanine, tryptophan) has been suggested to contribute to

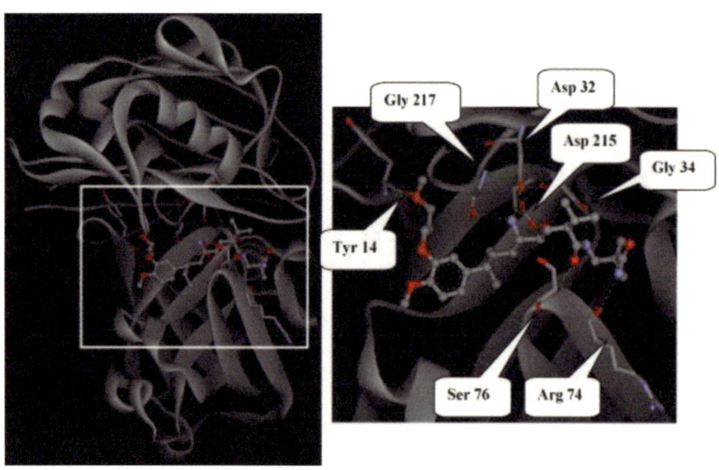

Figure 1. Binding mode of aliskiren as produced from crystallographic data. The protein backbone is shown in ribbons. Residues of the binding site are displayed as gray sticks and aliskiren as ball and sticks. The right panel shows a zoom in the active site and the formed H-bonds with aliskiren [58].

Origin	Treatment	Identified sequences	Renin inhibitory activity *in vitro* IC50	Antihypertensive effects *in vivo*, SHRs	Reference
Bovine serum albumin	Papain, <1 kDa MWCO fraction of the hydrolysate	SLR	1.18 mg/ml 7.29 mM	ΔSBP−32 mmHg after 8 h of oral administration, 200 mg/kg bw nd	[36]
Bovine blood globulins	Papain		1.18 mg/ml	nd	[39]
Bovine fibrinogen	Papain, <1 kDa MWCO fraction of the hydrolysate	YR SLR	32% at 1 mg/ml 8.78 mM 7.29 mM	nd nd nd	[38]
Bovine and porcine hemoglobin, collagen and serum albumin	Papain, pepsin, thermolysin	APPH, IIY, PPL, PPG, PFG, IPP, LPP	15–28% at 1 mg/ml	nd	[37]
Chicken skin protein	Alcalase, pepsin + pancreatin		1.6–2.2 mg/ml	ΔSBP −31.33 mmHg after 6 h of oral administration, 100 mg/kg bw	[52]
Cod muscle proteins	pepsin + trypsin + chymotrypsin RP-HPLC fraction of the hydrolysate		43% at 1 mg/ml 63% at 1 mg/ml	ΔSBP −19 mmHg after 2 h of oral administration, 200 mg/kg bw ΔSBP −40 mmHg after 2 h of oral administration, 30 mg/kg bw	[26]
Kidney bean protein	Alcalase, <1 kDa and 5–10 kDa MWCO fractions of the hydrolysate		40% at 1 mg/ml	nd	[48]
Flaxseed protein	Pepsin, ficin, trypsin, papain, thermolysin, pancreatin, and Alcalase Trypsin-pronase	Cationic, R-rich peptides	1.22–2.81 mg/ml 44.5% at 7.5 mg/ml	nd ΔSBP −17.9 mmHg after 2 h of oral administration 200 mg/kg bw	[71, 73]
Red seaweed (Palmaria palmata) protein	Papain	IRLIIVLMPILMA	42% at 1 mg/ml 3.344 mM	ΔSBP −34 mmHg after 24 h of oral administration, 50 mg/kg bw ΔSBP −33 mmHg after 24 h of oral administration, 3 mg/kg bw	[21, 22]
Hemp seed protein	Pepsin + pancreatin	WYT, SVYT, IPAGV	0.81 mg/ml 0.054 mM (WYT), 0.063 mM (SVYT), 0.093 mM (IPAGV)	ΔSBP −30 mmHg after 8 h of oral administration, 200 mg/kg bw ΔSBP −13.36 mmHg after 4 h of oral administration, 30 mg/kg bw	[29, 30]

Origin	Treatment	Identified sequences	Renin inhibitory activity *in vitro* IC50	Antihypertensive effects *in vivo*, SHRs	Reference
Hemp seed protein	Alcalase, pepsin, papain, pepsin + pancreatin		0.08–0.24 mg/ml	ΔSBP −25.33 mmHg after 4 h of oral administration, 200 mg/kg bw	[44]
Pea protein	Thermolysin, <3kDa MWCO fraction of the hydrolysate		17% at 1 mg/ml	ΔSBP −19 mmHg after 4 h of oral administration, 200 mg/kg bw ΔSBP −29 mmHg after 8 weeks of oral administration to Han:SPRD-*cy*, 0.1% of diet. Renal expression of renin mRNA levels was reduced significantly. ΔSBP −6 mmHg in a 3-week human intervention trial	[41]
African yam bean seed	Alcalase RP-HPLC fraction of the hydrolysate		35% at 1 mg/ml 55% at 1mg/ml		[1]
Rapeseed and canola protein	Alcalase, pepsin, trypsin, pancreatin Alcalase Pepsin + pancreatin	RALP, LY, TF GHS	15.80% at 1 mg/ml 0.968 mM (RALP), 1.868 mM (LY), 3.061 mM (TF) 0.320 mM	ΔSBP −25 mmHg (pepsin) and −34 mmHg (Alcalase) after 4 h of oral administration, 200 mg/kg bw ΔSBP −12 mmHg (TF), −26 mmHg (LY) and −16 mmHg (RALP) after 6 h of oral administration, 30 mg/kg bw ΔSBP −17 mmHg after 6 h of oral administration, 30 mg/kg bw	[2, 30, 31]

Table 1. Food protein-derived renin inhibitory peptides and antihypertensive effects *in vivo*.

higher renin inhibitory activity of dipeptides [71]. For example, dipeptides Leu-Tyr, Ile-Trp, and Thr-Phe have been reported to inhibit renin activity with IC50 values of 1.8, 2.3, and 3.7 mM, respectively [30]. The structures of these peptides mostly agree with the characteristics proposed to contribute to renin inhibition. The importance of C-terminal bulky hydrophobic amino acid residue was also observed by changing the position of amino acids residues from Thr-Phe to Phe-Thr, which resulted to substantial decrease in renin inhibition [30, 71]. However, highly hydrophilic peptides, such as Gly-His-Ser, have also been reported to inhibit renin with IC50 value of 1.09 mM [31]. Also, a cationic tetrapeptide Arg-Ala-Leu-Pro and a 13-amino acid residue, Ile-Arg-Leu-Ile-Ile-Val-Leu-Met-Pro-Ile-Leu-Met-Ala, have also shown rather high renin inhibitory potency [22, 30]. The highest renin inhibitory activity among the reported food protein-derived peptides thus far is 0.054 mM for Trp-Tyr-Thr produced from hemp seed protein [27]). Taken together, more research is needed to gain more knowledge on detailed SAR for designing potential renin inhibitory peptide sequences as physiological antihypertensive agents.

Quantitative computational tools are increasingly applied in medicinal and pharmaceutical drug discovery. At present, the relationship of peptide structure and bioactivity, especially the enzyme inhibitors of ACE are known in some extent. The knowledge of the active peptide sequences enables utilization of quantitative structure-activity relationship modeling (QSAR) for evaluating the crucial physicochemical features of the peptide for the effective bioactivity. A small number of QSAR studies have been carried out on ACE-inhibitory peptides [59, 66] however, no studies have been carried out with seeking potential renin inhibitory peptides.

4. Bioavailability

To induce health effects *in vivo*, peptides need to reach the physiological target organs in intact and active conformation. Considering the renin inhibition, there are three main barriers and hydrolytic threats on the way to the *in vivo* outcome: the digestive proteinases in the gastrointestinal tract, enzymes in the site of absorption, and serum peptidases in the circulation. Thus far, the published data concerning the bioavailability of the peptides, which have shown *in vitro* renin inhibitory activity, are very limited. This makes it very difficult to predict the *in vivo* antihypertensive effect of the *in vitro* renin inhibitory peptides. However, some structural characteristics have been shown to correlate with the bioavailability of, e.g., ACE-inhibitory peptides. These general peptidic characteristics can be considered with renin inhibitory peptides as well.

At first, after oral ingestion bioactive peptides need to resist the hydrolytic actions in stomach by pepsin and pancreatic peptidases, including trypsin, elastase, and chymotrypsin, and further, carboxypeptidases in the small intestine. Several different methods have been applied to model the gastrointestinal digestion *in vitro*. Most of the methods not only concern utilization of commercial porcine enzyme mixtures (e.g., Refs. [42, 46, 75]) but also human digestive liquids have been utilized [19, 49]. Due to the variation in the methods, the comparison of the results across the studies is difficult and thus, a harmonization of the various *in vitro* methods would be important. A consensus for a static process to model the digestion of plant secondary metabolites has been constructed based on *in vivo* data [3]. Indeed, the future research should focus more on the *in vivo* bioavailability of the peptides and based on the correlation with *in vivo* data, a harmonized *in vitro* method could be proposed.

The peptides are exposed to peptidolytic digestion also on the brush border membrane of the intestine. There are number of peptidases with varying specificities bound on the intestinal epithelial cells. It has been suggested that dipeptide and tripeptide tend to resist the gastric and duodenal digestion and also the hydrolytic action of peptidases at the brush border membrane. These small peptides can be absorbed by active transcellular transport or by passive process [63]. To study the absorption *in vitro,* the monolayer of intestinal cell lines, such as Caco-2 cells, simulating intestinal epithelium, is commonly utilized. Clinical data concerning the bioavailability of bioactive peptides are very restricted; however, ACE-inhibitory lactotripeptides, Ile-Pro-Pro and Val-Pro-Pro, have been detected in human and animal circulatory system after oral ingestion [25].

5. Effects of food protein-derived renin inhibitory peptides *in vitro* and *in vivo*

The most widely utilized method for assessing the renin inhibitory potential *in vitro* is a fluorometric assay utilizing a human recombinant renin (Cayman Chemical, MI, USA). Recent data indicate that some food protein-derived hydrolysates and peptides possess *in vitro* renin inhibitory activity. Inhibiting activity against human recombinant renin has been reported, for instance, for hemp seed, pea, bovine blood, and chicken skin protein-derived hydrolysates produced by various food grade proteases (**Table 1**).

Among the protein hydrolysates, the highest renin inhibitory activities have been reported for hemp seed protein hydrolysates with IC_{50} values of 0.08–0.81 mg/ml [27, 44]. These activities are at the same level with the synthetic renin inhibitor Z-Arg-Arg-Pro-Phe-His-Sta-Ile-His-Lys-(Boc)-OMe [22]. Alcalase has yielded to very active renin-inhibiting hydrolysates (e.g., Refs. [2, 30]), and also pancreatin and papain have produced high renin inhibitory activity (e.g., Refs. [21, 27]). Papain has also exhibited good prospects *in silico* in releasing renin inhibitory peptides from, for instance, bovine fibrinogen [37]. Moreover, simulated food protein hydrolysis with gastrointestinal enzymes has also resulted in products with renin inhibitory activities [27, 51]. Taken together, the efficiency of the protease to release renin inhibitory peptides seems to depend on the parent protein matrix. Thus, *in silico* tools are recommended to be utilized prior to the *in vitro* experiments to predict the efficacy of proteases with the particular protein matrixes.

Spontaneously hypertensive rats (SHR) are widely used animal model to assess the antihypertensive effects by *in vivo* experiments. This animal model is applied in short- and long-term manners, for example, to study the antihypertensive effects of milk protein-derived peptides [18, 23]. Recently, food protein-derived renin-inhibiting peptides and protein hydrolysates have induced antihypertensive effects when orally administered to spontaneously hypertensive rats. Decreases in SBP by 19–33 mmHg have been reported for instance, for enzymatic hydrolysates of chicken skin, red seaweed (*Palmaria palmata*), hemp seed, and pea protein (**Table 1**). Generally, the purified renin inhibitory peptides and RP-HPLC fractions have exerted the antihypertensive activities at lower dosage (30 mg/kg bw) compared to the crude protein hydrolysates and membrane-filtrated fractions, which has shown similar antihypertensive effects with 100–200 mg/kg bw (**Table 1**). Hydrolysates and peptides have shown dual inhibition against renin and ACE, or modulation capacity on the RAAS gene expression. Thus, the antihypertensive effects are not solely due to the renin inhibition (e.g., Ref. [41]). For example, egg-derived pentapeptide RVPSL has been recently shown to decrease renin mRNA expression in the kidney of SHRs with a dosage of 50 mg/kg bw administered daily for 4 weeks [79]. Also, weakly active renin-inhibiting peptides have been shown to display physiological antihypertensive activity. A weakly active pea protein hydrolysate (19% renin inhibition at 1 mg/ml) exhibited SBP lowering effects in SHRs and in a kidney disease rat model and was found to downregulate renal expression of renin mRNA in the rat model (**Table 1**). Also, the pea protein hydrolysate showed antihypertensive effects in hypertensive humans in a 3-week intervention trial (**Table 1**). This indicates that antihypertensive food protein-derived peptides may be acting at the same time via multiple pathways at the protein level as well as at the gene level modulating the RAAS.

6. Production of food protein-derived renin inhibitory peptides

A general challenge is how to process the protein hydrolysates further into peptide products with high yield and biological efficacy. Careful choice of suitable enzymes and conditions such as temperature, hydrolysis time, degree of hydrolysis, and enzyme-substrate ratio are crucial for production of peptides with targeted bioactivities and functional properties. Hydrolysis process is recommended to be performed as a continuous process rather than traditional batch process to reduce the enzyme consumption and increase the efficacy [45, 76]. One advantage of enzymatic hydrolysis process is the feasibility in pilot and industrial scale production [6, 7, 28].

To enhance the bioactivity, the active peptides should be concentrated after protein hydrolysis. Size, net charge, and hydrophobicity of the peptides have an important role to select the most suitable techniques to enrich the active peptides. The commonly used techniques include ultrafiltration membranes and chromatographic techniques to obtain an uniform product with the desired range of molecular mass (e.g. [15]). For example, ultrafiltration with 1 kDa membrane has been utilized to concentrate renin inhibitory peptides from rapeseed protein hydrolysate into permeate [36, 38, 48]. In addition to separation based on molecular size, ultrafiltration can be applied to separate peptides according to the net charge. This electrodialysis-ultrafiltration can be utilized to separate anionic, cationic, and neutral peptides of corresponding size range [5, 16, 17]. Large-scale chromatographic methods, used in sugar recovery and wastewater treatments, have been used to enrich peptides from hydrolysates and to separate off ineffective peptides or further undesirable components of the hydrolysates, such as colors, abnormal flavors, and/or salts [10]. Large-scale food-grade processing protocols for designed peptides fractions are needed for further development. Understanding the structural characteristics of peptides with targeted bioactivity and exploitation of these characteristics is a crucial requirement for this approach.

7. Safety aspects of peptides

The term food allergy refers to an immune response directed toward food and affects approximately 8% of children and 1–2% of adults, and its frequency is increasing [35]. Most allergens reacting with IgE antibodies are proteins found in peanuts, soybeans, tree nuts, milk, egg, fish, crustaceans, and wheat [53, 70].

European Food Safety Authority (EFSA) encourages the use of *in silico* tools for initial prediction of potential allergens from food proteins [8]. Although the toxicity and the allergenicity of food products must be assessed also *in vitro* and *in vivo*, the *in silico* tools can be also used to predict the toxicity of peptides [29]. The available bioinformatics-based allergen prediction tools consist of two groups. The first group is based on searches for sequence similarities following the Codex alimentarius guidelines produced by the Food and Agriculture Organization (FAO) and the World Health Organization (WHO), which states that a "protein is potentially allergenic if it either has an identity of over six contiguous amino acids or a minimum of 35% sequence similarity when compared to known allergens" [13]. The second group utilizes databases aiming to identify conserved, allergenicity-related linear motifs [13]. AlgPred (http://www.imtech.res.in/raghava/algpred/) integrates different approaches by means to predict the allergenicity of proteins [62].

After ingestion of food, proteins are naturally hydrolyzed in the gastrointestinal digestion. The digestion often produces peptides with low MW and free amino acids, which are transported across the intestine wall [57]. Highly hydrolyzed proteins and peptides with low MW are not generally toxic and are known to be less allergenic than the native proteins and are widely used in the formulation of hypoallergenic infant foods [32]. However, toxic peptides have been identified from plant as well as animal origin, and they can result in acute, physiological effects, and death. Toxic peptides are usually rich in residues like Asn, Cysm His, and Pro, whereas nontoxic peptides contain dominantly residues Ala, Arg, Gln, Ile, Leu, Lys, Met, Phe, Thr, and Val. [53].

Altogether, the *in silico* assessment of toxicity is not enough, and *in vivo* studies in animal models should be carried out before human consumption. The *in vivo* assessment of the toxicity of food products must be carried out following the guidelines proposed by international authorities. Large quantities of scientific evidence and tests need to be carried out on vertebrate models and cell lines, or unicellular microbial species [47]. Multiple peptide toxicity studies have been carried out in animal models to date [12, 57].

8. Application

Intensive research on bioactive peptides being carried out around the world has already led to the introduction of a wide range of commercial products. The bioactive peptides offer an exciting opportunity in the area of the development of novel functional foods which in turn could contribute to the prevention and management of certain diseases, such as hypertension, type 2 diabetes, or obesity, and more broadly metabolic syndrome. The functional foods or food ingredients containing milk-derived bioactive peptides, such as the fermented milk Calpis, are already in the market [55]. The claims related to peptides are hypotensive properties, aiding mineral absorption, improving athletic performance, and reducing stress. Since 1991, the Ministry of Health and Welfare in Japan has awarded the status of *Food of Specific Health Use* (FOSHU) to foods with scientifically validated health claims. Since then, anti-hypertensive peptides, such as Val-Pro-Pro, Ile-Pro-Pro, Val-Tyr, have obtained FOSHU approval [55]. In Europe, applications for nutrition and health claims are submitted to the European Food Safety Authority (EFSA) under Regulation 1924/2006 and are evaluated by Dietetic Products, Nutrition and Allergies (NDA) panel of scientific experts [4]. There are three categories of health claims as defined by EU legislation. Article 13.1 claims are defined as new function or emerging science claims. Recently, the aspects concerning the scientific information needed for the use of a health claim in the functional food product labeling and marketing should include the scientific evidence on the beneficial effects of the product. The characterization of food components with *in vitro* and animal models is needed but they are not sufficient to substantiate the biological functionality in humans. Human studies to investigate the effects of food or food components on reliable markers, such as blood pressure and oxidative damage, are essential. There is still a lot of confusion within the food industry as to what evidence is required with the EU. Regarding the applications already processed, the Commission of European Communities has not yet authorized any claims relating to the effect of bioactive peptides in foods.

9. Conclusions

There is no doubt that the hydrolysis of proteins gives rise to diversity of peptides, some of them displaying remarkable functionalities relevant to human health. The research should encourage the industry to invest more in the added-value products with scientific evidence of health benefits. To this end, novel technologies are available to standardize and stabilize the concentrations of active peptides in the products by means of chromatographic, membrane separation techniques, and encapsulation. Important structure-function parameters of peptides are increasing constantly, which can greatly enhance the production and processing of peptides. With improved understanding of the structure-activity relationship, we may be able to design targeted enzyme hydrolysis strategies to release these peptides.

According to Foltz et al. [25], it appears that it is only valid to propose efficacy once the peptide exhibits reasonable proteolytic stability and physiologically relevant absorption, distribution, metabolism, and excretion profiles. In this field, more in-depth topics include the stability of the biological activity of peptides, during processing as well as *in vivo* in the body before being absorbed and transported to the target site. Greater understanding of the biological fate of peptides and the site of action will allow delivery or an effective dose and formulation of the peptides to ensure that they reach their target sites. Moreover, we need to gain better understanding of the relationship between these *in vitro* activities and, especially, long-term health benefits in humans and establish appropriate biomarkers of biological efficacy. For example, the extent of the antihypertensive effects has been suggested to depend on the nature of delivery system, dose, study duration, genetic background of the subjects, and stages of hypertension (reviewed in [72]). Furthermore, molecular studies are needed to assess the mechanisms by which bioactive peptides exert their activities in the body. To this end, it may be necessary to employ proteomic and metabolomic methods. By means of these novel nutrigenomic approaches, it is possible and, in future, perhaps essential to investigate the impact of peptides on the expression of genes and hence, endeavor to optimize the nutritional and health effects delivered by peptides.

The safety of all novel peptides intended for food or pharmaceutical uses should be tested in accordance with international and national food safety regulations. In cases of products intended to be marketed in the EU member states, the novel food legislation has to be observed. Other challenges with dietary bioactive peptides are posed by health claims, which in the EU countries are strictly regulated and require science-based documentation before approval by the European Commission. At present, there are worldwide efforts to harmonize these regulations so as to develop fair global food marketing and protect consumers against false or misleading product information.

Acknowledgements

The authors participate in "ScenoProt" project funded by the Strategic Research Funds from the Academy of Finland.

Author details

Anne Pihlanto* and Sari Mäkinen

*Address all correspondence to: anne.pihlanto@luke.fi

Natural Resources Institute Finland, Jokioinen, Finland

References

[1] Ajibola CF, Fashakin JB, Fagbemi TN, Aluko R. Renin and angiotensin converting enzyme inhibition with antioxidant properties of African yam bean protein hydrolysate and reverse-phase HPLC-separated peptide fractions. Food Research International. 2013;**52**:437–444

[2] Alashi AM, Blanchard CL, Mailer RJ, Agboola SO, Mawson AJ, He R, et al. Blood pressure lowering effects of Australian canola protein hydrolysates in spontaneously hypertensive rats. Food Research International. 2014;**55**: 281–287

[3] Alminger M, Aura AM, Bohn T, Dufour C, El SN, Gomes A, et al. In vitro models for studying secondary plant metabolite digestion and bioaccessibility. Comprehensive Reviews on Food Science Food Safety. 2014;**13**:413–436

[4] Anon. Regulation (EC) NO 1924/2006 of the European Parliament and of the Council of 20 December 20026 on Nutrition and Health Claims made on foods. Official Journal of the European Union. 2006;**12**:3–18

[5] Bazinet L, Firdaous L. Membrane processes and devices for separation of bioactive peptides. Recent Patents on Biotechnology. 2009;**3**:61–72

[6] Burks AW, Tang M, Sicherer S, Muraro A, Eigenmann PA, Ebisawa M, et al. ICON: Food allergy. Journal of Allergy and Clinical Immunology. 2012;**129**:906–920

[7] Chiang WE, Cordle CT, Thomas RL. Casein hydrolysate produced using a formed-in-place membrane reactor. Journal of Food Science. 1995;**60**:1349–1352

[8] Christer H, Andersson S, Arpaia D, Casacuberta J, Davies H, Jardin P, et al. Scientific opinion on the assessment of allergenicity of GM plants and microorganisms and derived food and feed. EFSA Journal. 2010;**8**:1700

[9] Coates L, Tuan HF, Tomanicek S. The catalytic mechanism of an aspartic proteinase explored with neutron and X-ray diffraction. Journal of American Chemical Society. 2008;**130**:7235–7237

[10] Danneel. Method for Producing Peptide Fractions and Use Thereof US 20140228542 A1. 2014

[11] De Gasparo M, Septh RC, Baltatu OC, Vanderheyden P. Brain RAS: Hypertension and beyond. International Journal of Hypertension. 2013:157–180

[12] Dent MP, O'Hagan S, Braun WH, Schaetti P, Marburger A, Vogel OA. 90-day subchronic toxicity study and reproductive toxicity studies on ACE-inhibiting lactotripeptide. Food and Chemical Toxicology. 2007;**45**:1468–1477

[13] Dimitrov I, Bangov I, Flower DR, Doytchinova I. AllerTOP v.2—A server for in silico prediction of allergens. Journal of Molecular Modeling. 2014;**20**:2278. DOI: 10.1007/s00894-014-2278-5

[14] Dunn BM. Structure and mechanism of the pepsin-like family of aspartic peptidases. Chemical Reviews. 2002;**102**:4431–4458

[15] Doyen A, Beaulieu L, Saucier L, Pouliot Y, Bazinet L. Impact of ultrafiltration membrane material on peptide separation from a snow crab byproduct hydrolysate by electrodialysis with ultrafiltration membranes. Journal of Agricultural and Food Chemistry. 2011a;**59**: 1784–1792

[16] Doyen A, Beaulieu L, Saucier L, Pouliot Y, Bazinet L. Demonstration of in vitro anticancer properties of peptide fractions from a snow crab by-products hydrolysate after separation by electrodialysis with ultrafiltration membranes. Separation and Purification Technology. 2011;**78**: 321–329

[17] Dziuba M, Darewicz M. Food proteins as precursors of bioactive peptides: Classification into families. Food Science and Technology International. 2007;**13**:393–404

[18] Erdmann K, Cheung BW, Schröder H. The possible roles of food-derived bioactive peptides in reducing the risk of cardiovascular disease. The Journal of Nutritional Biochemistry. 2008;**19**:643–654

[19] Eriksen EK, Holm H, Jensen E, Aaboe R, Devold TG, Jacobsen M, et al. Different digestion of caprine whey proteins by human and porcine gastrointestinal enzymes. British Journal Nutrition. 2010;**104**:374–381

[20] Fisher NDL, Hollenberg NK. Renin inhibition: What are the therapeutic opportunities? Journal of the American Society of Nephrology. 2005;**16**:592–599

[21] Fitzgerald C, Aluko RE, Hossain M, Rai DK, Hayes M. Potential of a renin inhibitory peptide from the red seaweed *Palmaria palmata* as a functional food ingredient following confirmation and characterization of a hypotensive effect in spontaneously hypertensive rats. Journal of Agricultural and Food Chemistry. 2014;**62**:8352–8356.

[22] Fitzgerald C, Mora-Soler L, Gallagher E, O'Connor P, Prieto J, Soler-Vila A, et al. Isolation and characterization of bioactive Pro-peptides with *in vitro* renin inhibitory activities from the macroalga Palmaria palmate. Journal of Agricultural and Food Chemistry. 2012;**60**:7421–7427.

[23] Fitzgerald RJ, Murray BA, Walsh DJ. Hypotensive peptides from milk proteins. Journal of Nutrition. 2004;**134**:980–988.

[24] Fogari R, Zoppi A. New class of agents for treatment of hypertension: Focus on direct renin inhibition. Vascular Health and Risk Management. 2010;**6**:869–882.

[25] Foltz M, Meynen EE, Bianco V, van Platerink C, Koning TM, Kloek J. Angiotensin converting enzyme inhibitory peptides from a lactotripeptide-enriched milk beverage are absorbed intact into the circulation. Journal of Nutrition. 2007;**137**:953–958

[26] Girgih AT, Nwachukwu ID, Hasan F, Fagbemi TN, Gil, T, Aluko RE. Kinetics of the inhibition of renin and angiotensin I-converting enzyme by cod (*Gadus morhua*) protein hydrolysates and their antihypertensive effects in spontaneously hypertensive rats. Food & Nutrition Research. 2007;**59**:e29788

[27] Girgih AT, Udenigwe CC, Li H, Adebiyi AP, Aluko, RE. Kinetics of enzyme inhibition and antihypertensive effects of hemp seed (*Cannabis sativa* L) protein hydrolysates. Journal of the American Oil Chemists Society. 2011;**88**:1767–1774

[28] Guérard F. Enzymatic methods for marine by-products recovery. In: Shahidi F editor. Maximizing the value of marine by-products. Cambridge: Woodward Publishing Limited. pp. 107–143

[29] Gupta S, Kapoor P, Chaudhary K, Gautam A, Kumar R, Raghava GPS. *In silico* approach for predicting toxicity of peptides and proteins. Plos One. 2013;**8**:e73957

[30] He R, Malomo SA, Alashi A, Girgih AT, Ju X, Aluko RE. Purification and hypotensive activity of rapeseed protein derived renin and angiotensin converting enzyme inhibitory peptides. Journal of Functional Foods. 2013a;**5**:781–789

[31] He R, Malomo SA, Girgih AT, Ju X, Aluko RE. Glycinyl-histidinyl-serine (GHS), a novel rapeseed protein-derived peptide has blood pressure-lowering effect in spontaneously hypertensive rats. Journal of Agricultural and Food Chemistry. 2013b;**61**:8396–402

[32] Høst A, Halken S. Hypoallergenic formulas–When, to whom and how long: After more than 15 years we know the right indication! Allergy. 2004;**59**:45–52

[33] Inoue H, Takahashi S, Fukui K, Miyake Y. Leucine zipper motif in porcine renin-binding protein (RnBP) and its relationship to the formation of an RnBP-renin heterodimer and an RnBP homodimer. The Journal of Biological Chemistry. 1991;**266**:11896–11900

[34] Jensen C, Herold P, Brunner HR. Aliskiren: The first renin inhibitor for clinical treatment. Nature Reviews Drug Discovery. 2008;**7**:399–410

[35] Kim KBWR, Lee SY, Song EJ, Kim KE, Ahn DH. Effect of heat and autoclave on allergenicity of porcine serum albumin. Food Science and Biotechnology. 2008;**20**:455–459

[36] Lafarga T, Aluko RE, Rai DK, O'Connor P, Hayes M. Identification of bioactive peptides from a papain hydrolysate of bovine serum albumin and assessment of an antihypertensive effect in spontaneously hypertensive rats. Food Research International. 2016a;**81**: 91–99

[37] Lafarga T, O'Connor P, Hayes M. Identification of novel dipeptidyl peptidase-IV and angiotensin-I-converting enzyme inhibitory peptides from meat proteins using *in silico* analysis. Peptides. 2014;**59**:53–62

[38] Lafarga T, Rai DK, O'Connor P, Hayes MA. Bovine fibrinogen-enriched fraction as a source of peptides with *in vitro* renin and angiotensin-I-converting enzyme inhibitory activities. Journal of Agricultural and Food Chemistry. 2015;**63**:8676–8684

[39] Lafarga T, Wilm M, Wynne K, Hayes M. Bioactive hydrolysates from bovine blood globulins: Generation, characterisation, and *in silico* prediction of toxicity and allergenicity. Journal of Functional Foods. 2016b;**24**:142–155

[40] Li H, Aluko RE. Identification and inhibitory properties of multifunctional peptides from pea protein hydrolysate. Journal of Agricultural and Food Chemistry. 2010;**58**:11471–11476

[41] Li H, Prairie N, Udenigwe CC, Adebiyi AP, Tappia PS, Aukema HM, et al. Blood pressure lowering effect of a pea protein hydrolysate in hypertensive rats and humans. Journal of Agricultural and Food Chemistry. 2011;**59**:9854–9860

[42] Lo WMY, Li-Chan ECY. Angiotensin I converting enzyme inhibitory peptides from in vitro Pepsin-Pancreatin digestion of soy protein. Journal of Agricultural and Food Chemistry. 2005;**53**:3369–3376

[43] Ma TW, Kam KKH, Yan BY, Lam YY. Renin–angiotensin–aldosterone system blockade for cardiovascular diseases: Current status. British Journal of Pharmacology. 2010;**160**: 1273–1292

[44] Malomo SA, Onuh JO, Girgih AT, Aluko RE. Structural and antihypertensive properties of enzymatic hemp seed protein hydrolysates. Nutrients. 2015;**7**:7616–7632

[45] Mannheim A, Cheryan M. Continuous hydrolysis of milk protein in a membrane reactor. Journal of Food Sciences. 1990;**55**:381–385

[46] Marambe HK, Shand PJ, Wanasundara JPD. Release of angiotensin I-converting enzyme inhibitory peptides from flaxseed (*Linum usitatissimum* L.) protein under simulated gastrointestinal digestion. Journal of Agricultural and Food Chemistry. 2011;**59**:9596–9604

[47] Marques A, Lourenço HM, Nunes ML, Roseiro C, Santos C, Barranco A, et al. New tools to assess toxicity, bioaccessibility and uptake of chemical contaminants in meat and seafood. Food Research International. 2011;**44**:510–522

[48] Mundi S, Aluko RE. Inhibitory properties of kidney bean protein hydrolysate and its membrane fractions against renin, angiotensin converting enzyme, and free radicals. Austin Journal of Nutrition and Food Sciences. 2014;**2**:e1008

[49] Mäkinen S, Johansson T, Vegarud G, Pihlava JM, Pihlanto A. Angiotensin I converting enzyme inhibitory and antioxidant properties of rapeseed hydrolysates. Journal of Functional Foods. 2012;**4**:575–583

[50] Norris R, FitzGerald R. Antihypertensive peptides from food proteins. Bioactive food peptides in health and disease, Dr. Blanca Hernández-Ledesma (Ed.), 2013. InTech, DOI: 10.5772/51710 Available from: https://www.intechopen.com/books/bioactive-food-peptides-in-health-and-disease/antihypertensive-peptides-from-food-proteins

[51] Onuh JO, Girgih AT, Aluko RE, Aliani M. Inhibitions of renin and angiotensin converting enzyme activities by enzymatic chicken skin protein hydrolysates. Food Research International. 2013;**53**:260–267

[52] Onuh JO, Girgih AT, Malomo SA, Aluko RE, Aliani M. Kinetics of in vitro renin and angiotensin converting enzyme inhibition by chicken skin protein hydrolysates and their blood pressure lowering effects in spontaneously hypertensive rats. Journal of Functional Foods. 2015;14:133–143

[53] Panda R, Tetteh AO, Pramod SN, Goodman RE. Enzymatic hydrolysis does not reduce the biological reactivity of soybean proteins for all allergic subjects. Journal of Agricultural and Food Chemistry. 2015;**63**:9629–9639

[54] Parving HH, Brenner BM, McMurray JJ, de Zeeuw D, Haffner SM, Solomon SD, et al. Cardiorenal end points in a trial of aliskiren for type 2 diabetes. New England Journal of Medicine. 2012;**367**:2204–2213

[55] Phelan M, Aherne A, FitzGerald RJ, O'Brien NM. Casein-derived bioactive peptides: Biological effects, industrial uses, safety aspects and regulatory status. International Dairy Journal. 2009;**19**:643–654

[56] Pihlanto A, Korhonen H. Bioactive peptides and proteins. Advanced Food Research. 2003;**47**:175–276

[57] Ponstein-Simarro Doorten AY, vd Wiel JAG, Jonker D. Safety evaluation of an IPP tripeptide-containing milk protein hydrolysate. Food and Chemical Toxicology. 2009a; **47**:55–61

[58] Politi A, Durdagi S, Moutevelis-Minakakis P, Kokotos G, Mavromoustakos T. Development of accurate binding affinity predictions of novel renin inhibitors through molecular docking studies. Journal of Molecular Graphics and Modelling. 2010;**29**:425–435

[59] Pripp AH. Initial proteolysis of milk proteins and its effect on formation of ACE-inhibitory peptides during gastrointestinal proteolysis: A bioinformatic, in silico approach. European Food Research and Technology. 2005;**221**:712–716

[60] Rahuel J, Priestle JP, Grutter MG. The crystal structures of recombinant glycosylated human renin alone and in complex with a transition state analog inhibitor. Journal of Structural Biology. 1991;**107**:227–236

[61] Rahuel JR, Rasetti V, Maibaum JJ, Rueger H, Goschke R, Cohen NC, et al. Structure-based drug design: The discovery of novel nonpeptide orally active inhibitors of human renin. Chemistry & Biology. 2000;**7**:493–504

[62] Saha S, Raghava GPS. AlgPred: Prediction of allergenic proteins and mapping of IgE epitopes. Nucleic Acids Research. 2006;**34**:W202–W209

[63] Shimizu M, Tsunogai M, Arai S. Transepithelial transport of oligopeptides in the human intestinal cell, caco-2. Peptides. 1997;**18**:681–687

[64] Singh BP, Vij S, Hati S. Functional significance of bioactive peptides derived from soybean. Peptides. 2014;**54**:171–179

[65] Sipahi I, Debanne SM, Rowland DY, Simon DI, Fang JC. Angiotensin receptor blockade and risk of cancer: Meta-analysis of randomised controlled trials. The Lancet Oncology. 2010;**11**:627–636

[66] Staessen JA, Li Y, Richart T. Oral renin inhibitors. Lancet. 2006;**368**:1449–1456

[67] Tabassum N. Aliskiren: A new renin inhibitor as antihypertensive. Journal of Applied Pharmaceutical Science. 2011;**1**:30–33

[68] Takahashi S, Kumagai M, Shindo S, Saito K, Kawamura Y. Renin inhibits N-acetly-D-glucosamine-2-epimerase (renin binding protein). Journal of Biochemistry. 2000;**128**:951–956

[69] Tice CM. Renin inhibitors. Annual Reports in Medicinal Chemistry. 2006;**41**:155–167

[70] Turnbull JL, Adams HN, Gorard DA. Review article: The diagnosis and management of food allergy and food intolerances. Alimentary Pharmacology & Therapeutics. 2015;**41**:3–25

[71] Udenigwe CC, Adebiyi AP, Doyen A, Li H, Bazinet L, Aluko RE. Low molecular weight flaxseed protein-derived arginine-containing peptides reduced blood pressure of spontaneously hypertensive rats faster than amino acid form of arginine and native flaxseed protein. Food Chemistry. 2012;**132**:468–475

[72] Udenigwe CC, Aluko RE. Food protein-derived bioactive peptides: production, processing, and potential health benefits. Journal of Food Science. 2012:**77**:R11-R24

[73] Udenigwe CC, Lin YS, Hou WC, Aluko RE. Kinetics of the inhibition of renin and angiotensin I-converting enzyme by flaxseed protein hydrolysate fractions. Journal of Functional Foods. 2009;**1**:199–207

[74] Verdecchia P, Angeli F, Mazzotta G, Martire P, Garofoli M, Gentile G, et al. Aliskiren versus ramipril in hypertension. Therapeutic Advances in Cardiovascular Disease. 2010;**4**:193–200

[75] Vermeirssen V, van Camp J, Decroos K, van Wijmelbeke L, Verstaete W. The impact of fermentation and in vitro digestion on the formation of angiotensin-I-converting enzyme inhibitory activity from pea and whey protein. Journal of Dairy Science. 2003;**56**:429–438

[76] Wang YK, He HL, Wang GF, Wu H, Zhou BC, Chen XL, Zhang YZ. Oyster (*Crassostrea gigas*) hydrolysates produced on a plant scale have antitumor activity and immunostimulating effects in BALB/c mice. Marine Drugs. 2010;**8**:255–268

[77] Wuerzner G, Azizi M. Renin inhibition with aliskiren. Clinical and Experimental Pharmacology and Physiology. 2008;**35**:426–430

[78] WHO World Health Organization. Cardiovascular Diseases (CVD's). Fact sheet N°317. 2011

[79] Yu Z, Yin Y, Zhao W, Chen F, Liu J. Antihypertensive effect of angiotensin-converting enzyme inhibitory peptide RVPSL on spontaneously hypertensive rats by regulating gene expression of the renin–angiotensin system. Journal of Agricultural and Food Chemistry. 2014;**62**:912–917